Forthcoming Volumes in the Surgical Techniques Atlas Series

Atlas of **Endocrine Surgical Techniques**
Edited by Quan-Yang Duh, MD

Atlas of **Surgical Techniques for the Upper Gastrointestinal Tract and Small Bowel**
Edited by Jeffrey Ponsky, MD, and Michael Rosen, MD

Atlas of **Thoracic Surgical Techniques**
Edited by Joseph B. Zwischenberger, MD

Atlas of **Minimally Invasive Surgical Techniques**
Edited by Stanley W. Ashley, MD, and Ashley Haralson Vernon, MD

Atlas of **Pediatric Surgical Techniques**
Edited by Dai H. Chung, MD, and Mike Kuang Sing Chen, MD

Atlas of **Trauma/Emergency Surgical Techniques**
Edited by William Cioffi, Jr., MD

Atlas of **Surgical Techniques for Colon, Rectum, and Anus**
Edited by James W. Fleshman, MD

Atlas of **Surgical Techniques for the Hepatobiliary Tract and Pancreas**
Edited by Reid B. Adams, MD

Atlas of
Breast Surgical Techniques

A Volume in the Surgical Techniques Atlas Series

Editor

V. Suzanne Klimberg, MD

Professor and Muriel Balsam Kohn Chair in Breast Surgical Oncology
Department of Surgery and Pathology
University of Arkansas for Medical Sciences
Director of Breast Cancer Program
Winthrop P. Rockefeller Cancer Institute
Little Rock, Arkansas

Series Editors

Courtney M. Townsend, Jr., MD

Professor and John Woods Harris Distinguished Chairman
Department of Surgery
The University of Texas Medical Branch
Galveston, Texas

B. Mark Evers, MD

Director, Lucille P. Markey Cancer Center
Professor and Vice-Chair for Research, UK Department of Surgery
Markey Cancer Center Director Chair
Physician-in-Chief, Oncology Service Line
University of Kentucky
Markey Cancer Center
Lexington, Kentucky

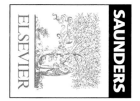

SAUNDERS

ELSEVIER

SAUNDERS
ELSEVIER

1600 John F. Kennedy Blvd.
Ste 1800
Philadelphia, PA 19103-2899

ATLAS OF BREAST SURGICAL TECHNIQUES   ISBN: 978-1-4160-4691-2

Copyright © 2010 by Saunders, an imprint of Elsevier Inc.

Notice

Knowledge and best practice in this field are constantly changing. As new research and experience broaden our knowledge, changes in practice, treatment, and drug therapy may become necessary or appropriate. Readers are advised to check the most current information provided (i) on procedures featured or (ii) by the manufacturer of each product to be administered, to verify the recommended dose or formula, the method and duration of administration, and contraindications. It is the responsibility of the practitioner, relying on their own experience and knowledge of the patient, to make diagnoses, to determine dosages and the best treatment for each individual patient, and to take all appropriate safety precautions. To the fullest extent of the law, neither the Publisher nor the Authors assume any liability for any injury and/or damage to persons or property arising out of or related to any use of the material contained in this book.

The Publisher

Library of Congress Cataloging-in-Publication Data
Atlas of breast surgical techniques / editor, V. Suzanne Klimberg.—1st ed.
      p. ; cm.—(Surgical techniques atlas series)
   Includes bibliographical references and index.
   ISBN 978-1-4160-4691-2 (hardcover : alk. paper)   1. Breast—Surgery—Atlases.
1. Klimberg, V. Suzanne.   II. Series: Surgical techniques atlas series.
   [DNLM: 1. Breast Diseases—surgery—Atlases.   2. Breast Neoplasms—surgery—Atlases.
WP 17 A8798 2010]
   RD667.5.A85 2010
   618.1'9059—dc22
                                                            2009022705

Acquisitions Editor: Judith Fletcher
Developmental Editor: Kristina Oberle
Publishing Services Manager: Anne Altepeter
Project Manager: Cindy Thoms
Design Direction: Steven Stave

Printed in China

Last digit is the print number: 9   8   7   6   5   4   3   2   1

CONTRIBUTORS

Benjamin O. Anderson, MD
Professor of Surgery, Department of Surgery,
    University of Washington School of Medicine;
    Director, Breast Health Clinic, Seattle Cancer Care
    Alliance, Seattle, Washington
    *Oncoplastic Approaches to the Partial Mastectomy for Breast
        Conservation Therapy*

Matilde M. Audisio
Art Foundation, Carmel College, St Helens,
    United Kingdom
    Radioisotope Occult Lesion Localization

Riccardo A. Audisio, MD, FRCS
Department of Surgery, St Helens and Knowsley
    University Hospitals NHS Trust, Liverpool,
    United Kingdom
    Radioisotope Occult Lesion Localization

Bettina Ballardini, MD
Assistant, Breast Unit and Plastic Surgery, Fondazione
    Salvatore Maugeri, Pavia, Italy
    Axillary Sentinel Lymph Node Biopsy

Donald P. Baumann, MD
Assistant Professor, Department of Plastic Surgery,
    The University of Texas, MD Anderson Cancer
    Center, Houston, Texas
    Tissue Breast Reconstruction

Peter D. Beitsch, MD, FACS
Director, Dallas Breast Center, Department of Surgery,
    Medical City Dallas Hospital, Dallas, Texas
    *MammoSite Balloon Catheter Placement and Other Brachytherapy
        Delivery Devices*

Keiva Bland, MD
Southfield, Michigan
    Needle Localization Breast Biopsy

Kirby I. Bland, MD
Fay Fletcher Kerner Professor and Chair, Deputy
    Director, Comprehensive Cancer Center, University
    of Alabama at Birmingham, Birmingham, Alabama
    Chest Wall Resection

Kristine E. Calhoun, MD
Assistant Professor, Department of Surgery, Division
    of Surgical Oncology, University of Washington,
    Seattle, Washington
    *Oncoplastic Approaches to the Partial Mastectomy for Breast
        Conservation Therapy*

Anees B. Chagpar, MD, MSc, MPH
Assistant Professor, Department of Surgery, University
    of Louisville, Louisville, Kentucky
    Cryoablation-Assisted Lumpectomy

Chin-Yau Chen, MD
National Yang-Ming University, Institute of
    Microbiology and Immunology, Taipei, Taiwan;
    National Yang-Ming University Hospital,
    Department of Surgery, I-Lan, Taiwan
    *Oncoplastic Approaches to the Partial Mastectomy for Breast
        Conservation Therapy*

Alice Chung, MD
Assistant Director, John Wayne Cancer Institute
    Breast Center, Santa Monica, California
    Mediastinal Sentinel Lymph Node Biopsy

William C. Dooley, MD
Professor, Department of Surgery and Surgical
    Oncology, The University of Oklahoma Health
    Sciences Center; Surgeon, Department of Surgery,
    The University of Oklahoma Medical Center,
    Oklahoma City, Oklahoma
    Breast Ductoscopy

Richard E. Fine, MD, FACS
Associate Clinical Professor, Department of Surgery,
    University of Tennessee, Chattanooga Unit,
    Chattanooga, Tennessee; Chairman, Breast Care
    Continuum Committee, Northwest Oncology
    Program, WellStar Kennestone Hospital; Director,
    Advanced Breast Care of Georgia, Marietta,
    Georgia
    Ultrasound-Guided Percutaneous Excisional Biopsy
    Stereotactic Breast Biopsy

R. Jobe Fix, MD
Professor, Department of Surgery, Division of Plastic
Surgery, The University of Alabama at Birmingham;
Attending Surgeon, Department of Surgery,
University of Alabama Hospital; The Children's
Hospital of Alabama; Veterans Administration
Medical Center; Birmingham, Alabama
Chest Wall Resection

Michael Andrew Henderson, MD, FRACS
Associate Professor, Surgery, University of Melbourne;
Surgeon, Division of Surgical Oncology,
Peter MacCallum Cancer Center, Melbourne,
Victoria, Australia
Targeted Intraoperative Radiation Therapy (TARGIT)

Julio Hochberg, MD
Professor of Surgery, Plastic Surgery, Marshfield
Clinic, Marshfield, Wisconsin
*Breast Reconstruction Postmastectomy with Tissue Expanders
and Alloderm*

John Harrison Howard, MD
Chief Resident, Department of Surgery, University of
Alabama at Birmingham Hospital, Birmingham,
Alabama
Chest Wall Resection

Nancy Klauber-DeMore, MD
Associate Professor of Surgery, Department of
Surgery, University of North Carolina at
Chapel Hill, Chapel Hill, North Carolina
In Vivo Intraoperative Radiation Therapy for Breast Cancer

V. Suzanne Klimberg, MD
Professor and Muriel Balsam Kohn Chair in Breast
Surgical Oncology, Department of Surgery and
Pathology, University of Arkansas for Medical
Sciences; Director of Breast Cancer Program,
Winthrop P. Rochefeller Cancer Institute,
Little Rock, Arkansas
Aspiration of a Breast Cyst
Incision and Drainage of an Abscess
Excisional Breast Biopsy of Palpable or Nonpalpable Lesions
Needle Localization Breast Biopsy
Excision Followed by Radiofrequency Ablation
Axillary Sentinel Lymph Node Biopsy
Axillary Lymph Node Dissection
Axillary Reverse Mapping
Simple Mastectomy
Simple Extended and Modified Radical Mastectomy

Steven J. Kronowitz, MD, FACS
Associate Professor, Department of Plastic Surgery,
The University of Texas, MD Anderson Cancer
Center, Houston, Texas
Tissue Breast Reconstruction

Gail S. Lebovic, MA, MD, FACS
President, American Society of Breast Disease;
Director of Women's Services, The Cooper Clinic,
Dallas, Texas
Utility of Reduction Mammoplasty Techniques in Oncoplastic Surgery

Jaime D. Lewis, MD
Resident, Department of Surgery, University of
Cincinnati College of Medicine, Cincinnati, Ohio
Forequarter Amputation

Jennifer B. Manders, MD
Medical Director of Oncoplastic Surgical Program,
Attending Physician, Department of Surgery, The
Jewish Hospital; Cincinnati Oncoplastic Surgery,
Cincinnati, Ohio
Forequarter Amputation

David R. McCready, MD, MSc, FRCSC, FACS
Professor of Surgery, Department of Surgery,
University of Toronto; Gattuso Chair in Breast
Surgical Oncology, Department of Surgical
Oncology, Princess Margaret Hospital, University
Health Network; Department of Surgery, Mount
Sinai Hospital, Toronto, Ontario, Canada
Targeted Intraoperative Radiation Therapy (TARGIT)

David W. Ollila, MD
Associate Professor of Surgery, Department of
Surgery, University of North Carolina at
Chapel Hill, Chapel Hill, North Carolina
In Vivo Intraoperative Radiation Therapy for Breast Cancer

Hodigere S.J. Ramesh, MS, FRCS, EBSQ
Department of Surgery, St. Helens & Knowsley
University Hospitals, NHS Trust, Liverpool,
United Kingdom
Radioisotope Occult Lesion Localization

Virgilio Sacchini, MD
Attending Surgeon, Memorial Sloan-Kettering Cancer
Center; Professor of Surgery, Weill Medical College
of Cornell University, New York, New York
Mediastinal Sentinel Lymph Node Biopsy

Carolyn I. Sartor, MD
Assistant Professor, Department of Radiation
Oncology, University of North Carolina at
Chapel Hill, Chapel Hill, North Carolina
In Vivo Intraoperative Radiation Therapy for Breast Cancer

Elizabeth A. Shaughnessy, MD, PhD
Associate Professor of Surgery, Department of
Surgery, Division of Surgical Oncology, University
of Cincinnati, Cincinnati, Ohio
Forequarter Amputation

Ching-Wei D. Tzeng, MD
General Surgery Resident, University of Alabama,
School of Medicine, Birmingham, Alabama
Chest Wall Resection

Kent C. Westbrook, MD
Distinguished Professor, University of Arkansas for
Medical Sciences, Little Rock, Arkansas
Needle Localization Breast Biopsy

James C. Yuen, MD
Professor of Surgery and Chief, Division of Plastic
Surgery, Department of Surgery, University of
Arkansas for Medical Sciences; John L. McClellan
Memorial Veterans Hospital, Little Rock, Arkansas
*Breast Reconstruction Postmastectomy with Tissue Expanders
and Alloderm*

Vittorio Zanini, MD
Chief of Department, Breast Unit and Plastic Surgery,
Fondazione Salvatore Maugeri, Pavia, Italy
Axillary Sentinel Lymph Node Biopsy

FOREWORD

"A picture is worth a thousand words."

Anonymous

This atlas is for practicing surgeons, surgical residents, and medical students for their review and preparation for surgical procedures. New procedures are developed and old ones are replaced as technologic and pharmacologic advances occur. The topics presented are contemporaneous surgical procedures with step-by-step illustrations, preoperative and postoperative considerations, and pearls and pitfalls, taken from the personal experience and surgical practices of the authors. Their results have been validated in their surgical practices involving many patients. Operative surgery remains a manual art in which the knowledge, judgment, and technical skill of the surgeon come together for the benefit of the patient. A technically perfect operation is the key to this success. Speed in operation comes from having a plan and devoting sufficient time to completion of each step, in order, one time. The surgeon must be dedicated to spending the time to do it right the first time; if not, there will never be enough time to do it right at any other time. Use this atlas; study it for your patients.

"An amateur practices until he gets it right; a professional practices until she can't get it wrong."

Anonymous

Courtney M. Townsend, Jr., MD
B. Mark Evers, MD

PREFACE

Surgical treatment of the breast is an underappreciated art. Although the anatomy of the breast and axilla is relatively simple, it can be very confusing during surgery because of the varied approaches and the fatty content of the axilla. This book tries to simplify the anatomy based on approach and surgical techniques.

I have heard many residents say how easy they thought breast surgery was. Yet even in these modern times as many as 40% of patients having lumpectomies emerge from their operation with close or positive margins and an increased risk for local recurrence. This atlas specifically teaches techniques that will improve the outcome for patients facing breast cancer. These include the latest techniques in intraoperative removal of tumors, ablation of margins, accurate sentinel lymph node identification and removal, axillary reverse mapping to prevent lymph-edema, and reconstruction techniques.

In surgery we usually do not say where we trained as much as we say who trained us. In breast surgery I trained with Copeland, Bland, and Westbrook, who are some of the great thinkers of our time and whose text and atlases, such as this one, are important in disseminating technical knowledge. We hope that this atlas will serve as a simplified compendium of breast disease and the latest and best techniques to treat it. This work is built on the shoulders of those who came before us.

V. Suzanne Klimberg, MD

Acknowledgment

Thank you to the family of Jack Diner for the use of his superb illustrations of breast and chest wall anatomy, which provided the inspiration for many of the major illustrations in this book.

CONTENTS

xiv   Contents

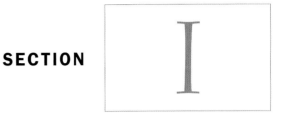
Excisional Biopsy/Partial Mastectomy

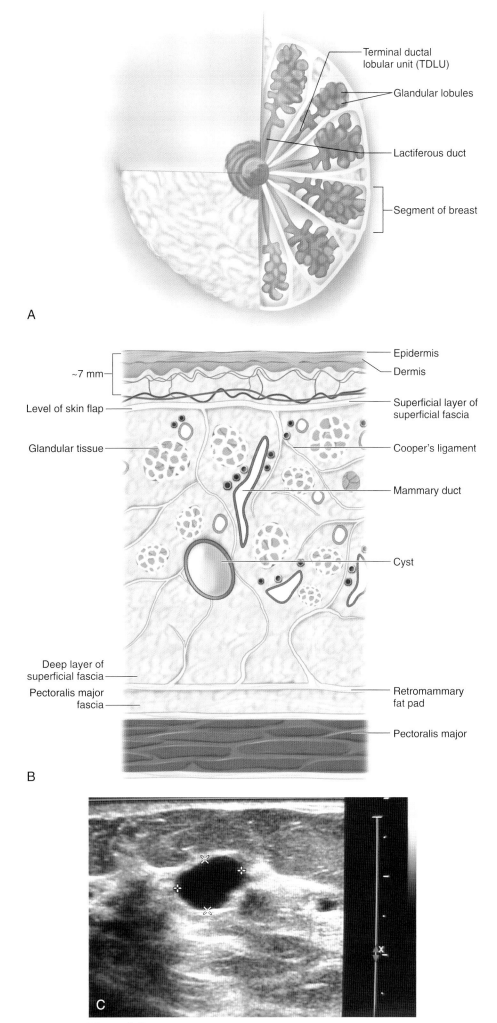

Figure 1-1

◆ Larger syringes are harder to handle but should be used when the cyst is larger than 2 cm in diameter. Avoid changing a full syringe in the middle of an aspiration, which can cause loss of positioning and bleeding.

2. Palpable Positioning

◆ Palpable positioning is not recommended and should be used only when US is not available.
◆ Position the patient flat on the table with a bump underneath the shoulder and the arm above the head. Occasionally there may be a reason to aspirate a cyst with the patient in the upright position. Although not wrong, this is not ideal. If you choose to aspirate in an upright position, make sure there is adequate assistance available should the patient faint.
◆ When cysts are located laterally or in the axilla, position the patient in a lateral decubitus position so the breast falls medially. This may work for inframammary lesions as well, but such lesions usually require additional retraction. Get a second assistant or use a sticky biodrape to retract and hold the breast in one position.

3. Positioning the Ultrasound Probe

◆ Position the US probe directly over the cyst with the cyst located at the side of the probe (not in the middle of the visible field), thus indicating the shortest possible distance to the cyst (Fig. 1-3). Before aspiration, fully scan through the cyst in all planes such that the full extent of the cyst and any septa are known and loculated areas can be aspirated. The notch on the US probe indicates the left side of the US field, so the entry path to the cyst can always be identified on the visible screen. Check positioning under the probe by placing a finger at the edge of transducer; the finger will shadow. If positioning is not accurate, an unaspirated area may be mistakenly interpreted as a solid component or an early recurrence of the cyst on follow-up scans.

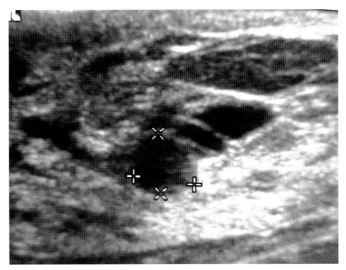

Figure 1-2

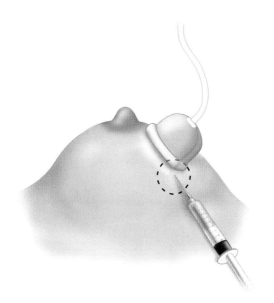

Figure 1-3

4. **Positioning of the Needle**

- ◆ Place the needle far enough away from the probe to allow entry of the needle in a plane parallel to the US probe and to the chest wall. Most of the pain with an aspiration is from needle entry. Place 1 mL of 1% lidocaine in the syringe before needle entry and anesthetize the skin only. Avoid injection of the subcutaneous tissues because the injectate itself may look like a cyst. The needle is best seen when exactly parallel to and centered under the probe. The tip of the needle should be in the center of the cyst (Fig. 1-4).
- ◆ Steady your hand on the patient to control movement and maintain the plane of entry. Loss of positioning may occur through excessive and unnecessary local anesthesia around the cyst itself. Needle planes less than parallel and greater than 45 degrees to the plane of the US probe, along with operator movement (in and out, side to side), cause loss of visualization.

Loss of Positioning

- ◆ If excessive anesthetic has been administered, put pressure on the breast and wait about 15 minutes for the anesthetic to diffuse, then relocalize. If there is difficulty getting the needle in the visible field, try looking only at the probe and the needle (not the US screen) so as to keep them exactly parallel on entry.

5. **Aspiration**

- ◆ Retract the syringe plunger as the needle enters the cyst. This usually results in complete and immediate aspiration of a simple cyst. Reposition the needle under direct US visualization to aspirate without fully withdrawing the needle from the skin (Fig. 1-5). Multiple sticks are unnecessary, may be painful, and increase the risk of bleeding and infection.

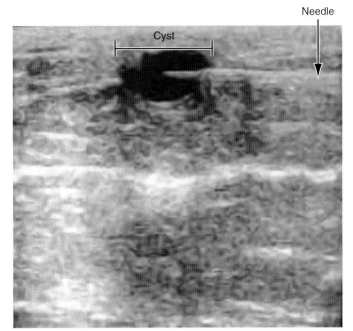

Figure 1-4

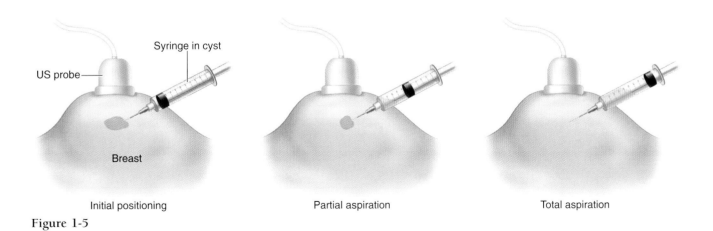

Figure 1-5

Step 4. Postoperative Care

- Clear aspirate from a completely aspirated cyst may be discarded. Cloudy, mucinous, bloody, or otherwise suspect fluid should be sent for cytology. However, the sensitivity for detecting cancer is low (<50%).
- In general, it is sufficient to hold 5 minutes of continuous pressure over the cyst location and the tract to the aspiration site. Ensure that the pressure is continuous; avoid periodic checking.
- For continued bleeding, first try continuous pressure for 15 minutes. If this is insufficient, it will be necessary to open the breast along the needle tract to ligate the bleeder.
- A dressing is usually not necessary. At most, a simple adhesive bandage is sufficient.
- If the cyst is completely aspirated, any pain should immediately subside. The patient should be followed for recurrence if detected by palpation in 1 month, or in 6 months if detected by mammography or US.
- If a cyst recurs immediately (<1 week), it will need excision. If recurrent after 1 month, it can be drained again. If the cyst recurs again, it should be excised (see Chapter 6, Excisional Breast Biopsy of Palpable or Nonpalpable Lesions).

Step 5. Pearls and Pitfalls

- Sometimes simple puncture of a cyst can result in rupture of the cyst into the surrounding tissue without resultant fluid in the syringe. This is not cause for concern.
- Sample a nonaspirating lesion with a core needle biopsy or excise using open excisional biopsy or percutaneous vacuum-assisted needle biopsy.
- Inability to aspirate a lesion or incomplete aspiration may be secondary to thick fluid or presence of a solid lesion. Bloody aspiration requires excisional biopsy because approximately 10% of such cases are carcinoma.
- Incomplete aspiration requires excisional biopsy to rule out cancer (~10%). Residual mass needs to be treated in the same way as any nodule (i.e., palpable suspect mass).
- Pneumothorax is rare (<1%) and is almost always a result of palpable aspiration. Avoid by keeping the angle of the needle parallel to the chest wall.

Bibliography

Smith DN, Kaelin CM, Korbin CD, et al: Impalpable breast cysts: Utility of cytologic examination of fluid obtained with radiologically guided aspiration. Radiology 1997;204:149-151.

2

INCISION AND DRAINAGE
OF AN ABSCESS

V. Suzanne Klimberg

Step 1. Surgical Anatomy

- Figure 2-1 provides sagittal and cross-sectional views of the relevant breast anatomy.

Step 2. Preoperative Considerations

- Most abscesses are subareolar. About one third are peripherally located.
- Incision and drainage of a breast abscess is always indicated. The difficult decision can be determining, at times, whether there really is an abscess present as opposed to simple cellulitis.
- Some advocate simple aspiration of an abscess and placing the patient on antibiotics. For small abscesses, this has a reported success rate of 50%.

Step 3. Operative Steps

1. Setup

- Preferentially, an incisional drainage is performed in the operating room under general anesthesia, although it may be possible to drain a small abscess in the outpatient setting.
- The patient is positioned in a supine or "lawn chair" position.
- Rarely, the abscess is in a lower or outer quadrant of the breast. Avoid awkward operative access by positioning such patients in the lateral decubitus position.

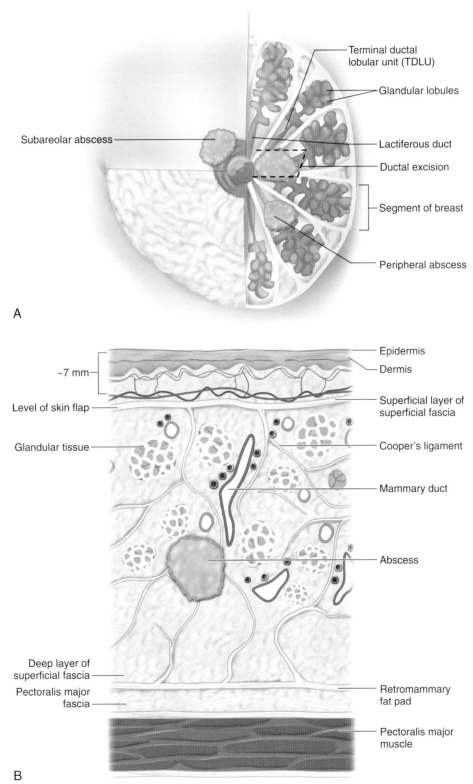

Terminal ductal lobular unit (TDLU)

Glandular lobules

Subareolar abscess

Lactiferous duct

Ductal excision

Segment of breast

Peripheral abscess

A

Epidermis

Dermis

~7 mm

Level of skin flap

Superficial layer of superficial fascia

Glandular tissue

Cooper's ligament

Mammary duct

Abscess

Deep layer of superficial fascia

Pectoralis major fascia

Retromammary fat pad

Pectoralis major muscle

B

Figure 2-1

2. Palpable Localization

- Palpate to locate the abscess (Fig. 2-2).
- Use palpable positioning only when ultrasonography needle positioning yields no abscess fluid.

3. Ultrasonographic Localization

- Use ultrasonography to attempt to locate the abscess's central cavity (Fig. 2-3). Visualization of the cavity is helpful, but failure to visualize the cavity does not rule out its presence.

4. Needle Localization

- Use a 20-gauge needle in aspiration position to find the abscess cavity. In this way, the course of the needle can be redirected without causing significant harm to the patient or tissues (Fig. 2-4).

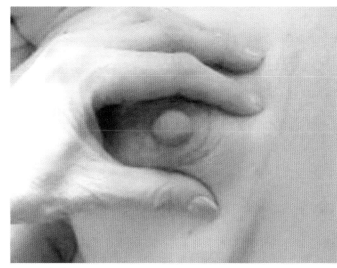

Figure 2-2

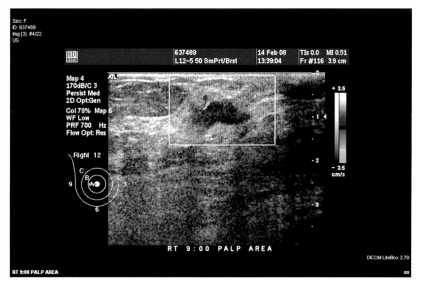

Figure 2-3

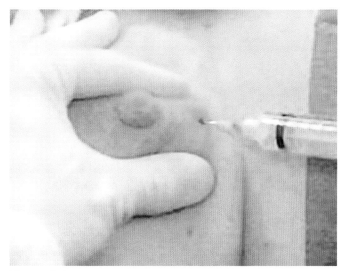

Figure 2-4

5. Incision along Needle Tract

- Once the abscess has been located, make an incision along the needle tract directly into the primary abscess.
- The abscess often is not located directly under the area of greatest erythema.
- Open directly over the abscess cavity (Fig. 2-5).
- Do not tunnel to the abscess cavity for cosmetic reasons. Not only will this delay healing, it may potentially prevent proper healing by allowing a pocket to re-form the abscess.
- If a hidden cancer is present, tunneling to a lesion may prevent breast conservation therapy for an incompletely resected lesion.
- Use a finger to break up any loculations in the cavity.
- Always be cognizant of the possibility of an unusual presentation of a cancer. Always take a biopsy of the cavity to rule out this possibility.
- For a subareolar abscess, make sure to remove the sinus tract as well as the segmental duct and extend the incision under the areola because subareolar abscesses can have multiple winding connections (Figs. 2-6 and 2-7). See also Fig. 2-1 for reference.

6. Dressing

- Place a sterile gauze inside the cavity with a fluffy dressing or absorbent pad on top to collect drainage.
- Have the patient take showers at home with the water directed into the wound to irrigate it. Vary the number of showers and dressings (usually three times a day) depending on how clean the wound appears.
- The patient does not need to use sterile gloves and saline to dress her own wound.
- The patient should wear a comfortable sports bra instead of tape to keep the dressings in place.

Step 4. Postoperative Care

- With the technique described here, the patient can easily take care of such a wound at home.
- It usually takes approximately 1 to 2 months for such a wound to heal. The larger the wound, the more time it takes to heal.
- Antibiotics are, in general, unnecessary unless a severe cellulitis is present. The only exception to this is the patient with previous radiation therapy. Once a wound is properly drained and cellulitis subsides, stop any antibiotics.
- Instruct the patient to wick the wound for as long as possible to allow the incision to heal from the inside and to avoid recurrent abscess.
- Continued or recurrent abscesses near the areola may represent a chronic subareolar abscess.

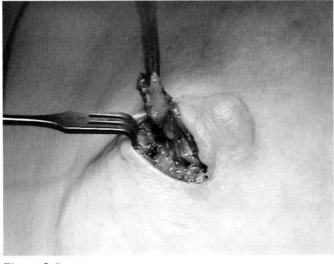

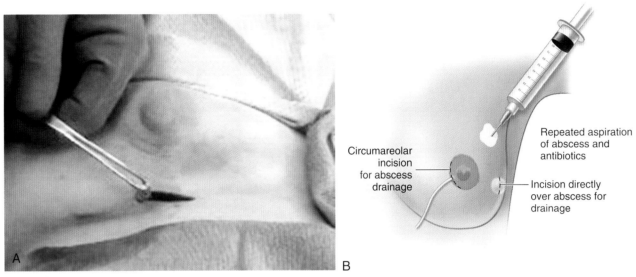

Circumareolar incision for abscess drainage

Repeated aspiration of abscess and antibiotics

Incision directly over abscess for drainage

Figure 2-5

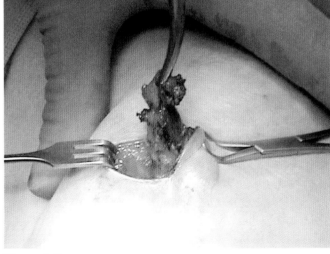

Figure 2-6   Figure 2-7

Step 5. Pearls and Pitfalls

- Antibiotics are sufficient treatment for simple cellulitis, but not an abscess. If cellulitis persists on intravenous antibiotics, reconsider the possibility of abscess (Fig. 2-8).
- Open the entire area over any abscess tunnel so that it may heal directly. Alternatively, make a counter-incision directly over the true abscess cavity and commit the patient to prolonged wet-to-dry dressings.
- If the intraoperative pathologic picture is suspect for cancer, resect the palpable area with overlying skin. Take additional shavings from the superior, inferior, medial, lateral, and posterior margins to attempt to clear the margin.
- If the wound appears "soupy," increase the number of dressing changes. As the wound starts to granulate, decrease the number of dressing changes.
- Do not "pack" the wound too tightly or you will inadvertently keep the wound open longer than necessary. Wicking the wound will keep the wound open while allowing good drainage.
- Prescribing antibiotics longer than necessary may result in resistant infection, candidiasis, or colitis.
- The abscess may recur if the opening of the wound is insufficient or is allowed to close before the abscess's cavity is resolved.
- When an abscess is near or under the areola, a diagnosis of chronic subareolar abscess should be entertained and treated appropriately with accompanying ductal excision. If the pathologic results indicate a chronic abscess, prescribe rotating antibiotics (doxycycline rotating with erythromycin), 1 week on and 3 weeks off. Strongly advise the patient to stop smoking and decrease her caffeine intake.
- Warn the patient that open drainage produces a significant scar, but that the scar can be revised at a later date.

Bibliography

Li S, Grant CS, Deguin A, Donohue J: Surgical management of recurrent subareolar abscesses: Mayo Clinic experience. Am J Surg 2006;192:528-529.
Scott BG, Silberfein EJ, Pham HQ, et al: Rate of malignancies in breast abscess and argument for ultrasound drainage. Am J Surg 2006;192:69-72.

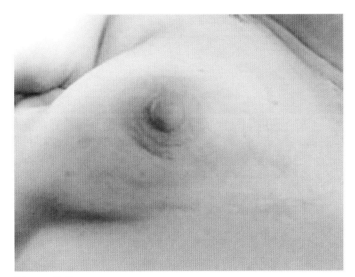

Figure 2-8

CHAPTER 3

ULTRASOUND-GUIDED PERCUTANEOUS EXCISIONAL BIOPSY

Richard E. Fine

Step 1. Surgical Anatomy

- A familiarity with normal breast ultrasound, along with the sonographic characteristics of benign and malignant lesions, is essential.
- Figure 3-1 demonstrates the normal ultrasound anatomy of the breast.
- Figure 3-2 illustrates the more common characteristics that distinguish benign from malignant lesions.

Step 2. Preoperative Considerations

- Repeat a diagnostic ultrasound to confirm the findings and interpretation of any outside studies.
- Document the lesion in terms of size and location (Fig. 3-3) in both the longitudinal and transverse planes.
- Perform a clinical breast examination to exclude associated palpable lesions.
- The patient should be presented with the risks and benefits of the procedure as well as the alternatives (i.e., open biopsy).

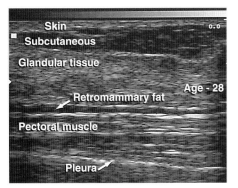

Figure 3-1

	Benign	**Malignant**

Margins

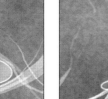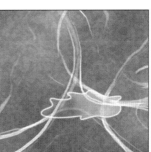

Smooth / sharp | Indistinct / jagged

Adjacent architecture

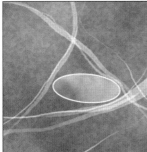

Grows within tissue planes | Disrupted

Shape

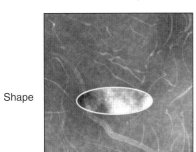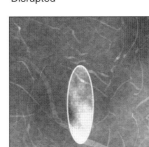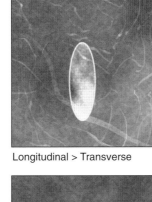

Transverse > Longitudinal | Longitudinal > Transverse

Retrotumoral effect

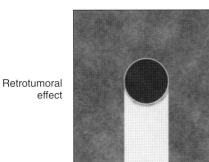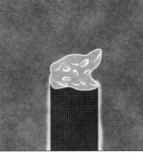

Posterior enhancement | Posterior shadowing

Figure 3-2

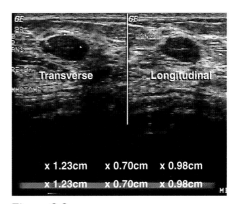

Figure 3-3

◆ The indications for percutaneous excisional biopsy with ultrasound guidance include but are not limited to the following:
  ▲ Nonoperative potential therapy for benign lesions: (1) diagnosis of probably benign and indeterminate masses (Breast Imaging Reporting and Data System [BI-RADS] scores 3 and 4; Fig. 3-4; see Fig. 3-3); (2) to remove palpability and/or image evidence of the lesion.
  ▲ Nonoperative potential therapy for malignant lesions: (1) suspect and highly suspect masses or densities (BI-RADS scores 4 and 5; Figs. 3-5 and 3-6); (2) lesions not larger than 1 cm, using a large intact sample device.
◆ The percutaneous excisional biopsy devices most commonly used include vacuum-assisted biopsy devices and large intact sample devices.
◆ Decisions regarding the choice of biopsy instrument are physician dependent and may be influenced by their desire to better preserve the histologic architecture for the pathologist. Figure 3-7 shows a pathologic section from a whole lesion removed intact.
◆ The patient should be questioned about allergies, the use of anticoagulants or aspirin, and a history of bleeding diathesis.

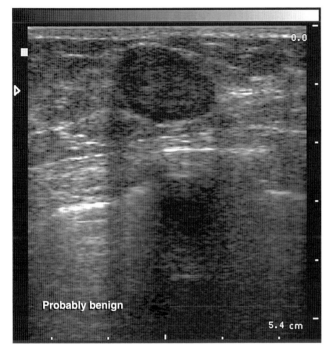

Figure 3-4

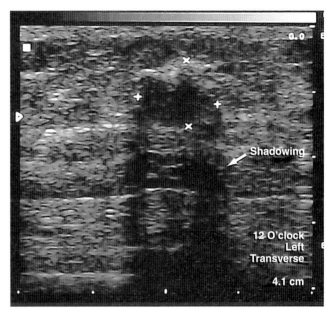

Figure 3-5

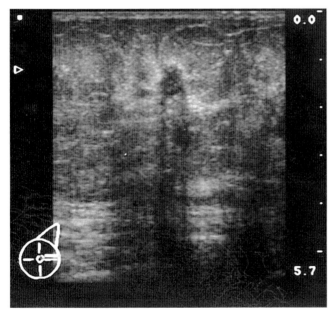

Figure 3-6

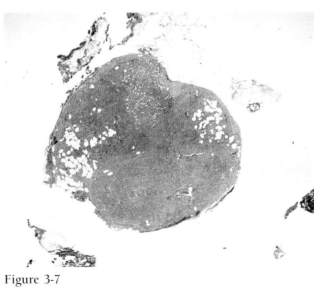

Figure 3-7

Step 3. Operative Steps

1. Preparation and Positioning

♦ The positions of the patient, the physician, and the equipment are essential to the success of the procedure. The patient is positioned supine on the procedure table with a pillow under the shoulder to tilt the patient's breast away from the physician (Fig. 3-8). The ultrasound equipment is positioned on the side opposite to that on which the surgeon is standing. The physician is then positioned with a direct line of sight that includes the biopsy instrument, the ultrasound transducer on the breast, and the ultrasound monitor (Fig. 3-9).

♦ The lesion is visualized and the ultrasound transducer is positioned to visualize the greatest diameter of the lesion and to place the lesion in the middle of the ultrasound monitor screen. The transducer is tilted away from the physician ("heel to toe") to allow the device insertion to be more parallel with the transducer face (Fig. 3-10).

2. Local Anesthetic and Incision

♦ The breast skin is prepared with an antiseptic and encircled with sterile towels or a disposable aperture drape. Individual packets of sterile ultrasound gel or povidone-iodine gel are available.

♦ Local anesthetic is injected at the site on the skin where the appropriate insertion has been determined (Fig. 3-11, A). The injection of deep local anesthetic into the breast parenchyma is performed under direct ultrasound visualization. Local anesthetic is placed on a tract leading beneath the lesion, as well as on the top and both sides of the lesion. Instillation of the local anesthetic may also be used to lift or separate the lesion from the chest wall or skin. Fig. 3-11, B shows the needle going under the lesion.

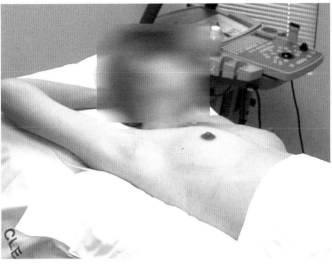

Figure 3-8

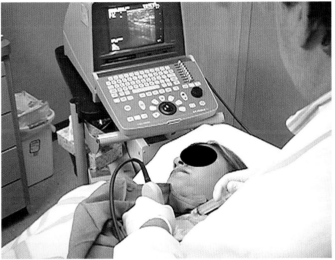

Figure 3-9

Figure 3-10

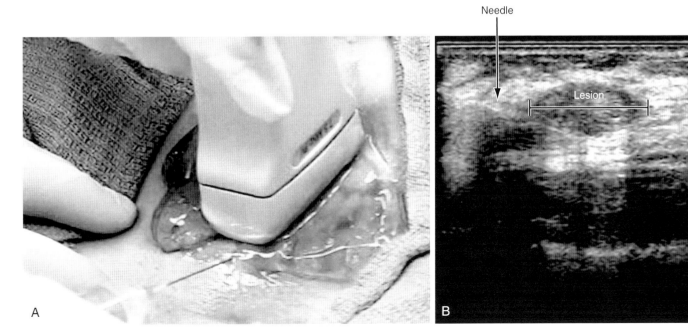

A

B

Figure 3-11

- The depth of the lesion on the ultrasound monitor is noted and the choice of incision site is chosen by visually triangulating the distance from the lateral edge of the transducer, which will allow the device to be inserted beneath the lesion (Fig. 3-12, also see Fig. 3-10).
- A small skin incision is made at the entry site for the biopsy device. The size of the incision is device dependent, but usually ranges from 3 to 8 mm in length.

3. Biopsy

- The biopsy device is manually inserted into the breast and guided beneath the lesion (Figs. 3-13, *A* and *B*). If the lesion is in close proximity to the chest wall, it may be beneficial to insert the large intact loop device slightly to the left (7 o'clock) to allow the loop to extend parallel to the chest before looping over the lesion.

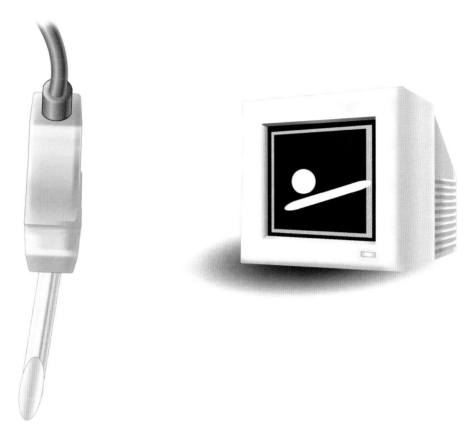

Figure 3-12

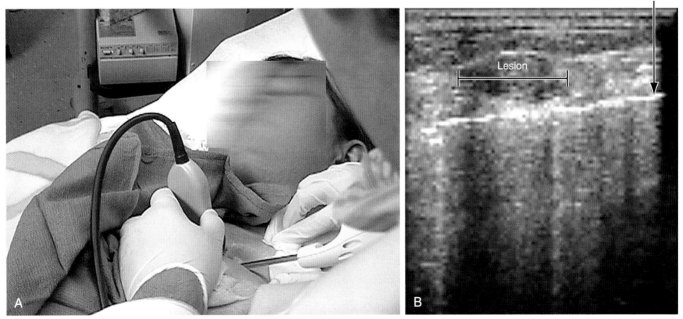

Figure 3-13

◆ The alignment of the image-detected abnormality with the biopsy device must be verified with a 90-degree cross-sectional view to ensure the lesion did not move or shift during device placement (Fig. 3-14, *A*). Both the vacuum-assisted and large intact sample loop devices are directional, allowing for slight offset from the device sampling area (Figs. 3-14, *B* and *C*).

◆ The image-detected lesion is adequately sampled for diagnosis and potential therapeutic removal. Because the devices have directional capabilities, the sampling pattern is adjusted based on the position of the device in relation to the lesion.

◆ With the vacuum-assisted device appropriately positioned, the lesion is excised in multiple cores, beginning at the deepest aspect and proceeding superficially both superiorly and inferiorly by rotating the position of the sampling aperture (Fig. 3-15).

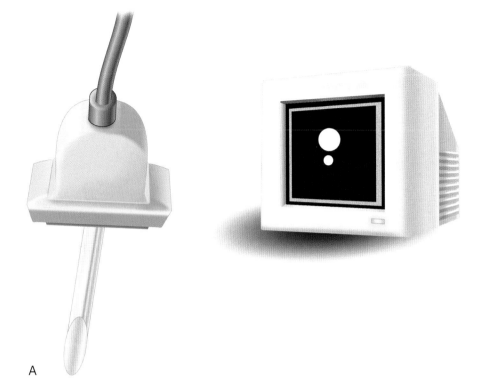

A

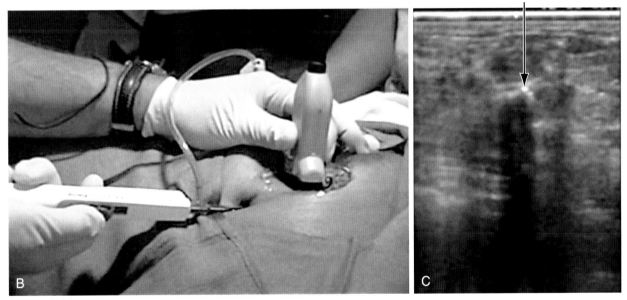

Needle in
transverse view

B   C

Figure 3-14

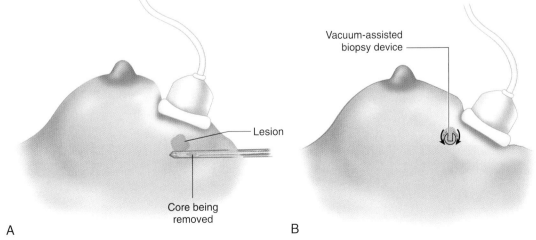

Vacuum-assisted
biopsy device

Lesion

Core being
removed

A   B

Figure 3-15

- Typical cores are shown in Figure 3-16.
- The large intact sample loop device has a radiofrequency-activated cutting loop that is brought out laterally (3 o'clock) and circumferentially rotated over the top of the lesion 180 degrees, followed by loop closure, which completes the excision with the lesion contained within a small attached sampling bag (Fig. 3-17). The device is withdrawn from the breast, maintaining loop closure, and the intact specimen is delivered (Fig. 3-18).

4. Postbiopsy

- If all imaging-detected aspects of the abnormality have been removed, consideration should be given to placing a marker that is both radiopaque and ultrasound visible. This ensures the ability to go back to the area for further intervention based on pathologic results (e.g., cancer, atypia, or discordant pathology). If the results are benign and concordant, the marker is then used to follow the patient with future imaging studies.

5. Closing

- Manual compression is used to obtain adequate hemostasis.
- The skin nick is closed with Steri-Strips and a Tegaderm dressing. Suture closure is rarely indicated.
- The patient is put in a compression wrap with an ice pack, if indicated.

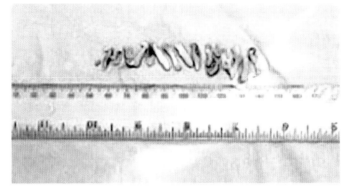

Figure 3-16

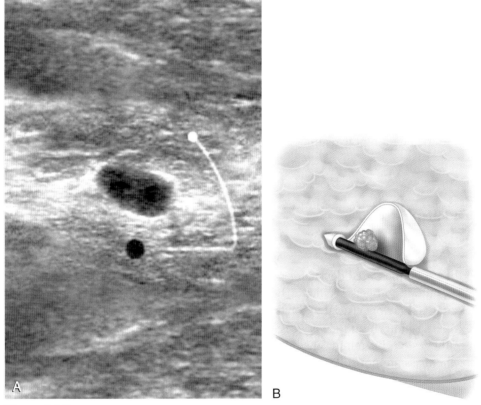

Figure 3-17

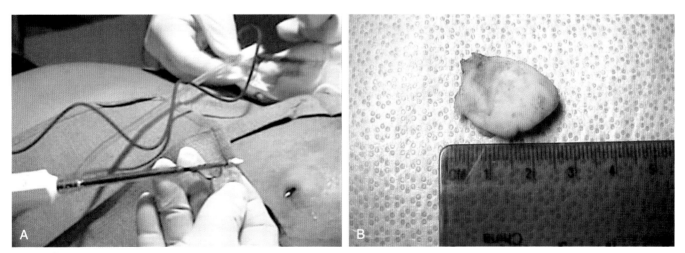

Figure 3-18

CHAPTER 4

STEREOTACTIC BREAST BIOPSY

Richard E. Fine

Step 1. Surgical Anatomy

- Familiarity with the normal mammogram, along with the morphologic features of those lesions that constitute an abnormal mammogram and indications for biopsy, is essential.
- Figure 4-1 demonstrates the radial lobar anatomy of the breast, comprising the parenchyma, fibrous network, and adipose elements.
- Figure 4-2 shows a histopathologic section of the normal terminal duct lobular unit (TDLU), the structure responsible for most of the mammographic abnormalities detected.
- Figure 4-3 illustrates the morphologic features of benign-appearing (Fig. 4-3, *A*) and malignant-appearing (Fig. 4-3, *B*) microcalcifications (the mammographic abnormality that is the most common indication for stereotactic breast biopsy). Benign lobular calcifications ("pearl-like," round, dense calcifications) form as spherical molds within the acini of the TDLU (see Fig. 4-3, *A*). Linear, casting calcifications with clefts associated with high-grade ductal carcinoma in situ (DCIS) follow the longitudinal mold of the duct and its branches (see Fig. 4-3, *B*).

Step 2. Preoperative Considerations

- Confirm that a complete diagnostic imaging work-up has been completed:
  - ▲ Special mammogram views (compression for masses or magnification for calcifications)
  - ▲ Breast ultrasonography
- Perform a clinical breast examination.
- The patient should be presented with the risks and benefits of the procedure as well as alternatives.

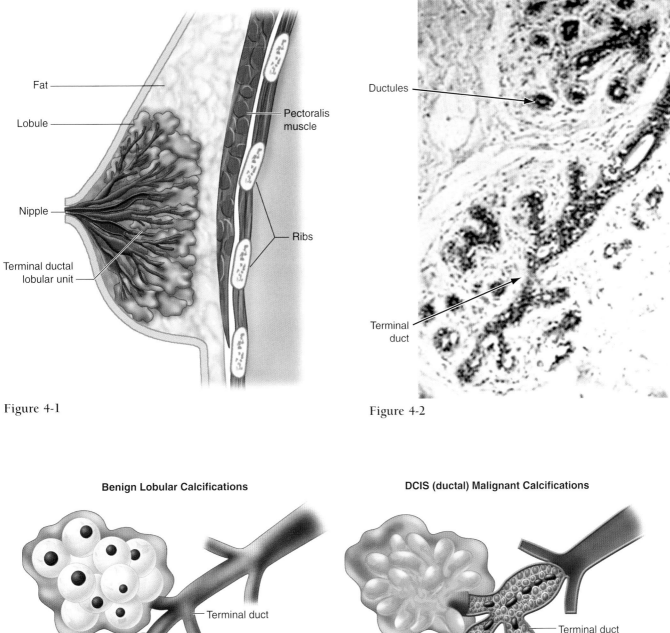

Figure 4-1

Figure 4-2

Benign Lobular Calcifications

DCIS (ductal) Malignant Calcifications

A

B

Figure 4-3

- The indications for image-guided breast biopsy with stereotactic guidance include, but are not limited to, the following:
  - ▲ Highly suspect microcalcifications or densities (Breast Imaging Reporting and Data System [BI-RADS] score 5) to confirm the diagnosis and facilitate treatment (Fig. 4-4)
  - ▲ Indeterminate or suspect microcalcifications or densities (BI-RADS 4; Fig. 4-5)
  - ▲ Probably benign microcalcifications or densities (BI-RADS 3) when there are valid clinical indications, including but not limited to a patient with a strong family history, difficult clinical and imaging examination, or a patient with a high level of anxiety
  - ▲ Multifocal or multicentric lesions to facilitate treatment planning
- BI-RADS 2 lesions are benign, as are the coarse calcifications seen in Figure 4-5, and do not require biopsy.
- The diagnostic biopsy devices most commonly used include but are not limited to the automated needle core device, vacuum-assisted biopsy devices (most common), and the large intact sample device.
- Decisions regarding the choice of biopsy instrument are physician dependent and may be influenced by the extent of lesion removal desired, which can be controversial.
- The patient should be questioned about allergies, the use of anticoagulants or aspirin, and a history of bleeding diathesis.
- The patient's weight and tolerance to remaining prone for the procedure are assessed for appropriateness of the procedure for that patient.

Step 3. Operative Steps

1. Preparation and Positioning

- Review the mammogram with the stereotactic technologist to establish the proper approach to the breast (cranial-caudal, medial-lateral, lateral-medial, or caudal-cranial).
- A cranial-caudal approach could be used for a lesion in the superior portion of the breast; however, if the lesion is lateral in the breast, a lateral-medial approach may be preferred because the lesion may be lower in the breast than it appears on the mediolateral oblique mammogram view. A medial lesion would require a medial-lateral or cranial-caudal approach. On the Lorad Multicare Platinum Stereotactic Table (Hologic, Inc., Bedford, MA), a lesion in the inferior aspect of the breast can be accessed using the caudal-cranial approach.
- The patient is positioned on the prone stereotactic table for visualization of the image-detected abnormality in a manner that affords the shortest distance to the lesion, but also taking into consideration the approach that best demonstrates the lesion (Fig. 4-6).

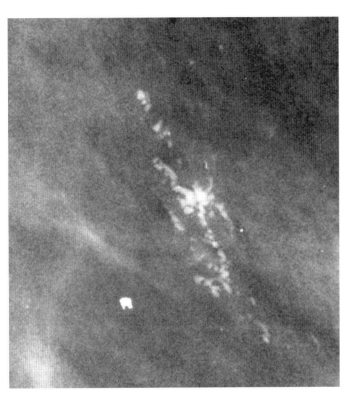

Figure 4-4

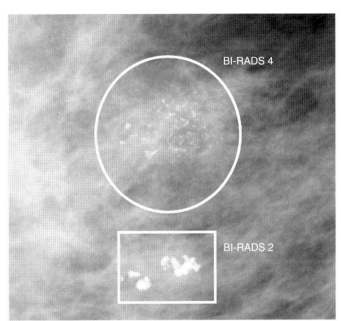

Figure 4-5

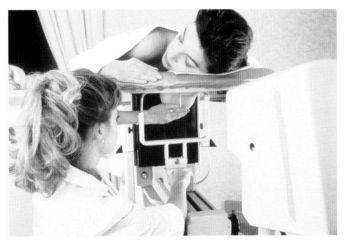

Figure 4-6

- A scout x-ray image in acquired. Regardless of the approach to the breast (cranial-caudal, medial-lateral, lateral-medial, or caudal-cranial), this image is taken perpendicular to the compressed breast. Figure 4-7 is a diagrammatic representation of a lesion detected on the prone cartesian stereotactic biopsy system. Figure 4-8, *A* is a scout image of calcifications for a vacuum-assisted biopsy procedure. Figure 4-8, *B* is a scout image for a procedure using a large intact sample loop device.

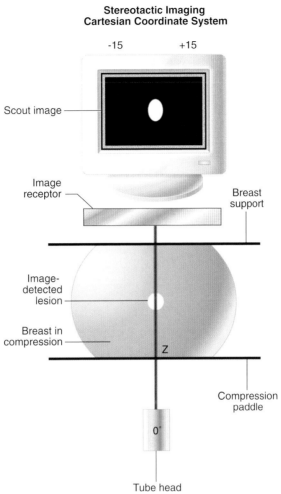

Figure 4-7

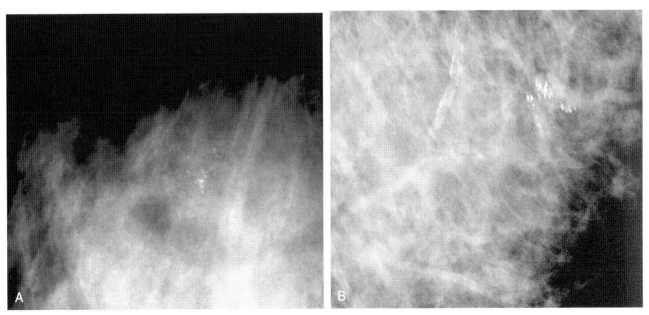

Figure 4-8

◆ The scout image is addressed to confirm appropriate position of the abnormality within the middle one third of the image. If the lesion is not within the middle third of the scout image, it may be thrown out of view on one of the two 15-degree stereotactic images, therefore making the lesion unavailable for targeting (Fig. 4-9).

◆ A stereotactic pair of images, −15 degrees and +15 degrees off center from the scout image, are taken. Figure 4-10 is a diagrammatic representation of the x-ray tube head movement on the prone cartesian stereotactic biopsy system. Figure 4-11, *A* is a stereopair image for a vacuum-assisted biopsy procedure. Figure 4-11, *B* is a stereopair image for a large intact sample loop device procedure.

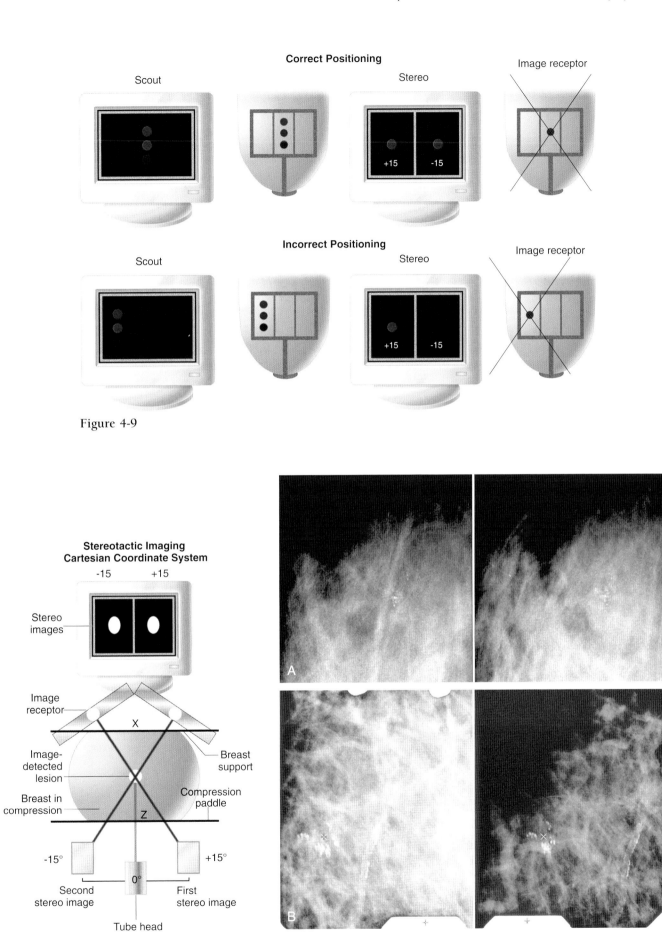

Correct Positioning

Scout   Stereo   Image receptor

+15   -15

Incorrect Positioning

Scout   Stereo   Image receptor

+15   -15

Figure 4-9

**Stereotactic Imaging
Cartesian Coordinate System**

-15   +15

Stereo
images

Image
receptor

X

Image-
detected
lesion

Breast
support

Breast in
compression

Compression
paddle

Z

-15°   +15°

0°

Second
stereo image

First
stereo image

Tube head

Figure 4-10

A

B

Figure 4-11

CHAPTER 1

ASPIRATION OF A BREAST CYST

V. Suzanne Klimberg

Step 1. Surgical Anatomy

- ◆ A cyst is a dilated duct (Fig. 1-1).
  - ▲ See also Fig. 1-3

Step 2. Preoperative Considerations

- ◆ A breast cyst should be aspirated if one cannot be sure it is a simple cyst (i.e., it is multiloculated [see Fig. 1-2] or has internal echoes on ultrasonography [US]), it is painful, or it shows signs of infection (see Chapter 2, Incision and Drainage of an Abscess).
- ◆ Most simple cysts, even when palpable, do not require aspiration. Explain to the patient that a simple cyst is simply a dilated duct to calm cancer phobia and avoid unnecessary cyst aspiration (Fig. 1-1, C).
- ◆ Unnecessary cyst aspiration may lead to hematoma or inadvertent infection of the cyst itself, requiring later open drainage.
- ◆ Hematoma requires only observation.

Step 3. Operative Steps

1. Setup

- ◆ Use a 20-gauge 2-inch needle, an alcohol pad, and a syringe compatible with the size of the cyst to be aspirated. A 20-gauge spinal needle may be used for deeper cysts. Usually a 5- to 10-mL syringe will suffice.

- The physician then places a target on the lesion in each of the stereotactic images using the computer mouse and the image monitor (Fig. 4-12). The system software then determines the accurate coordinates (horizontal, vertical, and depth) of the abnormality in the breast and transfers this information to the biopsy instrument stage.
- A unique procedure, referred to as *z-zero*, is performed at this time if using the Hologic Multicare Platinum Table. The stereotactic principles of this platform determine the depth of the lesion from the front compression paddle forward into the breast. Because each breast has a unique compression thickness, the system software must "know" where z equals zero for each device for the patient who is in compression. The device is placed on the biopsy instrument stage and motor driven to the predetermined z position, where it is then manually aligned with the reference point on the front compression paddle. The z-zero button then "zeros out" the device for this patient.
- With the biopsy device of choice properly positioned on the biopsy device stage, the physician uses the automated software to guide the needle or biopsy probe to the correct horizontal and vertical coordinates.
  - Because published studies have illustrated the limitations of automated Tru-cut biopsy needles with regard to diagnostic upgrading, the most common device used for stereotactic biopsy is the vacuum-assisted biopsy device (Fig. 4-13). A more recent category of stereotactic biopsy devices is the large intact sample loop device (Fig. 14-14). Early evidence with the intact sample device supports improved preservation of pathologic architecture and the potential for therapeutic application.
- The vertical or y value is adjusted so the biopsy instrument will be inserted beneath the lesion to be sampled (4 mm below for vacuum-assisted devices, and 8 mm below for the large intact sample loop device).
- The surgeon and mammographer position themselves on either side of the patient to direct the needles and remove specimens (Fig. 4-15).
- The needle/probe is advanced up to the skin surface for determination of the incision and device entrance site (Fig. 4-16).

2. Local Anesthetic and Incision

- The breast skin within the 5×5-cm opening on the front compression paddle is prepared with an antiseptic.
- Local anesthetic is injected at the site on the skin determined by aligning the needle tip at the calculated horizontal and vertical coordinates. The injection of deep local anesthetic into the breast parenchyma is based on physician preference and biopsy device type (see Fig. 4-16).
- A small skin incision is made at the entry site for the biopsy device. The size of the incision is device dependent, but usually ranges from 3 to 8 mm in length.

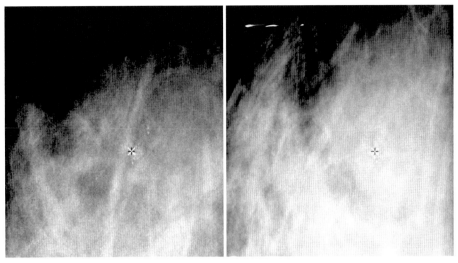

Figure 4-12

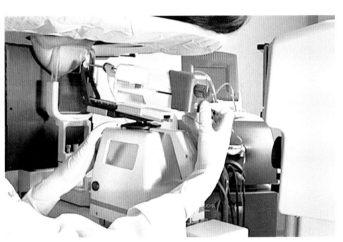

Figure 4-13

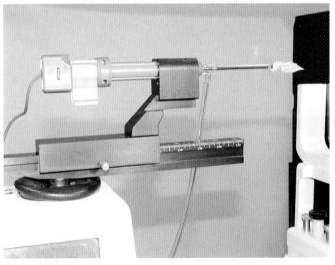

Figure 4-14

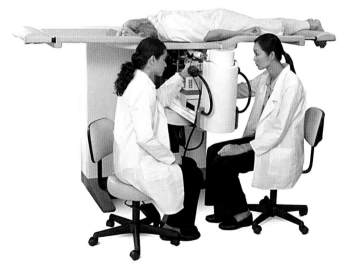

Figure 4-15

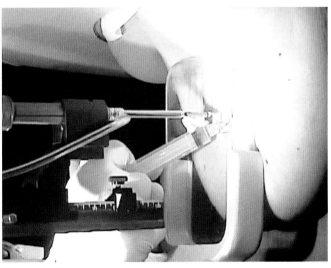

Figure 4-16

3. Biopsy

◆ The biopsy device is manually inserted into the breast to the predetermined depth (z value). Many of the biopsy devices have precalculated "pullback" depths that are based on the specific device's mechanics. Use of the pullback depth will center the imaged abnormality in that particular device's sampling area. Again, whether a biopsy device is advanced forward in the breast using the spring-loaded device driver or manually inserted to align the sampling aperture with the lesion is operator and device dependent.

◆ The alignment of the image-detected abnormality with the biopsy device must be verified with a pair of prestereotactic or poststereotactic images to confirm accurate placement of the biopsy device and to ensure the lesion did not move or shift during device placement. Figure 4-17 shows microcalcifications aligned with the sampling aperture of the vacuum-assisted biopsy device on 15-degree views.

◆ Figure 4-18 shows the large intact sample loop device positioned for radiofrequency activation and tissue cutting. Before obtaining the stereopair images, an additional scout image is obtained with the large intact sample loop device in the breast to verify the orientation of the device (clock position) in relation to the target lesion (see Fig. 4-18, *inset*).

◆ The image-detected lesion is adequately sampled for diagnosis and potential therapeutic removal. Because the devices have directional capabilities, the sampling pattern is adjusted based on the position of the device in relation to the lesion.

◆ The number of cores taken with a vacuum-assisted device averages 12 to 15 for the smaller (11- to 14-gauge) and 6 to 8 for the larger (7- to 9-gauge) devices, depending on the size of the lesion and the physician's preference as to whether to remove all image-based evidence of the lesion (Fig. 4-19).

◆ The loop on the large intact sample device is activated with radiofrequency (from a standard generator) and extended to a full loop height of 1.5 cm. The loop is then rotated in a counter-clockwise direction approximately 240 degrees and then pulled closed, trapping the tissue in the attached sample bag (Fig. 4-20). The *inset* in Figure 4-20 shows the resultant large intact sample.

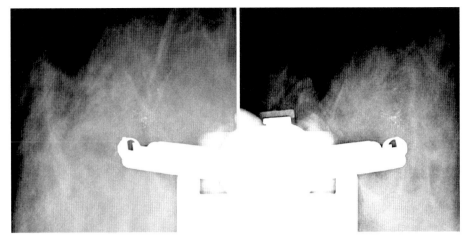

Figure 4-17

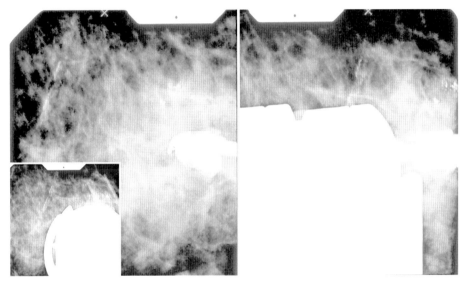

Figure 4-18

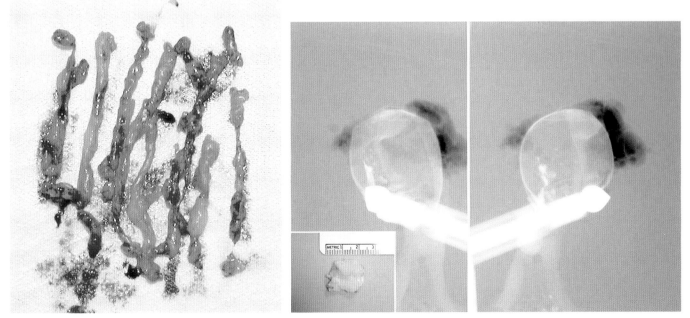

Figure 4-19

Figure 4-20

◆ Stereopair images are taken to assess the adequacy of the biopsy, which may be influenced by the goals of the physician in removing all image-based evidence of the lesion (Fig. 4-21).

4. Postbiopsy

◆ If all imaging-detected aspects of the abnormality have been removed, consideration should be given to placing a marker that is both radiopaque and ultrasound visible. This ensures the ability to go back to the area for further intervention based on pathologic results (e.g., cancer, atypia, or discordant pathology). If the results are benign and concordant, the marker is then used to follow the patient with future imaging studies. Stereotactic images are taken to confirm clip placement; Figure 4-22 is post vacuum-assisted device biopsy and Figure 4-23 is post large intact sample loop device biopsy.

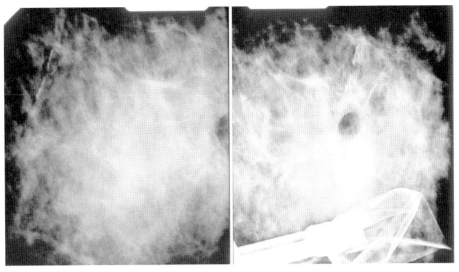

Figure 4-21

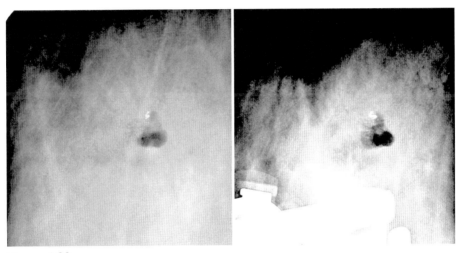

Figure 4-22

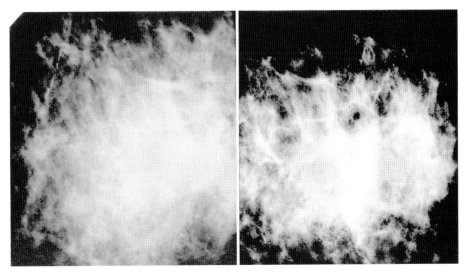

Figure 4-23

◆ A specimen radiograph is obtained to document appropriate sampling in cases where micro-calcifications were the target lesion. The presence of calcifications in the core sample increases the accuracy of the biopsy and makes it less likely the diagnosis will be upgraded. Figure 4-24 shows core samples from an 8-gauge vacuum-assisted device biopsy. Figure 4-25 is a specimen radiograph of a sample obtained with an intact sample loop device. Preservation of the histologic architecture is demonstrated in this low-power view of a pathology slide that clearly shows the three small hyalinizing fibroadenomas associated with the pattern of calcifications on the large intact specimen radiograph (Fig. 4-26).

5. Closing

◆ Manual compression for 10 minutes is used to obtain adequate hemostasis.
◆ The skin nick is closed with Steri-Strips and a Tegaderm dressing or skin glue. Suture closure is rarely indicated.
◆ For facilities that have access to mammography, a postprocedure mammogram is ideal to verify that there has been no clip migration.
◆ The patient is put in a compression wrap with an ice pack, if indicated (Fig. 4-27).

Step 4. Postoperative Care

◆ It is the physician's responsibility to confirm that the pathologic results are concordant with the impression of the radiologic imaging study. If a discordance is identified, further intervention is necessary and may include repeat biopsy or open surgical excision.
◆ An unexcised papilloma, atypical hyperplasia, or a diagnosis of malignancy requires the patient to be scheduled for definitive therapeutic surgery.
◆ If the diagnosis is of a benign nature, the patient should be placed on the appropriate follow-up protocol to include a repeat mammogram or ultrasonogram in 4 to 6 months.

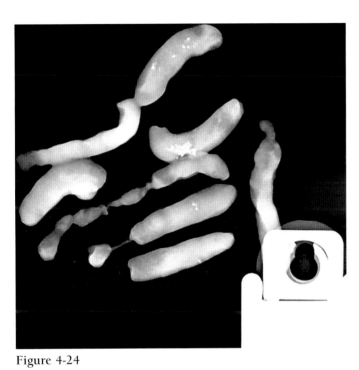

Figure 4-24

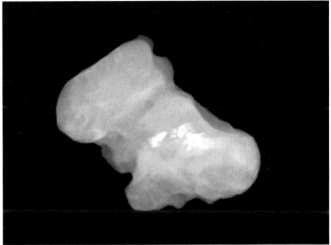

Figure 4-25

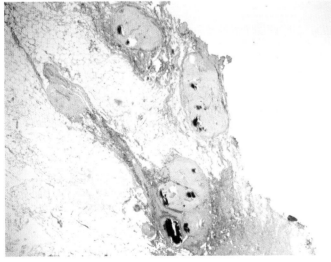

Figure 4-26

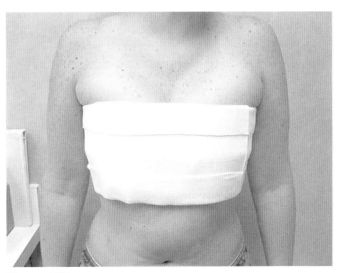

Figure 4-27

Step 5. Pearls and Pitfalls

- The most treacherous potential pitfall is performing a stereotactic biopsy on the wrong abnormality. Stereotactic biopsy imaging is limited to a 5 × 5-cm area of the breast, and there is a learning curve involved in identifying a lesion on a full film-screen mammogram and recognizing the same lesion on a magnified, digitized reproduction on the system monitor without seeing its relationship to the surrounding mammographic breast anatomy. It is the responsibility of the physician performing the biopsy (not the stereotactic technologist) to sample the correct abnormality. A postbiopsy mammogram can document removal.
- A common patient characteristic that may lead to a difficult biopsy is small breast size (compression thickness < 25 mm). With a small breast or a more posterior-positioned breast lesion, the biopsy device may impale the back side of the breast or compression paddle (negative stroke margin). The stereotactic table software allows the physician to confirm an adequate distance from the biopsy needle tip to the back compression paddle (stroke margin; Fig. 4-28).
- There are several methods to correct for a negative stroke margin. These include but are not limited to the following:
  - ▲ A different approach to the breast lesion (lateral vs. medial)
  - ▲ Manual insertion of the biopsy device without using automated firing
  - ▲ Use of a lateral arm. The lateral arm is attached at a 90-degree angle to the MammoTest (Siemens Medical, New York, NY) stereotactic table C-arm (parallel to the compression and image receptor paddles) to hold the biopsy device platform. The biopsy needle can then be inserted from the lateral or side approach.
  - ▲ Double-paddle technique. The double-paddle technique creates an air gap behind the breast with the use of a second compression paddle (with a 5 × 5-cm biopsy opening). The skin on the back of the breast may also protrude into the compression paddle opening, thus avoiding puncture.
- It is important for the physician to recognize targeting errors, where the target lesion has shifted position in relation to the sampling area of the biopsy device. Figure 4-29 illustrates a horizontal targeting error where the target lesion has shifted either to the right or the left of the biopsy instrument. The clock-face diagram shows how the directional capability of the biopsy device is used to adjust for such targeting errors.

Bibliography

American College of Radiology: BI-RADS—Mammography, 4th ed. In: ACR Breast Imaging Reporting and Data System, Breast Imaging Atlas. Reston, Va, American College of Radiology, 2003.

American Society of Breast Surgeons: Performance and Practice Guidelines for Stereotactic Breast Procedures. Available at www.breastsurgeons.org/PDF/StereoPerforGuidelines0807.pdf.

Burbank F: Stereotactic breast biopsy of atypical ductal hyperplasia and ductal carcinoma in situ lesions: Improved accuracy with directional vacuum-assisted biopsy. Radiology 1997;202:843-847.

Burbank F, Forcier N: Tissue marking clip for stereotactic breast biopsy: Initial placement accuracy, long-term stability and usefulness as a guide for wire localization. Radiology 1997;205:407-415.

Fine R: Image-directed breast biopsy. In Winchester DJ, Winchester DP (eds): Breast Cancer: Atlas of Clinical Oncology. Hamilton, Ontario, BC Decker, 2000, pp 65-88.

Fine RE, Boyd BA: Stereotactic breast biopsy: A practical approach. Am Surg 1996;62:96-102.

Kass R, Kumar G, Klimberg VS, et al: Clip migration. Am J Surg 2002;184:325-331.

Liberman L, Cohen MA, Dershaw DD, et al: Atypical ductal hyperplasia diagnosed at stereotaxic core biopsy of breast lesions: An indication for surgical biopsy. AJR Am J Roentgenol 1995;164:1111-1113.

Liberman LL, Dershaw DD, Rosen PR, et al: Stereotactic 14-gauge breast biopsy: How many core biopsy specimens are needed? Radiology 1994;192:793-795.

Liberman L, Dershaw DD, Rosen PP, et al: Stereotaxic core biopsy of breast carcinoma: Accuracy of predicting invasion. Radiology 1995;194:379-381.

Liberman LL, Evans WP, Dershaw DD, et al: Radiography of microcalcifications in stereotaxic mammary core biopsy specimens. Radiology 1994;190:223-225.

Meyer JE, Lester SC, Grenna TH, White FV: Occult breast calcifications sampled with large-core biopsy: Confirmation with radiography of the specimen. Radiology 1993;188:581-582.

Parker SH, Burbank F: State of the art: A practical approach to minimally invasive breast biopsy. Radiology 1996;200:11-20.

Parker SH, Lovin JD, Jobe WE, et al: Nonpalpable breast lesions: Stereotactic automated large-core biopsies. Radiology 1991;180:403-407.

Negative Stroke Margin

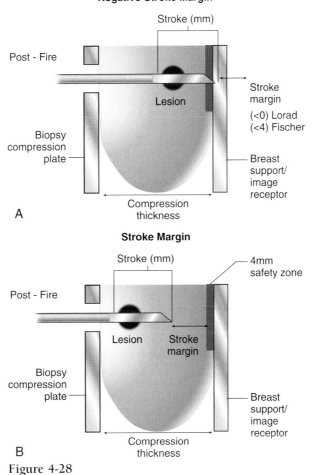

Figure 4-28

Horizontal Error

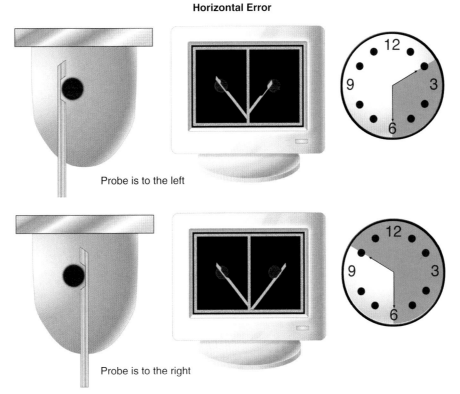

Figure 4-29

CHAPTER 5

BREAST DUCTOSCOPY

William C. Dooley

Step 1. Surgical Anatomy

- Breast ducts are numerous and lack predictable branching patterns (Fig. 5-1). Older texts describe 20 to 25 ducts exiting the nipple on the basis of histologic studies. Functional examinations during lactation and more modern attempts to cannulate ducts suggest the real number of complete ductal units that are functional and involved with breast cancer may be as little as 7 to 12 in many patients.
- The nonfunctional ducts may end in a saclike structure close to the areolar edge and give rise to the common periareolar abscess. These ducts are usually not connected to large regions of functional breast tissue.
- Usually two or three major ductal trees drain over two thirds of the breast volume. These are commonly associated with the outer few millimeters of the nipple papilla and anatomically form large coating regions such as in the upper outer quadrants. Central ductal units tend to be smaller and more teardrop-shaped in the distribution of their branches. All branches can be straightened out by simply pulling outward on the nipple papilla.

Step 2. Preoperative Considerations

- The most common indications for breast ductoscopy are to identify causes of pathologic nipple discharge and, if necessary, to direct the intraoperative excision of the suspect lesion (Fig. 5-2).
- Bloody or high-volume clear discharge usually is associated with relatively large and easy-to-cannulate ducts at the nipple papilla surface.
- Most Tis and T1 breast cancers (>90%) express fluid from the ductal orifice connected to the tumor. The volumes of fluid can be quite small. To best elicit fluid on the day of lumpectomy and be able to correctly identify the duct connecting to the cancer, it is important to keep the patient very well hydrated, warm the nipple region, give relaxation drugs, and massage the breast from periphery to center after careful dekeratinization of the nipple papilla surface. If fluid is not obtained, occasionally a nursing pump/nipple aspirator may be used.
- When obtaining preoperative core biopsies, it is important to sample the lesion from the back side to maintain the nipple-ductal connection for intraoperative ductoscopy.

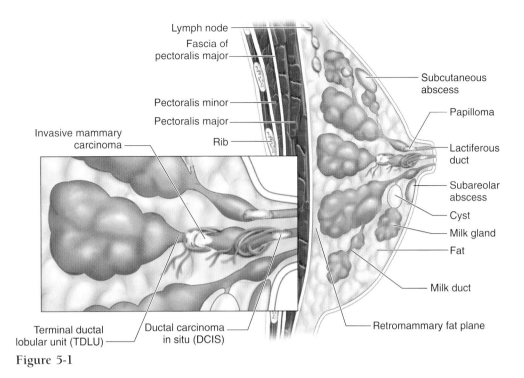

Lymph node
Fascia of pectoralis major
Pectoralis minor
Pectoralis major
Rib
Invasive mammary carcinoma
Subcutaneous abscess
Papilloma
Lactiferous duct
Subareolar abscess
Cyst
Milk gland
Fat
Milk duct
Terminal ductal lobular unit (TDLU)
Ductal carcinoma in situ (DCIS)
Retromammary fat plane

Figure 5-1

Muscle   Lobules   Ducts

Normal   Diseased

Micro-endoscope

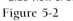
Side view of breast
Figure 5-2

Step 3. Operative Steps

1. Duct Selection and Cannulation

- ◆ Cleanse the nipple papilla (exfoliate using nonabrasive to remove keratin plugs).
- ◆ Have patient well hydrated and relaxed.
- ◆ Use sedation.
- ◆ Massage as if expressing at lactation using a thin, slippery lotion (e.g., Udderly Smooth Udder Cream; Redex Industries, Inc., Salem, OH; Fig. 5-3).
- ◆ Cannulate the fluid-producing duct (Fig. 5-4; the skin markings outline the area of abnormal findings). In case of pathologic discharge, use a 2-0 Prolene suture cut to a gentle taper; for breast cancer cases, the orifice will be smaller and produce much less fluid. In these cases, first inject Lymphazurin (Tyco Healthcare Group LP, Norwalk, CT) and local anesthetic in the region around the tumor to assist in selecting the correct low-volume duct. Cannulate with the 2-0 Prolene if possible or, if necessary, use more rigid introducers; the best current controllable tip is the Entree™ dilating trocar (ConMed EndoSurgery, Utica, NY; Fig. 5-5).
- ◆ Progressively dilate in Seldinger fashion over the 2-0 Prolene using 24-, 22-, and 20-gauge Angiocaths (Becton Dickinson Medical Surgical Systems, Sandy, UT; Fig. 5-6). With each Angiocath, inject 1 to 5 mL of local anesthetic into the duct for distention.

Centripetal Massage Methods

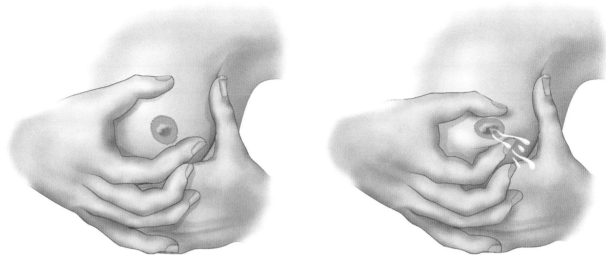

Figure 5-3

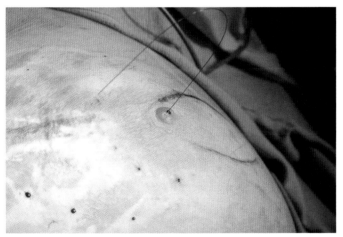

Figure 5-4

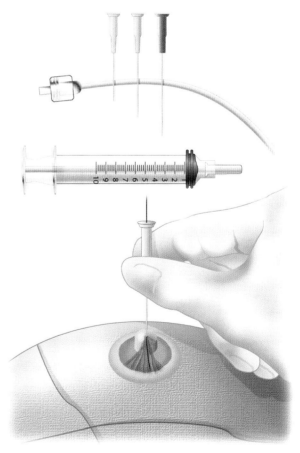

Figure 5-6

Entree™ Dilating trocar

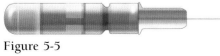

Figure 5-5

2. Ductoscopy—Diagnostic

* The endoscope sheath is introduced in Seldinger fashion, removing the hollow introducer and replacing it with the optical fibers of the scope. Ensure that the endoscope is well focused and white balanced before introducing it into the breast ducts (Fig. 5-7).
* The duct then can be distended using saline or a local anesthetic while preventing leakage by compressing the nipple papilla against the endoscope with the thumb and index finger.
* The endoscope is advanced as distention is obtained. Distraction of the nipple and gentle motion of the underlying breast mound can be used to negotiate the varying branches. The scope sheaths all come with markings to help keep track of depth.
* When you come to multiple branches, the largest-diameter branch usually leads to the most proliferative lesion.
* To find the position of the scope tip if an abnormality that needs excisional biopsy is seen, turn off all the overhead lights in the operating room and use the transillumination from the scope tip to identify the site for biopsy.

3. Ductoscopy—Therapeutic

* When directing breast cancer procedures, remember that the volume of expressed fluid may be small, making ductal cannulation more challenging. Do not perforate the ductal system, or efforts to distend the ducts will fail and ductoscopy will not be useful. Be gentle and expect that distention may take longer.
* The ductal orifice chosen should usually lie in the radial sector of the nipple papilla 100 to 110 degrees in either direction from the known lesion position in the breast (see Fig. 5-4). For example, if a known cancer is at 2:00 (i.e., 2 o'clock) and 5 cm out from the nipple papilla, the discharging orifice connecting to that cancer will be on the nipple papilla at 2:00 ± 100 to 110 degrees, or roughly between 9:45 to 4:45.
* Always direct the endoscope down the largest branches first because these are more likely to connect to the tumor.
* Once the obstructing tumor is found, mark the position by transillumination.
* Work your way backward, directing the endoscope down each smaller branch and marking the positions of intraductal luminal defects by transillumination on the breast surface.
* Leave the endoscope at the most proximal extent of nipple-ward progression of intraluminal disease.
* Design the excision of the subsegmental quadrant to include from scope tip to a pie-shaped wedge to the periphery of the breast from the known tumor. The width of this wedge is determined by the intraluminal disease foci identified in side branches.

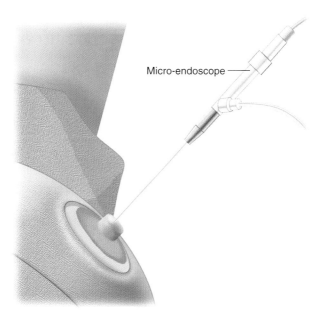

Micro-endoscope ———

Figure 5-7

Step 4. Postoperative Care

- These patients require no different care than that provided after any surgical breast-tissue excision. It is normal for bloody fluid to drain from the nipple for several days after ductoscopy, but rarely longer than 3 weeks.

Step 5. Pearls and Pitfalls

- Papillomas in the nipple papilla may make it hard for the surgeon to decide what he or she is initially looking at because the duct is full of material. Usually the duct is very dilated below the papilloma, so advance the endoscope until the normal duct is seen below the papilloma. If the papilloma is within 12 mm of the nipple papilla surface, it usually can be excised by removing the scope and, using a 3-mm skin punch biopsy, removing the ductal opening and pushing down in the direction in which the scope most easily advances. Usually a 15-mm or larger duct can be removed in this way. The hole does not need to be sutured because the circular muscle of the nipple papilla will pursestring the opening as soon as the local anesthetic wears off. It will bleed, however, much like a fingertip paper cut. Figure 5-8 shows a range of normal, benign, and malignant findings (ductal carcinoma in situ [DCIS]).
- Massaging the breast deeply in a centripetal fashion, using a smooth hydrating lotion, is the best way to express fluid (see Fig. 5-3).

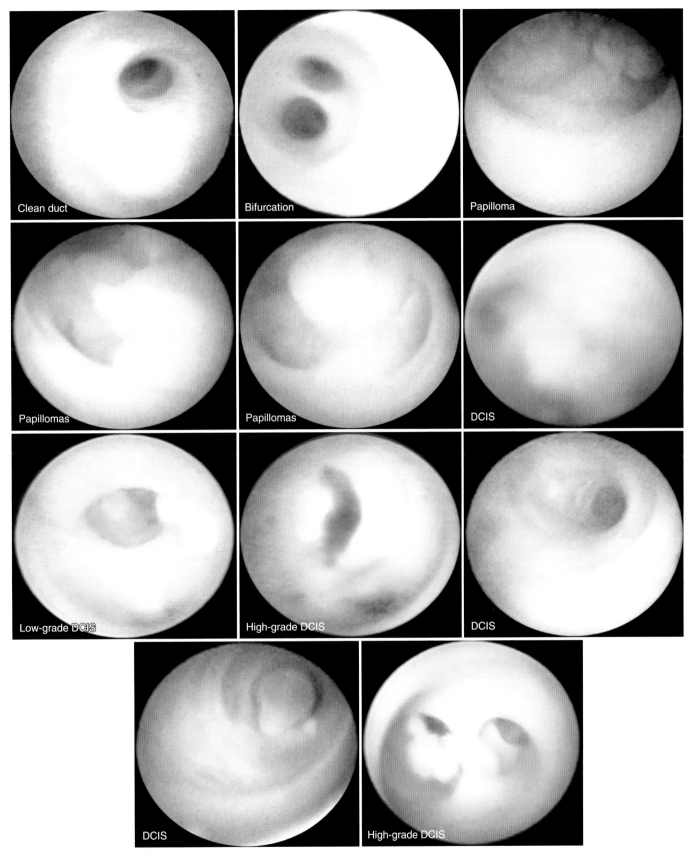

Figure 5-8

- ◆ Dekeratinizing agents should not contain shards of particulate material or be sticky and difficult to wash off because both can interfere with ductal orifice identification. A nipple aspirator may be used in difficult cases (Fig. 5-9).
- ◆ When the image dims, usually this means more proteinaceous secretions or blood may be present. It may be necessary to fill the ductal system with saline and empty it several times to get a clear image for complete ductoscopy.
- ◆ Cytologic study will identify cancer in less than one third of cases in which it has been seen endoscopically. Remember that excisional biopsy must still be the standard for correctly diagnosing an endoscopically visible lesion.
- ◆ Small, widely spaced lesions (<0.2 mm) are rarely malignant.
- ◆ Multiple proliferative lesions in the ductal wall are commonly associated with widespread DCIS or atypical ductal hyperplasia.

Bibliography

Dietz JR, Crowe JP, Grundfest S, et al: Directed duct excision by using mammary ductoscopy in patients with pathologic nipple discharge. Surgery 2002;132:582-587.

Dooley WC: Routine operative breast endoscopy for bloody nipple discharge. Ann Surg Oncol 2002;9:920-923.

Dooley WC: Routine operative breast endoscopy during lumpectomy. Ann Surg Oncol 2003;10:38-42.

Dooley WC, Francescatti D, Clark L, Webber G: Office-based breast ductoscopy for diagnosis. Am J Surg 2004;188:415-418.

Jacobs VR, Kiechle M, Plattner B, et al: Breast ductoscopy with a 0.55-mm mini-endoscope for direct visualization of intraductal lesions. J Minim Invasive Gynecol 2005;12:359-364.

Kim JA, Crowe JP, Woletz J, et al: Prospective study of intraoperative mammary ductoscopy in patients undergoing partial mastectomy for breast cancer. Am J Surg 2004;188:411-414.

Matsunaga T, Kawakami Y, Namba K, Fujii M: Intraductal biopsy for diagnosis and treatment of intraductal lesions of the breast. Cancer 2004;101:2164-2169.

Matsunaga T, Ohta D, Misaka T, et al: Mammary ductoscopy for diagnosis and treatment of intraductal lesions of the breast. Breast Cancer 2001;8:213-221.

Moncrief RM, Nayar R, Diaz LK, et al: A comparison of ductoscopy-guided and conventional surgical excision in women with spontaneous nipple discharge. Ann Surg 2005;241:575-581.

Okazaki A, Okazaki M, Asaishi K, et al: Fiberoptic ductoscopy of the breast: A new diagnostic procedure for nipple discharge. JPN J Clin Oncol 1991;21:188-193.

Sauter ER, Ehya H, Klein-Szanto AJ, et al: Fiberoptic ductoscopy findings in women with and without spontaneous nipple discharge. Cancer 2005;103:914-921.

Sauter ER, Ehya H, Schlatter L, MacGibbon B: Ductoscopic cytology to detect breast cancer. Cancer J 2004;10:33-41.

Sauter ER, Klein-Szanto A, Ehya H, MacGibbon B: Ductoscopic cytology and image analysis to detect breast carcinoma. Cancer 2004;101:1283-1292.

Sharma R, Dietz J, Wright H, et al: Comparative analysis of minimally invasive microductectomy versus major duct excision in patients with pathologic nipple discharge. Surgery 2005;138:591-596.

Yamamoto D, Senzaki H, Nakagawa H, et al: Detection of chromosomal aneusomy by fluorescence in situ hybridization for patients with nipple discharge. Cancer 2004;97:690-694.

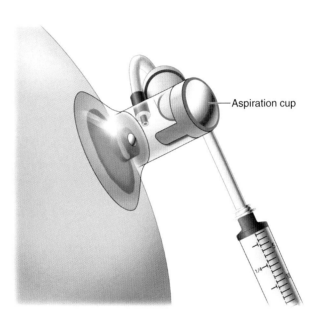

Aspiration cup

Figure 5-9

CHAPTER 6

Excisional Breast Biopsy of Palpable or Nonpalpable Lesions

V. Suzanne Klimberg

Step 1. Surgical Anatomy

- Figure 6-1 demonstrates the anatomic positions of various breast abnormalities.
- Figure 6-2 shows the subcutaneous anatomy of the breast.

Step 2. Preoperative Considerations

- It is preferable to obtain a definitive diagnosis through needle core biopsy before performing excisional breast biopsy (EBB).
- The so-called triple-negative test was developed to identify patients in whom EBB could be obviated and refers to a combination of results from physical examination, imaging (mammography or ultrasonography [US]), and pathology in palpable lesions less than 1 cm in diameter. When all three modalities indicate a benign lesion, the probability of a diagnostic error is less than 1%.
- Obtaining a preoperative diagnosis of cancer allows for a single definitive cancer operation (including axillary staging) in 75% to 100% of cases, compared with 25% to 40% of patients in whom the diagnosis has not been established before EBB.
- The indications for EBB include the following:
  - ▲ Any suspect new finding or change in follow-up clinical examination or imaging
  - ▲ A lesion that is almost certainly benign but is greater than 2 cm, painful, or recurring, or where the mass represents growing cysts or fibroadenomas
  - ▲ Solid masses with equivocal clinical or radiologic features, high-risk lesions, or discordant lesions
  - ▲ Patient preference
- Lesions diagnosed on core biopsy that have a significant risk of underestimating cancer characterized as high-risk, including atypical ductal or lobular hyperplasia, lobular carcinoma in situ, papilloma, and radial scar, should undergo EBB. Lesions diagnosed as malignant should undergo EBB or segmental mastectomy.

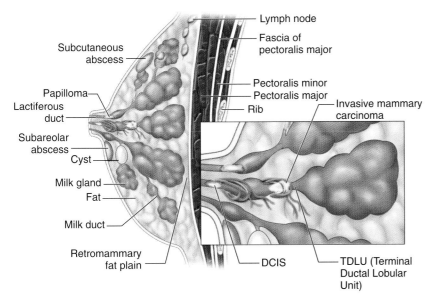

Figure 6-1

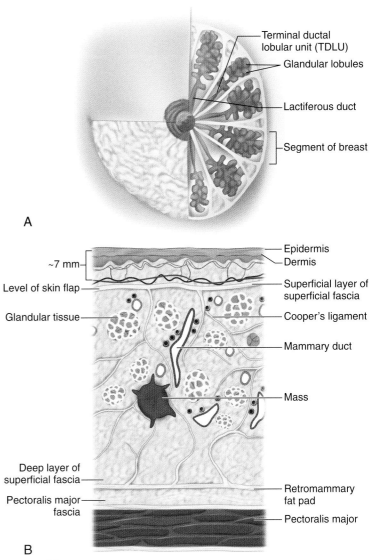

A

B

Figure 6-2

Step 3. Operative Steps

1. Setup

- Excision of palpable breast lesions can be performed under local anesthesia and sedation or general anesthesia. Local anesthesia using a mixture of short- and long-acting anesthetics with epinephrine is ideal. Supplemental sedation relaxes the patient during the procedure. Some have suggested that better margin clearance is obtained with general anesthesia.
- The patient's body should be juxtaposed to the edge of the table and the arm ipsilateral to the index lesion should be positioned at 90 degrees, such that the surgeon and assistant can stand close to the patient above or below the arm (Fig. 6-3).
- Padding under the upper arm should be level with the table and the wrist should be partially cocked back with padding. In a patient with a large, pendulous breast or lesion in the lower outer quadrant, a biodrape instead of an assistant can be used to hold the breast in an optimal position for EBB.

2. Intraoperative Localization

- Intraoperative localization can be accomplished simply by palpating the location and extent of the index lesion.
- US with a 7.5- or 10-MHz probe can be used to increase the accuracy of palpable lesion localization, or to localize the nonpalpable lesion (Fig. 6-4).

3. Incision

- Although it is desirable to place the EBB incision to obtain the best cosmetic result, consideration should be given to subsequent surgical procedures if the lesion is suspected to be malignant (Fig 6-5).
- Incisions along Langer's lines usually provide the best cosmesis in the upper pole of the breast.
- For large masses in the lower half of the breast, an incision along a Langer's line may produce a significant cosmetic deformity, pulling the nipple–areolar complex toward the inframammary crease on closure. Radial incisions are preferred in this circumstance. Others prefer radial incisions because cancer grows in a radial fashion (see Fig. 6-1). The edge of the dermis is then freed to facilitate retractor placement as well as optimal closure.

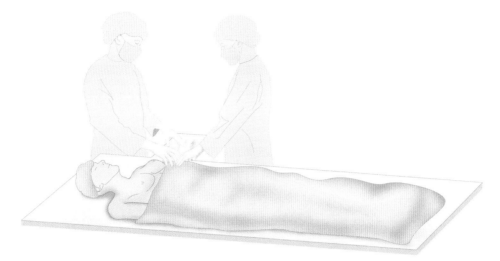

Figure 6-3

Incision lines

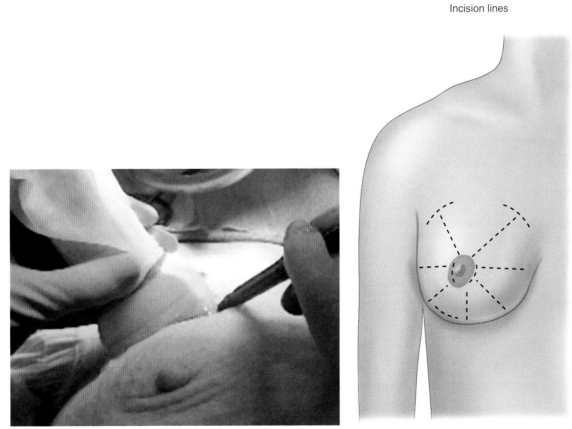

Figure 6-4

Figure 6-5

4. Margin Estimation

- The surgeon should aim for a 1-cm margin around a mass as determined by palpation and US guidance (Fig. 6-6).
- Figure 6-7 shows the US probe being used to determine how deep the EBB needs to be by placing it laterally in the wound.
- Intraoperative US can be used to visualize approximately 50% of nonpalpable lesions and can improve margin negativity with both palpable and nonpalpable lesions by a line-of-sight technique (see Fig. 6-6).

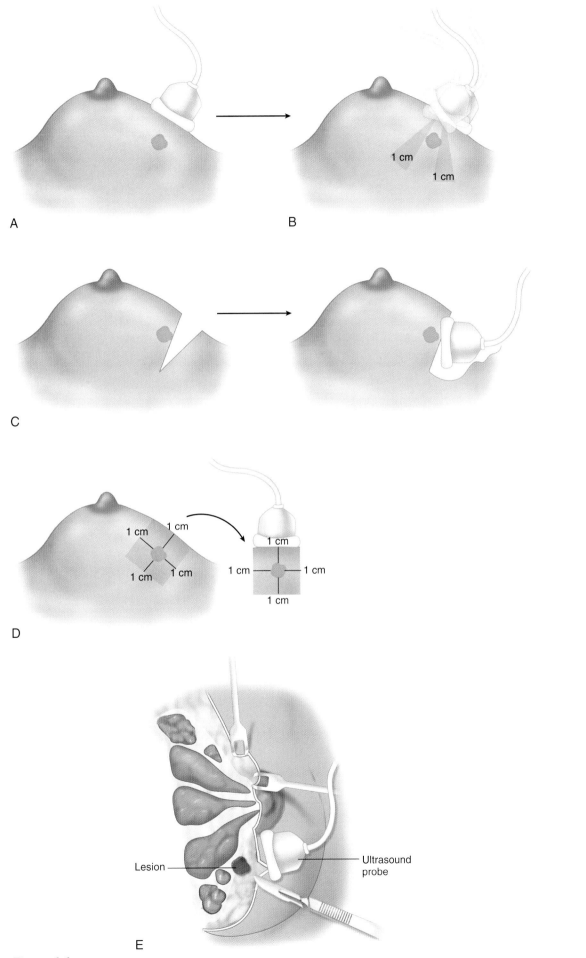

A

B

C

D

E

Figure 6-6

5. Specimen Imaging

◆ Once a lesion has been removed, inspect the mass to detect positive or close margins. This can be done by visual inspection or by specimen US (Fig. 6-8).
◆ Specimen US, using water on the specimen or submersion of the specimen in a bowl of water, can determine close or positive margins on all six sides of the specimen. Reexcision, if necessary, can then be directed to a specific margin.

6. Pathology Marking

◆ The specimen should be marked either while still in the patient or immediately after delivery from the wound in order not to confuse orientation.
◆ It is good practice to mark specimen orientation in the same way every time—for example, "superior" with a short stitch and "lateral" with a long stitch.
◆ In addition, ink from the marking pen can be used to mark the anterior surface (Fig. 6-9). It is not permanent and allows further orientation and ink marking during pathologic examination with six different colors (one for each side).

7. Palpation of Cavity

◆ Palpation of the cavity after removal of the primary lesion, even when margins appear negative, can sometimes find nodules or disease that was not initially apparent.

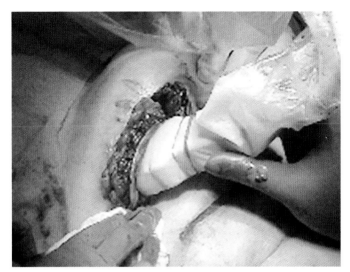

Figure 6-7

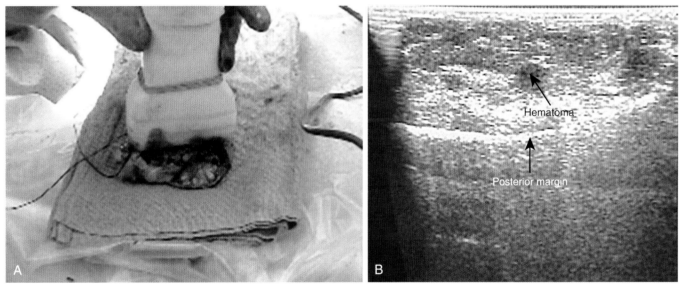

Figure 6-8

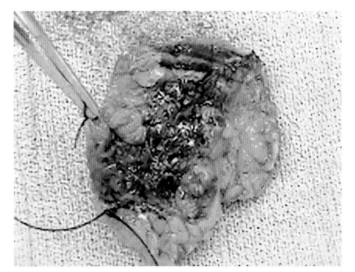

Figure 6-9

8. Shaved Margins

- If a particular margin is close, instead of performing a whole-site reexcision, the intraoperative pathology or permanent inked margins can be used to determine the specific involved margin (or margins), and the problem can be addressed using a shave technique (Fig. 6-10).
- Two clamps are placed approximately 1 cm above and on either side of the index lesion site.
- A flat, approximately 1-cm-thick slice of tissue is shaved from the involved margin (e.g., lateral), the new margin is marked with ink, and the specimen is sent for pathologic examination.

9. Hemostasis

- The breast is extremely vascular, so it is important to obtain excellent hemostasis using electrocautery and ties. A mixture of short- and long-acting local anesthesia containing epinephrine facilitates hemostasis and postoperative pain control.

10. Closure

- For the best cosmetic results, the subcutaneous tissue of the cavity just below the incision is closed. It is critical that the tissue thickness there be at least 7 mm (Fig. 6-11) in case partial breast irradiation is used later.
- Either a running or interrupted absorbable suture can be used to close the dermis. A subcuticular running stitch is best to close the skin.
- A drain is unnecessary and may adversely affect cosmesis.

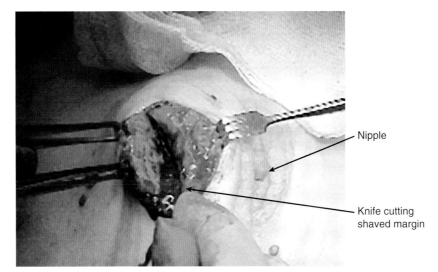

Nipple

Knife cutting shaved margin

Figure 6-10

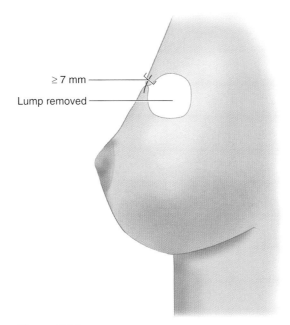

≥ 7 mm

Lump removed

Figure 6-11

Step 4. Postoperative Care

- A pressure dressing is not necessary. Glue or Steri-Strips oriented horizontally over the wound is sufficient.
- A sports bra is sufficient to stabilize the breast for at least the first 48 hours.

Step 5. Pearls and Pitfalls

- Too little padding under the upper arm can cause neuropraxia or neuralgia of the axillary nerve. Too little under the wrist can cause radial nerve praxis.
- Hematomas can be avoided by meticulous attention to hemostasis. Stick ties should be used for any major vessels or oozing, not simply electrocautery. A drain should be placed only if generalized oozing continues. Make sure to take patients off of any nonsteroidal anti-inflammatory drugs (for 7 to 10 days) because of their antiplatelet effects. Hematomas can occur for up to 10 days after surgery.
- Blisters from Steri-Strips not placed parallel to the plane of the incision or under tension can make scars more unsightly than the incision itself. Incision glue is a good alternative.
- Palpation followed by US of the cavity can sometimes help locate a missed lesion. Reexcision of the cavity can also be attempted if, based on reexamination of the mammogram, the operator is confident of the location of the missed lesion. If the lesion still cannot be located, the incision should be closed and a repeat mammogram taken; if the lesion is confirmed still to be present, it should be localized using needle localization and the patient taken directly back to the operating room.

Bibliography

Chalas E, Valea F: The gynecologist and surgical procedures for the breast disease. Clin Obstet Gynecol 1994;37:948-953.

Crow JP, Rim A, Patrick R, et al: A prospective review of the decline of excisional breast biopsy. Am J Surg 2002;184:353-355.

Kerlikowske K, Smith-Bindman R, Ljung BM, Grady D: Evaluation of abnormal mammography results and palpable breast abnormalities. Ann Intern Med 2004;139:274-284.

Schwartz GF, Veronesi U, Clough KB, et al: Consensus Conference on Breast Conservation. J Am Coll Surg 2006;203:198-207.

Vetto J, Pommier R, Schmidt W, et al: Diagnosis of palpable breast lesions in younger women by the modified triple test is accurate and cost-effective. Arch Surg 1996;131:967-974.

CHAPTER 7

NEEDLE LOCALIZATION BREAST BIOPSY

V. Suzanne Klimberg, Keiva Bland, and Kent C. Westbrook

Step 1. Surgical Anatomy

- ◆ Figure 7-1 demonstrates the anatomic positions of various breast abnormalities.
- ◆ Figure 7-2 shows the subcutaneous anatomy of the breast.

Step 2. Preoperative Considerations

- ◆ It is preferable to obtain a definitive diagnosis through needle core biopsy before performing excisional breast biopsy (EBB). Stereotactic biopsy guided by mammography is the preferred method of diagnosis if the lesion is not seen by ultrasonography (US).
- ◆ The indications for needle localization breast biopsy (NLBB) include the following:
  - ▲ Any suspect new finding or change in follow-up clinical examination or mammography not seen by US
  - ▲ Suspect calcification (five or more clustered calcifications), solid masses with equivocal clinical or mammographic features, high-risk lesions, or discordant lesions; or because of patient preference
  - ▲ Lesions diagnosed on core biopsy that have a significant risk of underestimating cancer characterized as high-risk, including atypical ductal or lobular hyperplasia, lobular carcinoma in situ, papilloma, and radial scar, should undergo NLBB if not palpable or can be excised by hematoma-directed ultrasound guidance (HUG) if visible on US. Lesions diagnosed as malignant should undergo segmental mastectomy.
- ◆ The needle for NLBB is placed while the patient is in the sitting position with the breast compressed by a plate that is numbered on one side and lettered on the other. The lesion is localized using a needle and wire, that, if possible, is placed behind the target lesion to facilitate excision (Fig. 7-3). Various needles are available to localize lesions, including the Kopans needle (checkmark wire), the Hawkins needle (multiple barbs and the only retractable wire for repositioning), and the Homer needle (J wire), which is the only virtually nontransectable needle.

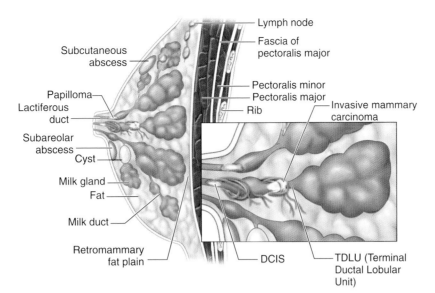

Subcutaneous abscess
Papilloma
Lactiferous duct
Subareolar abscess
Cyst
Milk gland
Fat
Milk duct
Retromammary fat plain

Lymph node
Fascia of pectoralis major
Pectoralis minor
Pectoralis major
Rib
Invasive mammary carcinoma
DCIS
TDLU (Terminal Ductal Lobular Unit)

Figure 7-1

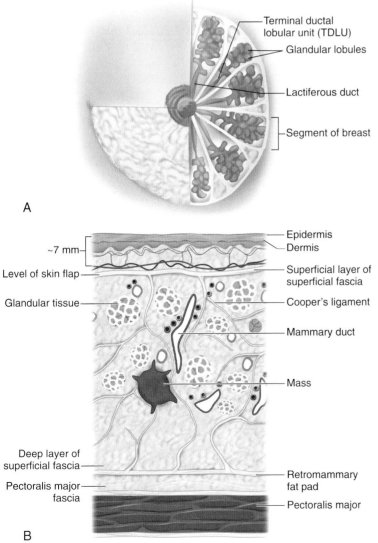

Terminal ductal lobular unit (TDLU)
Glandular lobules
Lactiferous duct
Segment of breast

A

Epidermis
Dermis
~7 mm
Level of skin flap
Glandular tissue
Superficial layer of superficial fascia
Cooper's ligament
Mammary duct
Mass
Deep layer of superficial fascia
Pectoralis major fascia
Retromammary fat pad
Pectoralis major

B

Figure 7-2

Needle wire
Index lesions circled
Needle wire
Cranial caudal view
Medical lateral view

Figure 7-3

♦ It is advisable to leave the needle over the wire so that the wire is strengthened and is more easily palpated and seen on US.
♦ The patient should be scheduled for excision as soon as feasible after placement because the wire and needle placement and the retained needle itself can be uncomfortable.

Step 3. Operative Steps

1. Setup

♦ As with the excision of palpable breast lesions, NLBB can be performed under local anesthesia with sedation or general anesthesia.
♦ The patient's body should be juxtaposed to the edge of the table and the arm ipsilateral to the index lesion should be positioned at 90 degrees, such that the surgeon and assistant can stand close to the patient above or below the arm (Fig. 7-4). Appropriate padding of the arm should be used.
♦ Care should be taken when removing bandages covering the extraneous portion of the wire and needle because it is easily dislodged.

2. Intraoperative Localization

♦ Intraoperative localization can be performed simply by palpating the needle (Fig. 7-5).
♦ US with a 7.5- or 10-MHz probe provides additional accuracy; the tip of the needle wire can be difficult to palpate; if necessary, US can be used to find the tip and excise the needle and wire.

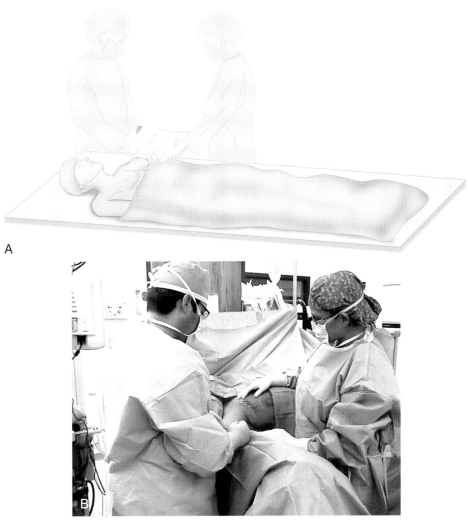

Figure 7-4

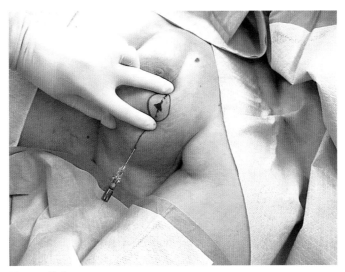

Figure 7-5

3. Incision

◆ Although it is desirable to place the EBB incision to obtain the best cosmetic result, such as through an incision in the inframammary fold and following the needle wire down to the tip of the needle (Fig. 7-6), most often the lesion is accessed by making an incision directly over the tip of the palpable wire or next to the needle and wire and following it down to the tip to find the target lesion (Fig. 7-7).

◆ For large masses in the lower half of the breast, incision along a Langer's line may produce a significant cosmetic deformity, pulling the nipple–areolar complex toward the inframammary crease on closure. Radial incisions are preferred in this circumstance. Others prefer radial incisions because cancer grows in a radial fashion along the ductal system (see Fig. 7-1). The edge of the dermis is then freed to facilitate retractor placement as well as optimal closure.

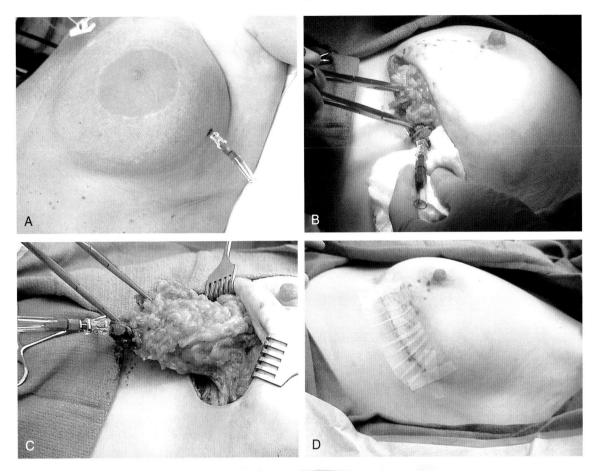

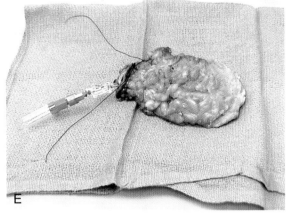

Figure 7-6

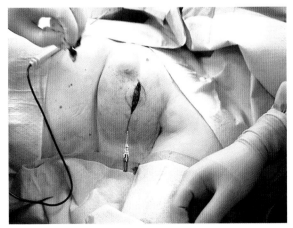

Figure 7-7

4. Excision

- After making the incision, a clamp should be used to secure the hub of the needle wire construct proximal to the targeted lesion (Figs. 7-8 and 7-9).
- Rakes can then be used to open up the wound over the lesion (Fig. 7-9), with the goal of removing a cylinder of tissue around the wire (Fig. 7-10).
- Ideally, the wire should be placed behind the index lesion so that the surgeon can cut along the needle wire posteriorly, in effect marking the posterior extent of the resection.
- A clamp is used to secure the tissue distal to the tip of the needle wire (Fig. 7-11).
- The tissue surrounding the needle–wire is then lifted out of the wound, with dissection continuing to take a cylinder of tissue around the needle wire (Fig. 7-12).

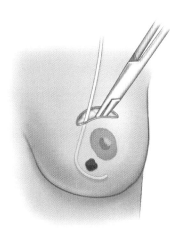

Figure 7-8

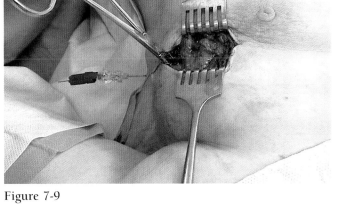

Figure 7-9

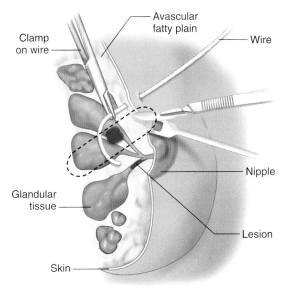

Figure 7-10

Clamp on wire

Avascular fatty plain

Wire

Nipple

Glandular tissue

Lesion

Skin

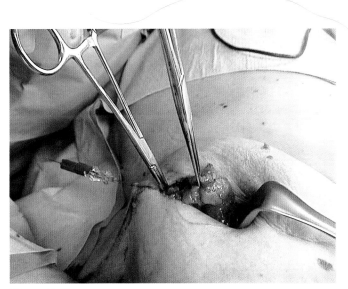

Figure 7-11

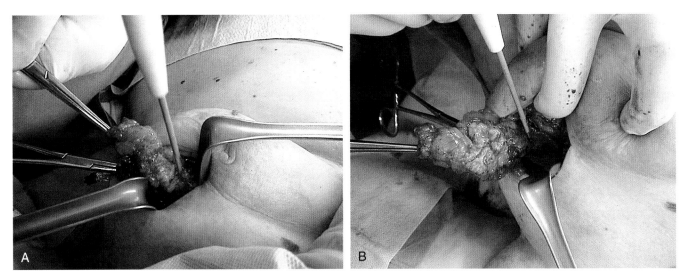

A   B

Figure 7-12

- Once the dissection has reached the proximal clamp, the lock on the wire is released (Fig. 7-13) and the needle removed, leaving the wire in place with the proximal clamp on it (Fig. 7-14).
- The clamp is then loosened and the wire is exited through the wound (Fig. 7-15).

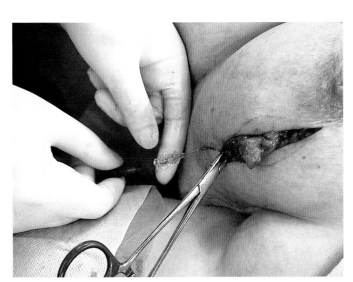

Figure 7-13

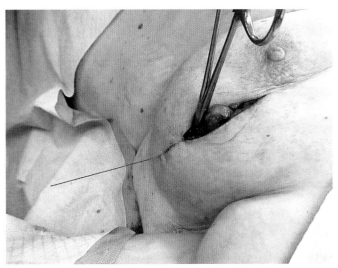

Figure 7-14

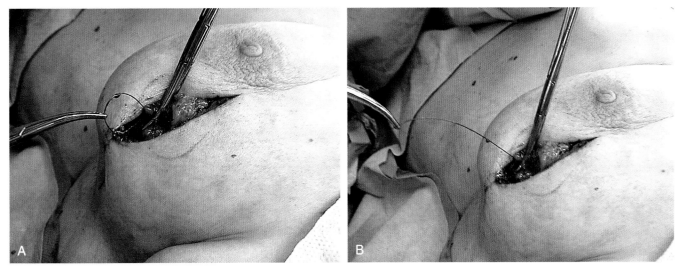

Figure 7-15

♦ The dissection is then completed, delivering the specimen with wire intact through the wound (Fig. 7-16).

5. Margin Estimation

♦ The surgeon should aim for a cylindrical 1-cm margin around the mass and wire (see Fig. 7-10).

6. Specimen Imaging

♦ Once the lesion has been removed, inspect the mass to detect positive or close margins. This can be done by visual inspection.

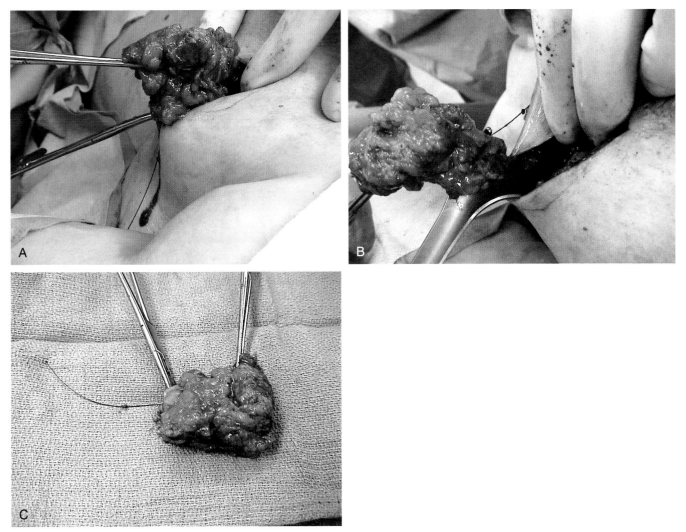

Figure 7-16

◆ Plain radiography of the specimen confirms that the targeted lesion and calcifications were removed and shows how close they were to a margin (Fig. 7-17). Although specimen radiography cannot confirm completely negative margins because it is taken in only one plane, it does confirm a positive one.

7. Pathology Marking

◆ The specimen should be marked as described in Chapter 6 (Fig. 7-18), with a superior short stitch, a lateral long stitch, and ink anteriorly.

8. Palpation of Cavity

◆ Palpation of the cavity after removal of the primary lesion, even when margins appear negative, can sometimes find nodules or disease that was not initially apparent.

9. Shaved Margins

◆ If a particular margin is close, instead of performing a whole-site reexcision, the intraoperative pathology or permanent inked margins can be used to determine the specific involved margin (or margins), and the problem can be addressed using a shave technique in which a 1-cm thickness from each wall of the cavity is removed sequentially (Fig. 7-19).

10. Hemostasis

◆ The breast is extremely vascular, so it is important to obtain excellent hemostasis using electrocautery and ties. A mixture of short- and long-acting local anesthesia containing epinephrine facilitates hemostasis and postoperative pain control.

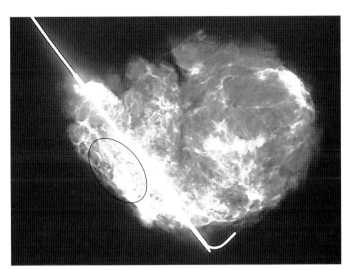

Figure 7-17

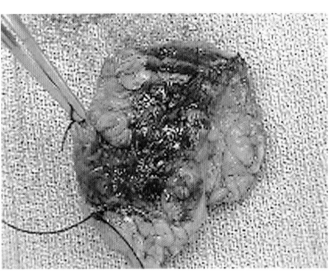

Figure 7-18

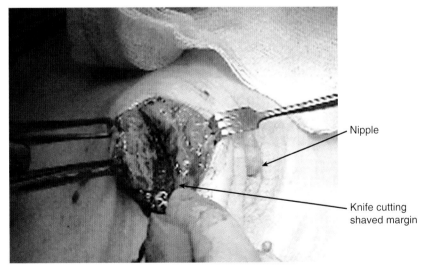

Nipple

Knife cutting
shaved margin

Figure 7-19

11. Closure

- For the best cosmetic results, the subcutaneous tissue of the cavity just below the incision is closed. It is critical that the tissue thickness left there be at least 7 mm (Fig. 7-20) in case partial breast irradiation is used later.
- Either a running or interrupted absorbable suture can be used to close the dermis. A subcuticular running stitch is best to close the skin.
- A drain is unnecessary and may adversely affect cosmesis.

Step 4. Postoperative Care

- A pressure dressing is not necessary. Glue or Steri-Strips over the wound is sufficient.
- A sports bra is sufficient to stabilize the breast for at least the first 48 hours.

Step 5. Pearls and Pitfalls

- Four to 9% of lesions can be missed with NLBB. When removing a lesion, the surgeon should always try to visualize where he or she would reexcise if the lesion were missed the first time. Palpation and then US of the cavity can sometimes help locate a missed lesion. Reexcision of the cavity can also be attempted if, based on reexamination of the mammogram, the operator is confident of the location of the missed lesion. If the lesion still cannot be located, the patient should be closed and a repeat mammogram taken; if the lesion is confirmed still to be present, it should be relocalized using needle localization and the patient taken directly back to the operating room.

Bibliography

Chalas, Valea F: The gynecologist and surgical procedures for the breast disease. Clin Obstet Gynecol 1994;37:948-953.
Crow JP, Rim A, Patrick R, et al: A prospective review of the decline of excisional breast biopsy. Am J Surg 2002;184:353-355.
Kerlikowske K, Smith-Bindman R, Ljung BM, Grady D: Evaluation of abnormal mammography results and palpable breast abnormalities. Ann Intern Med 2004;139:274-284.
Schwartz GF, Veronesi U, Clough KB, et al: Consensus Conference on Breast Conservation. J Am Coll Surg 2006;203:198-207.
Vetto J, Pommier R, Schmidt W, et al: Diagnosis of palpable breast lesions in younger women by the modified triple test is accurate and cost-effective. Arch Surg 1996;131:967-974.

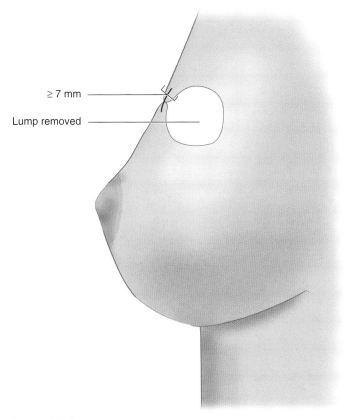

≥ 7 mm

Lump removed

Figure 7-20

CHAPTER 8

RADIOISOTOPE OCCULT LESION LOCALIZATION

Hodigere S.J. Ramesh, Matilde M. Audisio,
and Riccardo A. Audisio

Step 1. Surgical Anatomy

- ◆ Familiarity with the ultrasonographic characteristics of the normal breast as well as those of benign and malignant lesions is essential (see also Chapter 3).
- ◆ Figure 8-1 demonstrates the normal ultrasonographic anatomy of the breast.
- ◆ Figure 8-2 illustrates the more common characteristics that distinguish benign from malignant lesions.

Step 2. Preoperative Considerations

- ◆ Indications for radioisotope occult lesion localization (ROLL) include the following:
  - ▲ Microcalcifications
  - ▲ Parenchymal distortions (i.e., radial scars, atypical hyperplasia)
  - ▲ Nonpalpable, suspect soft tissue masses
  - ▲ Impalpable cancers after neoadjuvant chemotherapy
  - ▲ Foreign bodies in soft tissue
- ◆ ROLL is performed for the diagnostic excision biopsy of suspect lesions as well as the therapeutic excision of a proven cancer. The aim is to remove cancerous tissue with clear resection margins within the smallest possible amount of glandular tissue, to achieve excellent cosmetic results. ROLL is frequently performed under general anesthesia as a day case. Initial diagnostic imaging (i.e., mammography, ultrasonography) should be available at the time of localization and in the operating room to plan the surgical approach and to compare with the specimen radiograph to confirm excision of the target lesion.

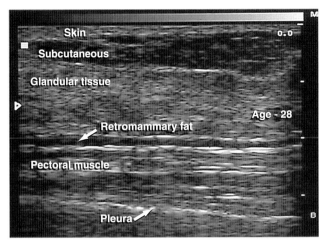

Figure 8-1

	Benign	Malignant
Margins	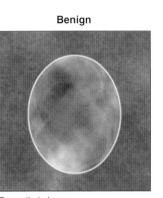 Smooth / sharp	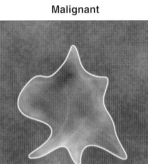 Indistinct / jagged
Adjacent architecture	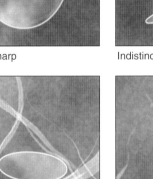 Grows within tissue planes	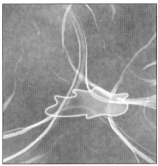 Disrupted
Shape	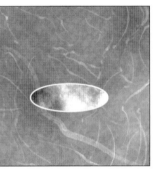 Transverse > Longitudinal	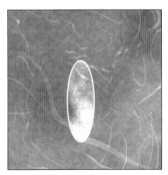 Longitudinal > Transverse
Retrotumoral effect	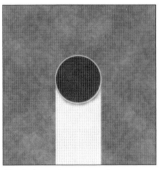 Posterior enhancement	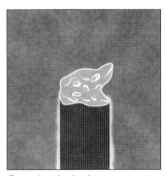 Posterior shadowing

Figure 8-2

- The nonpalpable lesion can be targeted mammographically or ultrasonographically, such as the lesion shown in Figure 8-3.
- Technetium-99m–labeled (half-life of 6 hours) macroaggregate is freshly prepared by radio-pharmacy and delivered a few hours before localization. The localization fluid (0.2 mL) is delivered in a preloaded, sterile-packed syringe in a protective lead case (Fig. 8-4). Care should be taken to shake the preloaded syringe gently to mix the macroaggregates before injection.
- The absorbed radiation dose to hospital personnel is low and requires neither radiation protection control nor classification of exposed workers as class A or B. Special containers for radioactive wastes are necessary in the administration room but not in the operating room, where possible contamination is negligible. In cases when a surgeon performs 100 procedures per year, a finger dose (FD) dose of approximately 1 mSv is received, which is well within the annual dose limit of 150 mSv. Annual whole-body dosage of assisting staff may reach 0.04 mSv, compared with an annual limit of 6 mSv. These low doses indicate that no additional radiation protection measures are necessary, although they may be required by law.
- Localization is performed by a trained radiologist in the radiology department. After reviewing initial diagnostic imaging and case notes, the radiologist injects 0.2 mL ^{99m}Tc-labeled nanocolloid into the core of the lesion under ultrasonographic or stereotactic guidance 1 to 4 hours before surgery. The radiation dosage delivered is 1 MBq, equivalent to 0.02 mSv (=1 chest radiograph). The lesion is most frequently localized by ultrasonography (~75%; Fig. 8-5; also see Fig. 8-3); stereotaxis may be used when the lesion is not visible on ultrasonography (~25%).
- A final check for radioactive signal is made in the anesthesia room while the patient is in a sitting as well as a supine position; this not only ensures the working status of the system (gamma camera and radioisotope) but provides a final opportunity to plan, discuss, and mark the most appropriate surgical approach to the lesion while the patient is awake (Fig. 8-6).
- General anesthesia is recommended, although local anesthesia may be considered in a suitable candidate.

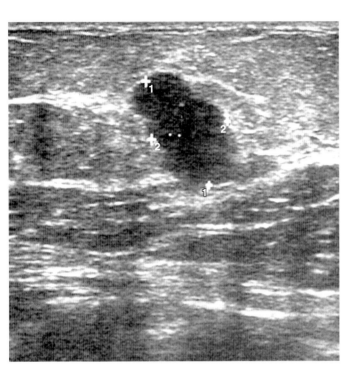

Figure 8-3

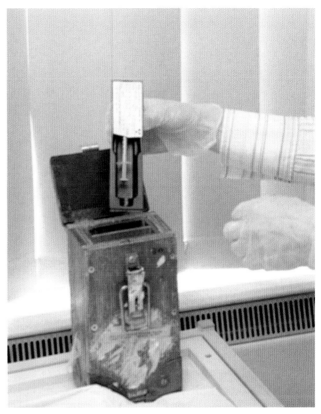

Figure 8-4

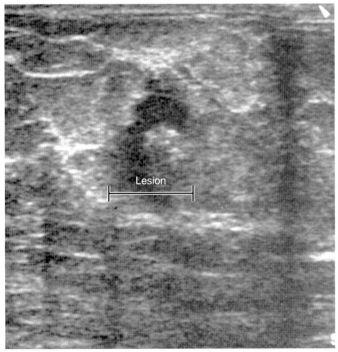

Figure 8-5

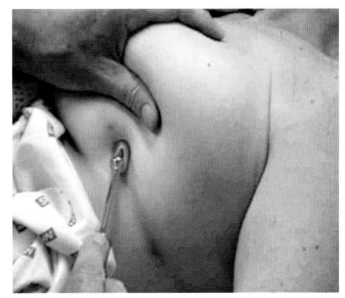

Figure 8-6

Step 3. Operative Steps

1. Patient Position

- The patient is positioned supine on the operating table with the arm ipsilateral to the lesion abducted to expose the outer breast quadrants and fully extended at the elbow, resting on a well-padded arm board (Fig. 8-7).

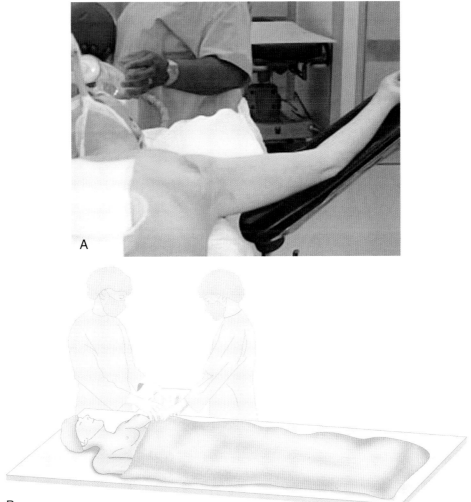

Figure 8-7

2. Incisions

◆ The appropriate skin incision is chosen to facilitate surgical removal in accordance with onco-logic principles while providing the best cosmetic results. ROLL allows great flexibility in approaching the lesion, bearing in mind that the incision line should fall within the boundaries of a subsequent mastectomy or lumpectomy, should such a procedure become necessary. Whenever possible, it is our preference to use an inframammary incision for lesions in the lower quadrants (Fig. 8-8), a periareolar incision for lesions in the central quadrant (Fig. 8-9),

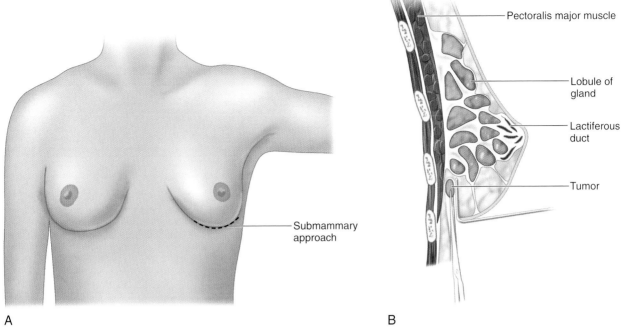

A

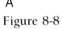

Figure 8-8

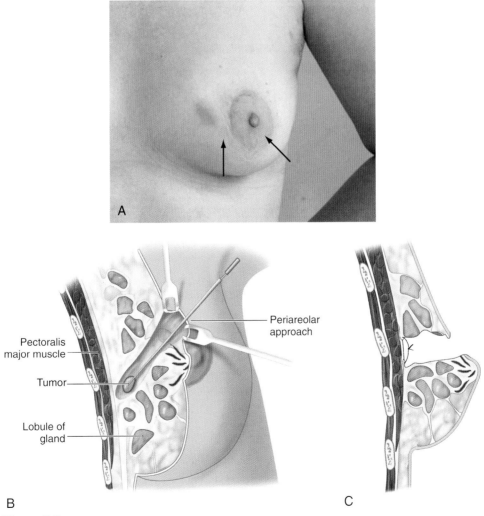

Figure 8-9

or an axillary incision for lesions in the upper-outer quadrant (Fig. 8-10). These incision lines provide excellent cosmetic results.

♦ Skin incisions paralleling Langer's lines result in thin, cosmetically acceptable scars for peripheral lesions requiring a direct anterior approach (Fig. 8-11).

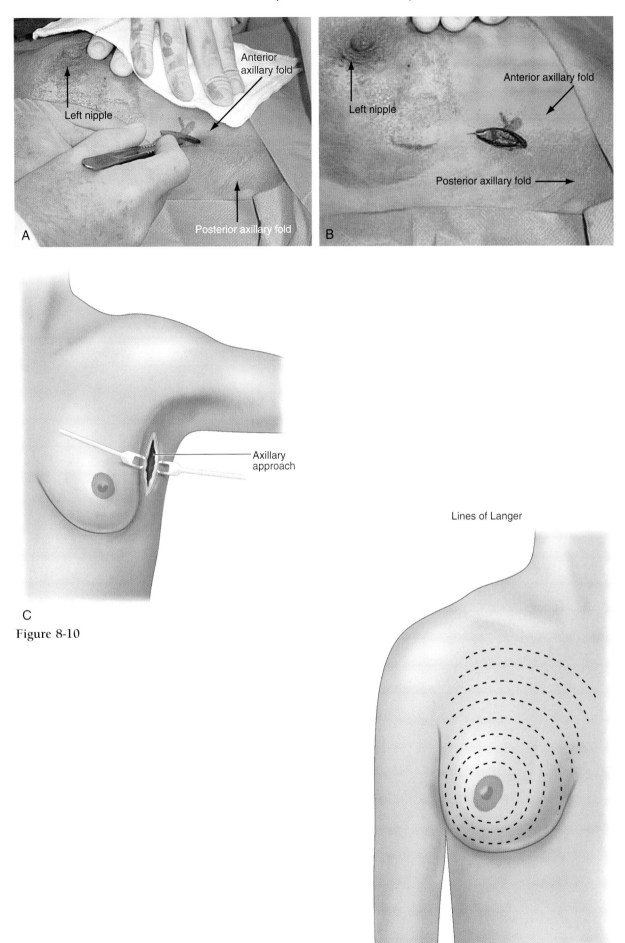

Figure 8-10

Figure 8-11

3. Targeting the Lesion

◆ The gamma camera with a mounted collimator is wrapped in a sterile polythene cover (Fig. 8-12). The collimator filters the stream of gamma rays so that only those from the injection site traveling parallel to the probe tip are scanned. Without a collimator, rays from all directions are recorded and localization may be more difficult.

◆ The most intense area of radioactivity (i.e., center of targeted lesion) is identified with the gamma probe by listening for audible signal at the injection site (Fig. 8-13).

◆ After the skin is incised, a check for gamma signal facilitates choosing the most direct approach to the lesion.

4. Excision and Marking of Index Lesion

◆ Excision biopsy is carried out following audible gamma signals and using finger palpation of the tissue being excised. The wound is deepened to include the pectoral fascia, aiming to achieve 5 to 10 mm of healthy margins encasing the neoplastic lesion. The localized tissue is checked for signal before being dissected from the glandular tissue (Fig. 8-14).

◆ Excision of the target lesion is confirmed by the absence of residual signal in the cavity (Fig. 8-15).

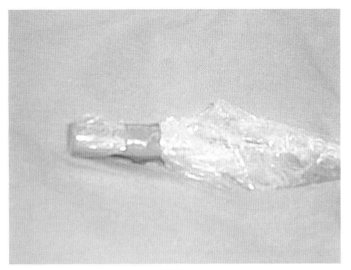

Figure 8-12

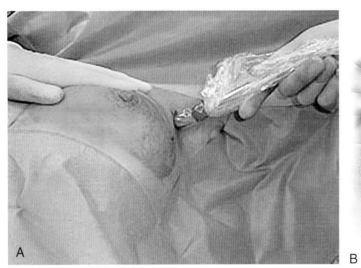

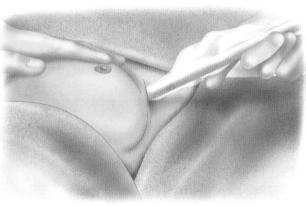

Figure 8-13

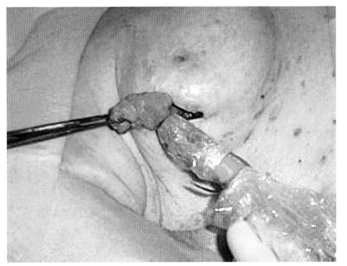

Figure 8-14

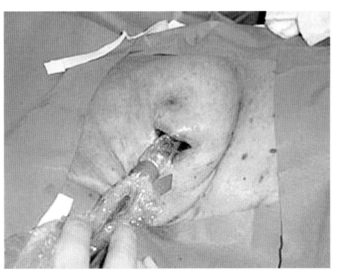

Figure 8-15

◆ The specimen is then marked with standard orientation stitches for pathologic examination, and checked once again for presence of radioactive signal (Fig. 8-16).

5. Specimen Radiography

◆ Specimen radiography ensures that the lesion is present within the excised tissue; the presence of healthy tissue margins may provide reassurance as to the oncologic adequacy of the removal, although this must be confirmed by pathology (Fig. 8-17).

6. Closure

◆ Meticulous hemostasis is ensured. Drainage of the breast cavity is not necessary.
◆ The excisional cavity is obliterated by approximating the breast plate overlying the pectoral fascia with 2-0 Vicryl absorbable stitches. Stitches in the fat are avoided (see Fig. 8-9, *C*).
◆ Skin edges are approximated with continuous subcuticular absorbable 3-0 Vicryl Rapide stitches (Fig. 8-18).
◆ The wound edges may be reinforced with ¼-inch Steri-Strips (Fig. 8-19). Breathable dressings or pressure dressings are avoided.
◆ See Chapter 6 for a detailed explanation of excisional breast biopsy.

Step 4. Postoperative Care

◆ Patients are encouraged to resume normal activity on the evening of surgery. Postoperative assessment should include evaluation of the wound for hematoma formation.

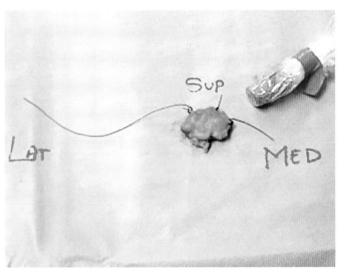

Figure 8-16

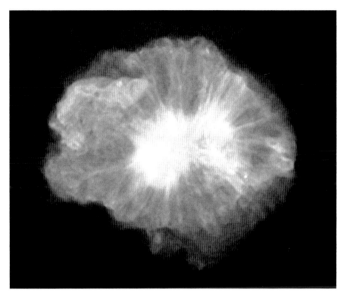

Figure 8-17

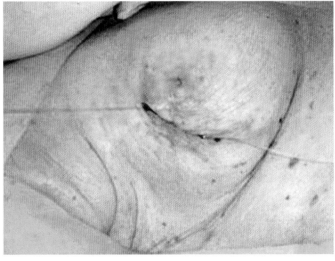

Figure 8-18

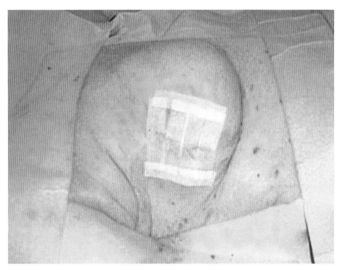

Figure 8-19

Step 5. Pearls and Pitfalls

1. Pearls

- The breast tissue should constantly be felt for consistency throughout the procedure. Biopsy of suspect areas, despite absence of gamma signals, should be considered.
- Hot signals do not define the extent of cancer; ROLL should be regarded only as a localization aid.
- Bilateral nonpalpable breast cancers can be simultaneously localized without any adverse effects.
- ROLL can be combined with sentinel lymph node biopsy (SNOLL).

2. Pitfalls

- Check for allergic reactions (i.e., to albumin).
- The collimator should be mounted on the tip of the gamma camera. Failure to do so may result in inability to obtain accurate signals.
- Shake the syringe before use. Macroaggregates tend to adhere to the walls of the plastic syringe. The inadequate mixing of such components could result in inability to obtain signals.
- Spillage of injectate along the needle tract should be avoided. The plunger of the syringe is pushed to the end of the barrel only when the radiologist is certain about the needle tip position within the lesion to be injected. Spillage along the needle tract can mislead the surgeon by giving false-positive signals.
- Ensure that the radioisotope is injected into the lesion. In our experience, 1% to 2% of radioisotope injections resulted in failed localization. The availability of an alternative method of localization is recommended in the rare event the radioisotope technique fails.
- Small, contained hematomas can be managed conservatively. Large, expanding hematomas may need open surgical drainage and antibiotics. Allergic reactions to the radioisotope or macroaggregates, although possible, have not yet been reported with ROLL.

Bibliography

Audisio RA, Nadeem R, Harris O, et al: Radioguided occult lesion localisation (ROLL) is available in the UK for impalpable breast lesions. Ann R Coll Surg 2005;87:92-95.

De Cicco C, Pizzamiglio M, Trifiro G, et al: Radioguided occult lesion localisation (ROLL) and surgical biopsy in breast cancer: Technical aspects. Q J Nucl Med 2002;46:145-151.

Feggi L, Basaglia E, Corcione S, et al: An original approach in the diagnosis of early breast cancer: Use of the same radiopharmaceutical for both non-palpable lesions and sentinel node localisation. Eur J Nucl Med 2001;28:1589-1596.

Ferrari M, Cremonesi M, Sacco E, et al: Radiation protection in the use of tracers in radioguided breast surgery. Radiol Med (Torino) 1998;96:607-611.

Gennari R, Galimberti V, De Cicco C, et al: Use of technetium-99m-labeled colloid albumin for preoperative and intraoperative localization of nonpalpable breast lesions. J Am Coll Surg 200;190:692-698.

Luini A, Zurrida S, Galimberti V, Paganelli G: Radioguided surgery of occult breast lesions. Eur J Cancer 1998;34:204-205.

Luini A, Zurrida S, Paganelli G, et al: Comparison of radioguided excision with wire localization of occult breast lesions. Br J Surg 1999;86:522-525.

Nadeem R, Chagla LS, Harris O, et al: Occult breast lesions: A comparison between radioguided occult lesion localisation (ROLL) vs. wire-guided lumpectomy (WGL). Breast 2005;14:283-289.

Nadeem R, Chagla LS, Harris O, et al: Tumour localisation with metal coil before the administration of neo-adjuvant chemotherapy. Breast 2005;14:403-407.

Rampaul RS, Dudley NJ, Thompson JZ, et al: Radioisotope for occult lesion localisation (ROLL) of the breast does not require extra radiation protection procedures. Breast 2003;12:150-152.

Ronka R, Krogerus L, Leppanen E, et al: Radio-guided occult lesion localization in patients undergoing breast-conserving surgery and sentinel node biopsy. Am J Surg 2004;187:491-496.

Thind CR, Desmond S, Harris O, et al: Radio-guided localization of clinically occult breast lesions (ROLL): A DGH experience. Clin Radiol 2005;60:681-686.

CHAPTER 9

CRYOABLATION-ASSISTED LUMPECTOMY

Anees B. Chagpar

Step 1. Surgical Anatomy

- Familiarity with the ultrasonographic characteristics of the normal breast, as well as those of benign and malignant lesions, is essential.
- Figures 9-1 and 9-2 demonstrate the normal anatomy of the breast and its ultrasonographic appearance.
- Figure 9-3 illustrates the more common characteristics that distinguish benign from malignant lesions.

Step 2. Preoperative Considerations

1. Appropriate Patient Selection

- Only patients who have relatively small (<18 mm), unifocal tumors should be offered this technique. Because the cryoprobe needle has a freezing length of 4 cm, it would be difficult to obtain clear margins in patients with tumors larger than 2 cm.
- The lesion must be visible on ultrasonography.
- Ideally the mass should be neither very superficial nor very deep in the breast.
- There are only limited data for the use of this technique in patients with ductal carcinoma in situ.
- The technique should be avoided in patients with invasive lobular carcinomas.

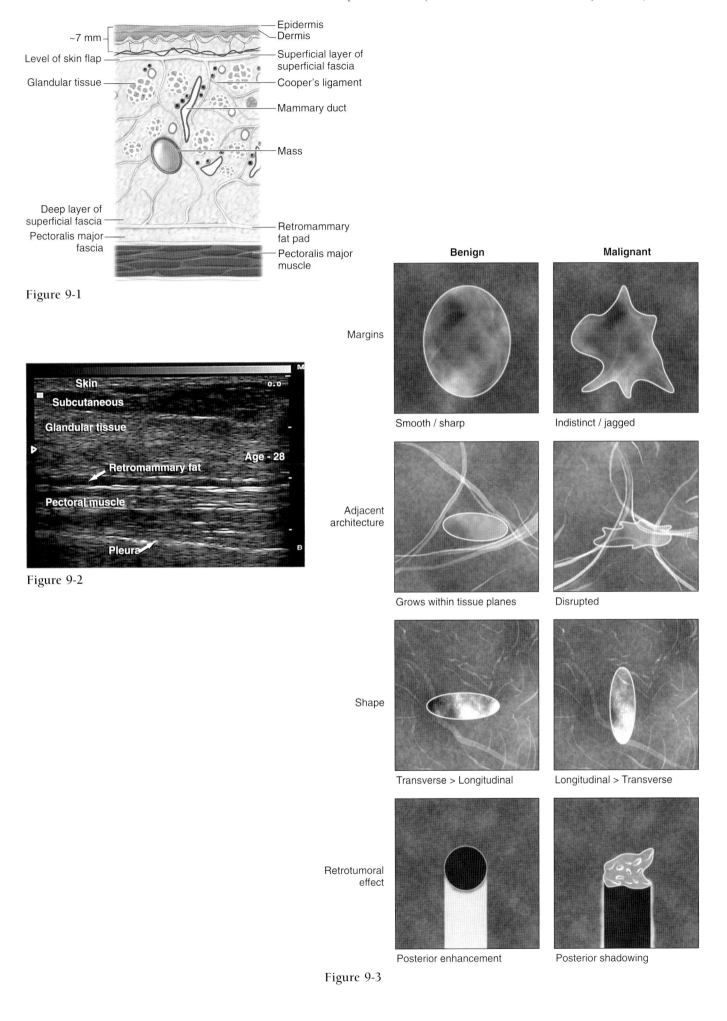

Figure 9-1

Figure 9-2

Figure 9-3

2. Preoperative Diagnostic Core Needle Biopsy for Receptors and Markers

◆ Freezing interferes with immunohistochemical and fluorescence in situ hybridization techniques for hormone receptor and her-2-*neu* analysis. Also, tumor grade may be difficult to discern after cryotherapy. Therefore, it is critical to obtain a preoperative core needle biopsy both for diagnosis and receptor analysis.

3. Equipment Needed

◆ The following equipment is required:
  ▲ Intraoperative ultrasonography
  ▲ Cryoprobe needle
  ▲ Local anesthetic or saline for infiltration
  ▲ Usual equipment needed for lumpectomy

Step 3. Operative Steps

1. Anesthesia, Patient Positioning, Draping

◆ This procedure can be done under general anesthesia or conscious sedation with monitored anesthesia care.
◆ The patient is positioned supine and draped in the usual fashion as is done for a lumpectomy (Fig. 9-4).

2. Ultrasonography

◆ The mass is visualized using intraoperative ultrasonography in both longitudinal and transverse axes (Fig. 9-5).
◆ The mass is measured in each axis and the largest measurement of the mass is noted.

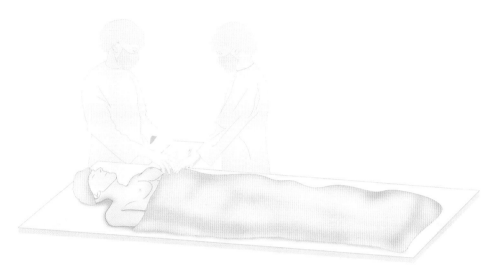

Figure 9-4

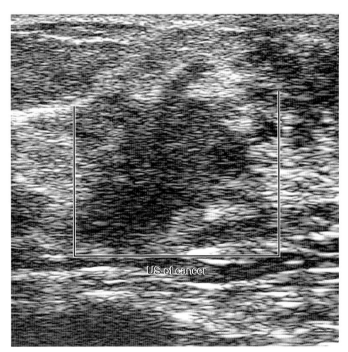

US of cancer

Figure 9-5

3. Placement of Probe

- While holding the ultrasound probe to visualize the mass in one hand, a small incision is made with the other hand along the long axis of the transducer.
- The cryoprobe needle is inserted toward the mass under ultrasonographic guidance, keeping the probe parallel to the transducer (Fig. 9-6).
- The ultrasonogram demonstrates the longitudinal approach and placement of the cryoprobe needle in the targeted mass (Fig. 9-7).
- Ensure that the probe is placed in the center of the lesion by scanning in the transverse axis. The probe should be visible as a bright white spot in the middle of the lesion (Fig. 9-8).

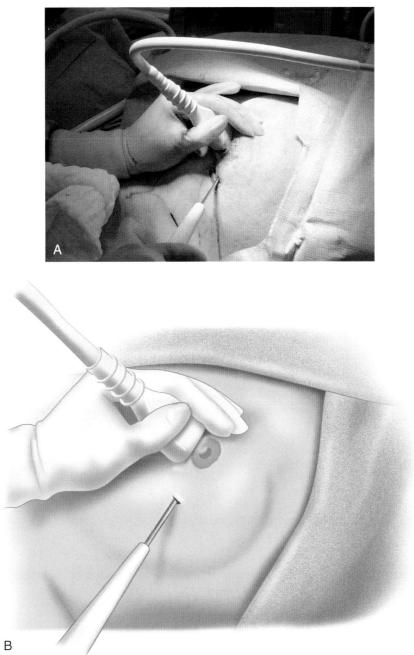

Figure 9-6

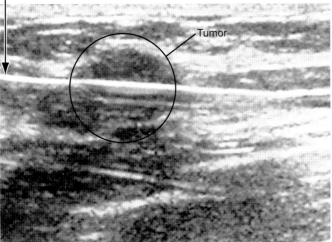

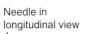

Figure 9-7

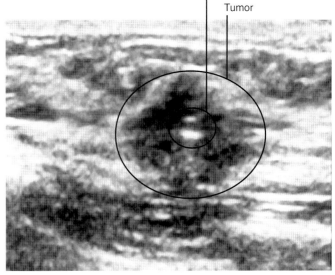

Figure 9-8

4. **Measurements**

- The probe's freeze zone has a standard length (usually 4 cm). Therefore, one cannot create a longer iceball than this, and the shortest axis will be the depth of the iceball, which will change with the duration of the freezing.
- In determining the appropriate depth of the freeze zone, some have considered an 8-mm margin around the lesion acceptable. Therefore, to determine the depth of freezing required, add the size of the mass and the extra margin you wish to cover multiplied by two (for the proximal and distal margins). For example, if the mass is 15 mm and an 8-mm margin is desired, the total depth of the freeze zone should be 15 mm + (8 mm × 2) = 31 mm (Fig. 9-9).
- The mass should be centered in the freeze zone of the probe.
  - ▲ To do this, calculate the distance beyond the edge of the lesion where the tip of the probe should be placed by subtracting the largest dimension of the lesion from the length of the freeze zone of the probe, and dividing by two.
  - ▲ The standard freeze length for a probe is 4 cm. If the lesion measures 15 mm, in order to center the lesion in terms of length one would aim to have (40 − 15)/2 = 12.5 mm of probe distal to the edge of the mass (see Fig. 9-9).
- The probe should be placed in the center of the lesion's vertical axis.
- If the lesion is not perfectly centered, the freeze depth can be modified accordingly. By scanning in the transverse plane, the longest distance from the probe to the edge of the lesion can be determined. For example, Figure 9-10 demonstrates a 15-mm lesion in which the probe is placed too far inferiorly—there is 9 mm from the probe to the top of the lesion. Multiply this distance by two (as though the probe was in the middle), which gives 18 mm. Given that this new measurement is greater than the true longest dimension of the lesion (15 mm), the depth of the iceball should be calculated using the larger measurement: 18 mm + (2 × 8-mm margin) = 36-mm iceball (see Fig. 9-10).

5. **Growth of Iceball**

- Once the probe is in position and the desired length of the iceball is calculated, the probe is set to high freeze; argon gas delivered to the probe achieves temperatures of −160° C, thereby immobilizing the lesion. The freeze process is monitored using real-time ultrasonography until the iceball reaches the predefined length (Fig. 9-11).
- Once the iceball reaches this length, the probe is turned to low freeze, which maintains the size of the iceball. The iceball is maintained at low freeze until it is excised. The freeze may then be turned off to allow the iceball to slide off the probe.

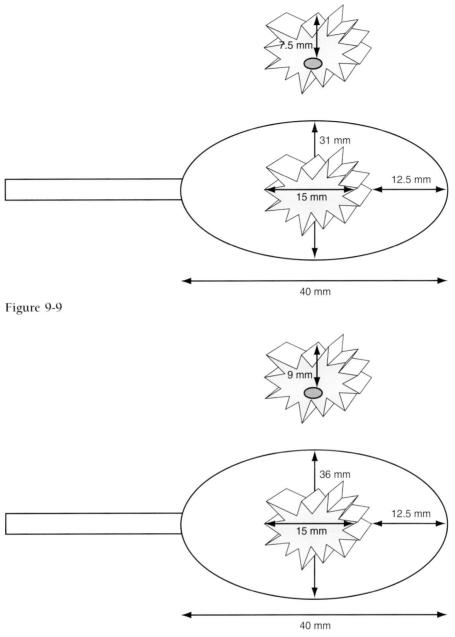

Figure 9-9

Figure 9-10

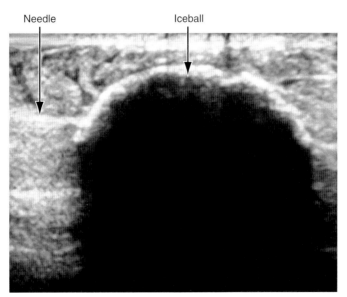

Figure 9-11

6. **Infiltration of Local Anesthetic or Saline**

♦ As the iceball grows, local anesthetic or saline can be injected to ensure the iceball does not encroach on the skin or pectoralis muscle (Fig. 9-12).

7. **Incision**

♦ An incision is made in the usual fashion over the now palpable mass (see Chapter 6 for a complete discussion of excisional breast biopsy).

8. **Excision of Iceball**

♦ Electrocautery is used to dissect around the palpable mass.
♦ The probe can be used as a lever, allowing the mass to be removed like a lollipop (Fig. 9-13).
♦ The freeze is turned off and the mass is oriented and removed off the probe.
♦ The probe is removed.
♦ The cavity is irrigated, meticulous hemostasis is achieved, and closure proceeds in the usual fashion (see Chapter 6).

Step 4. Postoperative Care

♦ Essentially, the postoperative care for patients undergoing cryoablation-assisted lumpectomy is the same as for patients undergoing a conventional lumpectomy.
♦ Care should be taken to inspect the skin after the procedure because frostbite can be noted.

Needle injecting saline
between iceball and skin

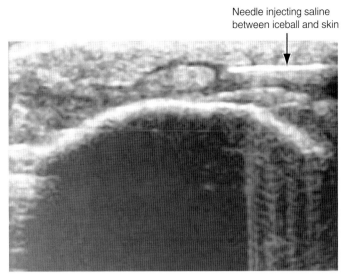

Figure 9-12

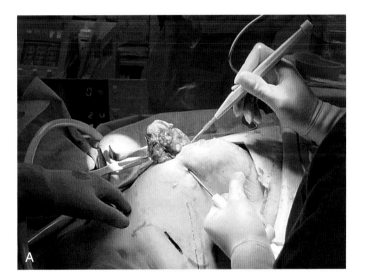

A

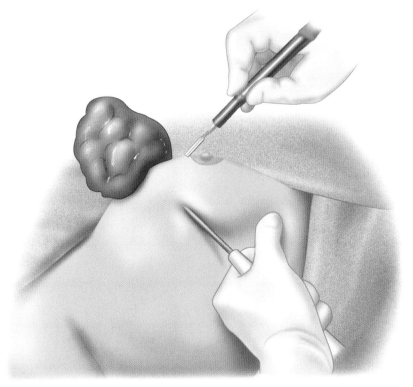

B

Figure 9-13

Step 5. Pearls and Pitfalls

1. Preoperative

♦ Appropriate patient selection is critical.
♦ Ensure that an adequate core-needle biopsy has been obtained for preoperative diagnosis and receptor studies.

2. Intraoperative

♦ Measurements are critical in this procedure. If the probe is eccentrically placed on the transverse view, this should be taken into consideration when calculating the maximum dimension of the iceball (see Fig. 9-10).
♦ Infiltration of local anesthetic to increase the space between the iceball and the skin or pectoralis muscle not only prevents freezing of the skin or muscle but helps with postoperative pain.
♦ Because the probe freezing can take up to 20 minutes, it is efficient to start with the sentinel node biopsy, which is often performed as a concomitant procedure, and perform the cryoablation-assisted lumpectomy while waiting for the intraoperative evaluation of the sentinel nodes. The surgeon can close the sentinel node incision while the iceball grows.
♦ The iceball often takes a spherical or elliptical shape that facilitates conformation and placement of a MammoSite (Cytyc Surgical Products, Marlborough, MA) brachytherapy balloon, if planned.

3. Postoperative

♦ Pathologists may find it more difficult to assess tumor grade and hormone receptor status with the iceball specimen. However, margins are assessed in the usual fashion.

Bibliography

Sabel MS, Kaufman CS, Whitworth P, et al: Cryoablation of early-stage breast cancer: Work-in-progress report of a multi-institutional trial. Ann Surg Oncol 2004;11:542-549.
Simmons RM: Ablative techniques in the treatment of benign and malignant breast disease. J Am Coll Surg 2003;197:334-338.
Tafra L, Fine R, Whitworth P, et al: Prospective randomized study comparing cryo-assisted and needle-wire localization of ultrasound-visible breast tumors. Am J Surg 2006;192:462-470.
Tafra L, Smith SJ, Woodward JE, et al: Pilot trial of cryoprobe-assisted breast-conserving surgery for small ultrasound-visible cancers. Ann Surg Oncol 2003;10:1018-1024.

EXCISION FOLLOWED BY RADIOFREQUENCY ABLATION

V. Suzanne Klimberg

Step 1. Surgical Anatomy

- When performing excision followed by radiofrequency ablation (eRFA), knowledge of the prior position of the tumor within the lumpectomy cavity and its relationship to the skin and the chest wall is key to positioning the radiofrequency (RF) probe for appropriate ablation of the tumor bed margin (Fig. 10-1).
- Figure 10-2 illustrates the eRFA concept.

Step 2. Preoperative Considerations

- The indications for RFA after lumpectomy for cancer (invasive or noninvasive) include the following:
  - ▲ To increase margin width without resecting additional tissue
  - ▲ To ablate occult disease in patients who cannot be treated with radiation therapy (e.g., collagen vascular disease, comorbid diseases, prior radiation therapy for conservative breast cancer treatment), who refuse radiation therapy, or in whom such therapy is of questionable value.

Step 3. Operative Steps

1. Setup

- Excision of breast lesions as well as RFA can be performed under local anesthesia with or without sedative, or general anesthesia. Local anesthesia using a mixture of short- and long-acting anesthetics with epinephrine is ideal.

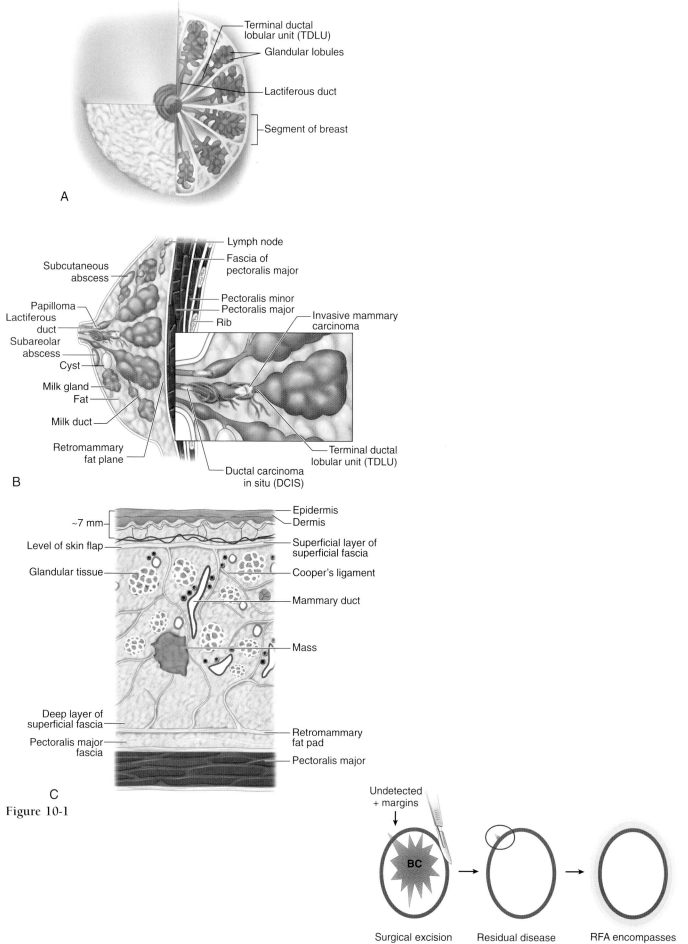

A

B

C

Figure 10-1

Figure 10-2

◆ The patient's body should be positioned the same as for the immediate prior lumpectomy, juxtaposed to the edge of the table with the ipsilateral arm at 90 degrees, such that the surgeon and assistant can stand close to the patient above or below the arm (see Fig. 6-3).

2. Preparation of the Bed for Radiofrequency Ablation

◆ After achieving hemostasis, place a pursestring suture in the cavity at the level of the previous tumor and bring the cavity together so that the opening is approximately 1 to 2 cm in diameter (Fig. 10-3).

3. Positioning the Radiofrequency Probe

◆ Deploy the RF probe in the tumor bed so that the tines enter the breast tissue of the lumpectomy bed to a depth of 1 cm (Figs. 10-4 and 10-5).
◆ Place sutures in the skin to pull it away from the area of ablation (Fig. 10-6).

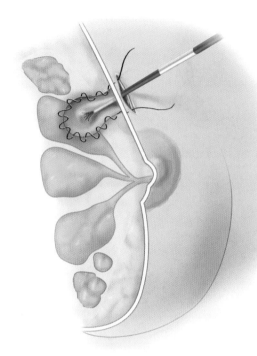

Figure 10-3

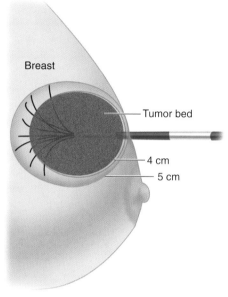

Figure 10-4

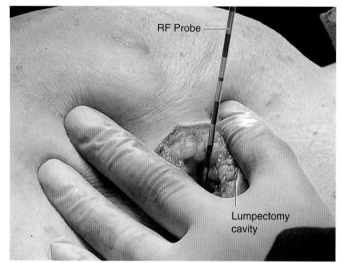

Figure 10-5

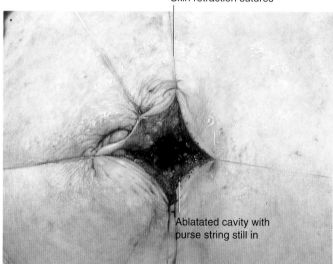

Figure 10-6

4. Ablation

◆ The RF probe is activated to 100° C for 15 minutes.
◆ After the ablation, wait 30 seconds. If the temperature of the probe goes below 55° C, ablate at 100° C for 5 more minutes.

5. Imaging the Ablation Zone

◆ Use Doppler ultrasonography to determine the width of ablation and to ensure the ablation zone does not jeopardize the skin. The ablation zone lights up on Doppler secondary to off-gassing of nitrogen as the tissue is heated (Fig. 10-7). If necessary, retract the RF probe to protect the skin.

6. Removing the Radiofrequency Probe

◆ Once the ablation is completed, remove the RF probe.
◆ Irrigate the wound to remove debris.
◆ Use electrocautery for hemostasis.

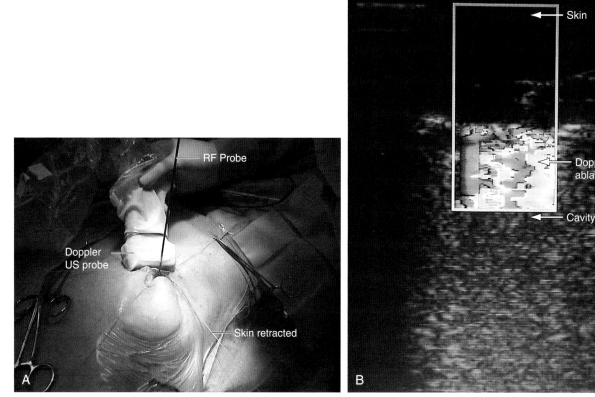

Figure 10-7

7. Confirming the Margin of Ablation

- The surgeon new to eRFA may want to confirm depth of ablation by using a 6-mm punch biopsy to at least a 1-cm depth on the superior, inferior, medial, lateral, and posterior margins. Pathologic study with hematoxylin and eosin stain, proliferating cell nuclear antigen (PCNA), or a vital stain will confirm successful ablation.

8. Closure

- Only the superficial subcutaneous tissue ($\geq$7 mm) is closed (see Fig. 6-11).
- Either a running or interrupted absorbable suture can be used to close the dermis. A subcuticular running stitch is best for closing the skin.
- A drain is unnecessary unless good intraoperative hemostasis cannot be achieved.

Step 4. Postoperative Care

- A pressure dressing is not necessary. Glue or Steri-Strips oriented horizontally over the wound is sufficient.
- A sports bra is sufficient to stabilize the breast for at least the first 48 hours.

Step 5. Pearls and Pitfalls

- It is necessary only to ablate the area where the tumor was sitting.
- When excising a tumor in preparation for eRFA, make the incision directly over the tumor.
- Excise the tumor with the intent of obtaining tumor-free margins.
- Ensure that the cavity wall is not too thin (≤1 cm) before deploying the RF probe.
- Ensure that the skin is kept away from the probe so that steam from the ablation does not burn the skin.
- A step ablation (overlapping a deep with a more superficial ablation) can be performed if the tumor bed span is greater than the depth of a single ablation.

Bibliography

Bland KL, Gass J, Klimberg VS: Radiofrequency, cryoablation, and other modalities for breast cancer ablation. Surg Clin North Am 2007;87:539-550.
Klimberg VS, Kepple J, Shafirstein G, et al: eRFA: Excision followed by RFA—a new technique to improve local control in breast cancer. Ann Surg Oncol 2006;13:1422-1433.

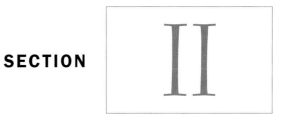

Lymph Node Biopsy

CHAPTER 11

Axillary Sentinel Lymph Node Biopsy

V. Suzanne Klimberg

Step 1. Surgical Anatomy

- ◆ Figure 11-1 shows the anatomic structures that must be considered with an axillary sentinel lymph node biopsy (SLNB).

Step 2. Preoperative Considerations

- ◆ The indications for SLNB include the following:
  - ▲ Use SLNB for patients with lesions clinically less than stage T2, clinically negative nodes, and no metastases.
  - ▲ Consider using SLNB in stage T3 lesions, locally advanced tumors, or multicentric cancers, but there are few data and such patients should be enrolled in available clinical trials.
  - ▲ The concordance of SLN with axillary lymph node dissection (ALND) results is much less for patients with significant disturbance of the breast, such as previous axillary surgery, pre-operative radiation or chemotherapy, or large upper outer quadrant excisions (ones that would block major lymphatics to the axilla). Use SLNB cautiously in such patients.
  - ▲ Consider using SLNB alone for aggressive (ductal carcinoma in situ [DCIS]) or large (>2.5 cm) lesions instead of a level I dissection.

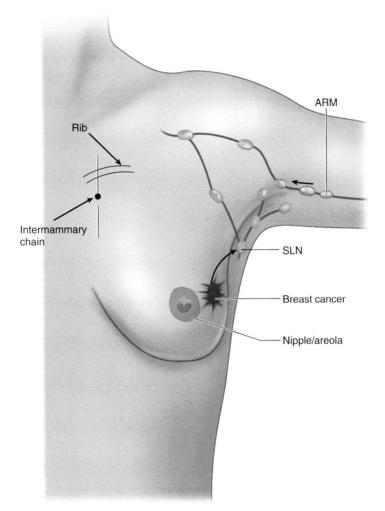

Figure 11-1

Step 3. Operative Steps

1. Setup

- Available materials for the localization and biopsy of the SLN include blue dye (1% isosulfan blue [Lymphazurin], dilute methylene blue, and vital blue dye) and technetium-99m (^{99m}Tc) sulfur colloid (filtered or unfiltered) or ^{99m}Tc albumin. The materials may be used alone or in combination.
- The timing and location of the injection can be varied until you find the technique that works well for you and your institution's facilities. Avoid local anesthesia because it may disturb the migration properties of the tracers. If the injection is given before general anesthesia, the patient should assume the supine position to avoid injury from a fainting episode.

2. Injection of Radiocolloid

- The surgeon or the radiologist can inject the ^{99m}Tc tracer in the nuclear medicine suite or other radiation safety-approved areas (Fig. 11-2).
- The tracer can be injected intraoperatively or up to 24 hours before surgery, with similar good results.
- Injection methods include peritumoral, within about 1 cm of the tumor (such intraparenchymal injections can be guided by palpation or ultrasonography); intratumoral; dermal (intradermal or subdermal); subareolar; and combinations thereof (Fig. 11-3).
- Radiotracer is the only way to locate the SLN before incision, and can identify SLNs located outside the axilla (8% of cases; e.g., internal mammary, supraclavicular, thyroid).
- Radiation exposure is minimal even for the busy surgeon and far less for other staff.

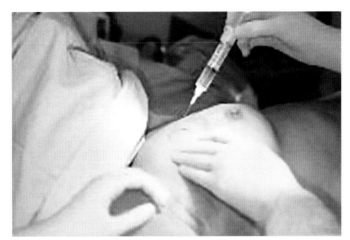

Figure 11-2

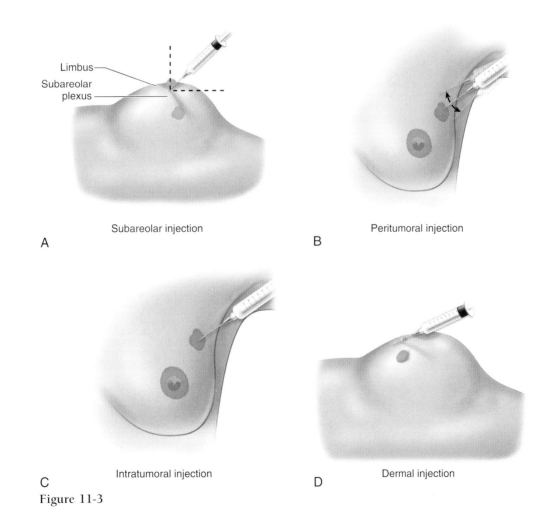

A   Subareolar injection

B   Peritumoral injection

C   Intratumoral injection

D   Dermal injection

Figure 11-3

3. Injection of Blue Dye

♦ Injection methods for the blue dye are similar to those for the radiotracer. Inject the dye approximately 5 minutes before the procedure for outer quadrant lesions using subareolar, peritumoral, or intratumoral placement, or dermally when there is an upper outer scar (Fig. 11-4). Inject 10 to 15 minutes before the procedure if injecting intraparenchymally for inner quadrant tumors.

♦ If 20 minutes or more has elapsed since the injection of blue dye and the biopsy procedure has not yet begun, consider injecting another dose.

♦ Inform the anesthesiologist when the blue dye is injected because it may cause a decrease in the patient's oxygen saturation. Likewise, recovery room personnel and family members should be notified about blue dye injection because the oxygen saturation will continue to be low and the patient will appear ashen.

♦ Life-threatening allergic reactions, some delayed for several hours, have been reported with the injection of blue dye. The anesthesiologist should be alert for a rise in peak airway pressures, and the surgeon for the appearance of a blue rash (Fig. 11-5). Most allergic reactions can be avoided by not using blue dye in patients with allergies to cosmetics that contain blue dyes.

4. Mapping a Zone of Diffusion

♦ Map out a zone of diffusion using the hand-held gamma probe. Adjust the gamma probe's sensitivity so the zone of diffusion does not overlap with any lymph node basins.

♦ If the zone of diffusion overlaps any of the lymph node–bearing areas, the location of the true SLN may be obscured. In the largest multicenter trial, all false-negative SLNs were from peritumoral injections in the upper outer quadrant, presumably because the zone of diffusion overlapped the true SLN (Fig. 11-6).

♦ Avoid overlap by decreasing the sensitivity of the gamma probe or use a collimator on the gamma probe to decrease the influence of scatter.

5. Preincision Localization of Sentinel Lymph Node

♦ Check for radiotracer migration to and location of the SLN by preoperative lymphoscintigraphy, bearing in mind this technique's low sensitivity (Fig. 11-7).

♦ A hand-held gamma probe is very sensitive for intraoperative location of the SLN. Some studies indicate that approximately 8% of SLNs are located outside the axilla proper (level II and III, internal mammary, supraclavicular, thyroid, pectoralis, intramammary, upper abdomen).

♦ Scan and mark any "hot spots" before incision.

♦ If the SLN cannot be localized before incision, inject approximately 40 mL of injectable saline in the same manner in which the ^{99m}Tc was injected. Massage 5 minutes and try again. If there still is no localization, proceed with skin incision in the axilla.

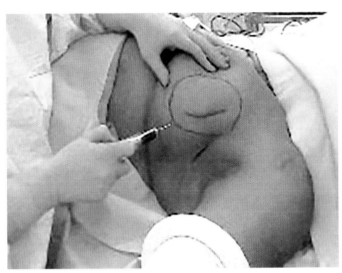

Figure 11-4

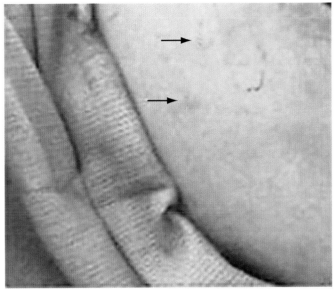

Figure 11-5

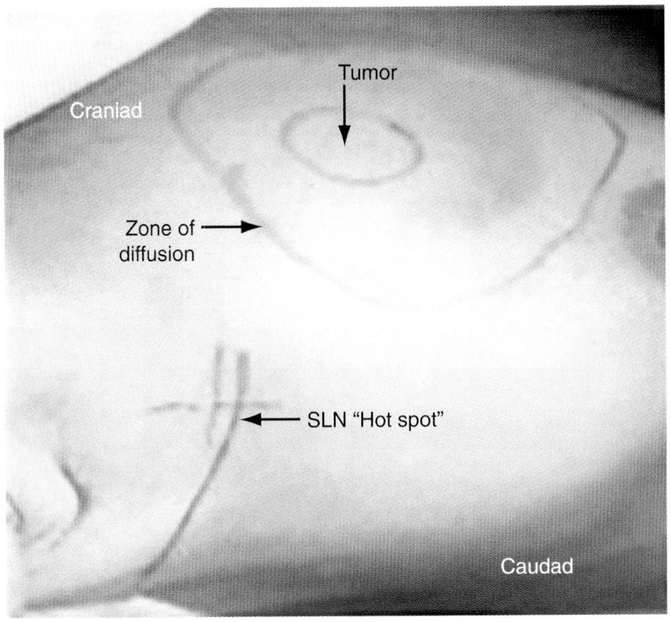

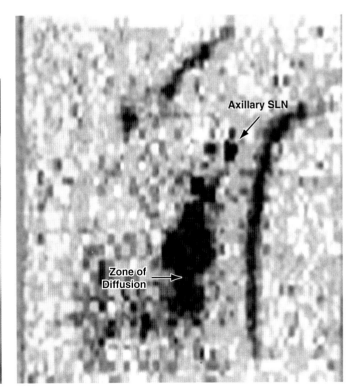

Figure 11-6

Figure 11-7

6. Background Count

- Once a potential SLN has been located, take a background count 1 to 2 cm away from the hot spot. A ratio of hot spot-to-background counts of 10 to 1 establishes SLN localization.

7. Skin Incision

- Make a 2- to 3-cm incision directly over the hot spot, wherever it is located. If no radiotracer has been used or it has failed to localize the SLN, make the skin incision just below the hairline in the anterior axillary line, posterior and perpendicular to the pectoralis major (PM; Fig. 11-8).
- Use either cautery or blunt dissection through the subcutaneous tissue (Fig. 11-9, *A*) down to the axillary fascia (Fig. 11-9, *B*), with retractors to provide exposure.

8. Incision of Axillary Fascia

- Incise both layers of axillary fascia parallel to the plane of the incision. Disregard any blue dye above the fascia because all the axillary lymph nodes are located under the fascia.

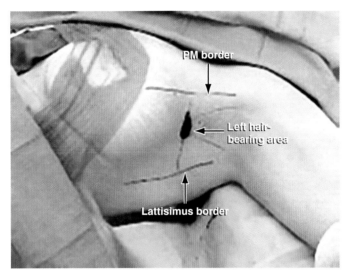

Figure 11-8

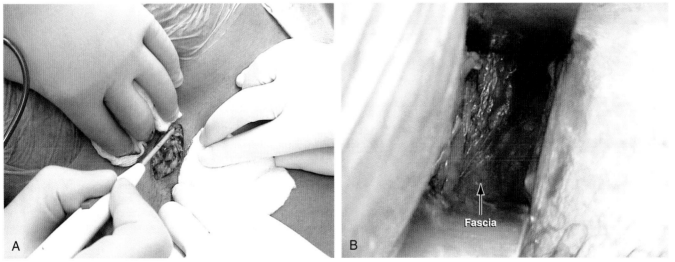

Figure 11-9

9. Line-of-Sight Dissection

♦ With dual injection of blue dye and radiotracer, the SLN may be "hot" (radioactive), blue, both, or only palpable. All are indications of sentinel status, so such nodes should be harvested. The gamma probe is inserted into the wound and slowly rocked back and forth in all directions to find the "hottest" (i.e., increased counts) direction in which to proceed. As you dissect through the fatty plane of the axilla, keep bringing the gamma probe (GP) in and out of the wound, constantly checking direction ("line of sight"; Fig. 11-10).

♦ As the dissection proceeds down toward the SLN, the counts should get higher. If you dissect away from the SLN, the counts will decrease. Make sure you have not dissected past the SLN or retracted the SLN after repositioning of instruments. If you still cannot find the SLN, remove all retractors and start over from the skin down.

10. Excision of Sentinel Lymph Node(s)

♦ Once the axillary fascia is incised, care should be taken not to disturb any blue lymphatics (Fig. 11-11). Blue lymphatics should be followed to their destination, using the GP as well if radiotracer was injected. Dissect down to but do not lift up the SLN to avoid misidentification of the SLN.

♦ Avoid skeletonizing the SLN. Metastases are not uncommonly found in the vessel leading to the fat around the SLN. Gently dissect parallel to the plane of the lymphatic, following it to a blue SLN, and use a noncrushing Allis clamp to secure the SLN (Fig. 11-12).

♦ Once either a hot and/or blue node is found, it may be excised using the surgeon's preferred technique, as long as care is taken to tie, clip, or cauterize the leading lymphatic vessel.

♦ Unligated lymphatics may lead to a lymphocele (lymph collection) in the lymph node dissection bed.

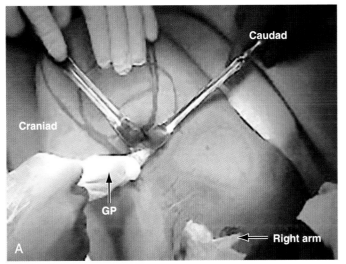

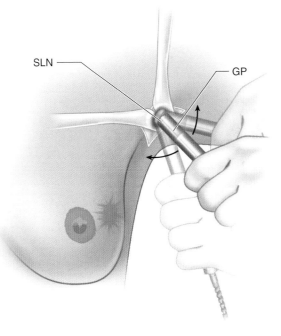

Figure 11-10

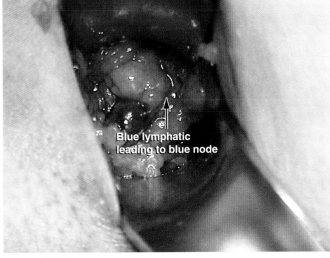

Figure 11-11

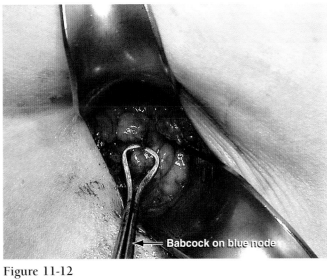

Figure 11-12

11. Ex Vivo Count

◆ Take counts on all lymph nodes removed.
◆ Direct the GP up and away from the patient and press the SLN onto the tip of the probe (Fig. 11-13).

12. Palpation of Axillary Bed

◆ Palpate the bed of dissection to locate any suspect palpable lymph nodes. Theoretically, lymph nodes blocked by tumor could divert the tracer to an alternate lymph node.

13. Bed Count

◆ Take a final bed count after all SLNs have been removed. If the bed count is higher than 10% of the background count, make a thorough search for additional SLNs. If there is sufficient overlap with the zone of diffusion, it may be impossible to obtain a bed count lower than 10% of the SLN count.

14. Pathology

◆ Intraoperative techniques for evaluation of the SLN include touch preparation or imprint cytology and frozen section.

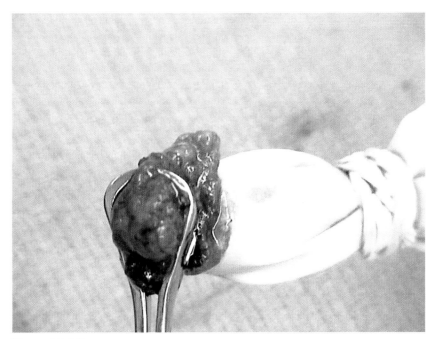

Figure 11-13

15. Intraoperative Assessment of Sentinel Lymph Node

- If it is available, use touch preparation cytology, which involves "stamping" the cut SLN pieces (3-mm cuts for SLNs > 5 mm) onto a glass slide and performing a hematoxylin and eosin (H&E) stain.
- Use frozen section cautiously on one or multiple pieces of the SLN.
- Touch preparation is faster and in general equally as or more accurate than frozen section, and does not run the risk of missing a diagnosis of micrometastasis.
- The College of American Pathologists does not recommend the use of special cytokeratin stains, except when suspicion is raised but not confirmed by final H&E staining.

16. Hemostasis

- Achieve hemostasis with clip, tie, or electrocautery, but take care when deep in the axilla to avoid the thoracodorsal or long thoracic nerve. Use nonparalyzing anesthesia to aid in recognizing impending nerve injury.

17. Closure

- Close the axillary or other fascia in layers with 3-0 absorbable sutures (Fig. 11-14). Lack of closure of the axillary fascia encourages formation of a lymphocele. However, there is no need for a drain.

18. Dressing

- Steri-Strips parallel to the incision or wound glue are sufficient. Such a dressing allows the patient to shower immediately after surgery. There is no need for a drain or pressure dressing.

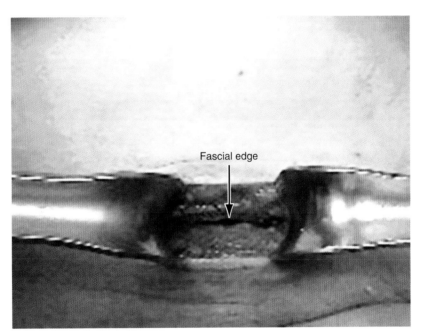

Figure 11-14

Step 4. Postoperative Care

- Caution the patient against significant arm movement or any exercise that would jostle the breast and axilla.
- As soon as the wound is healed (average, <1 week), mobilize the patient's arm to regain range of motion. Frozen shoulder occurs with SLNB in less than 1% of patients and is usually associated with reconstruction or mastectomy, in which the patient has been immobilized for longer periods. Avoid this risk by starting the patient on range-of-motion exercises on the first postoperative visit. Consult occupational therapy if the arm is not fully mobile at 1 month.

Step 5. Pearls and Pitfalls

- If a blue dye reaction is suspected, give the patient 50 mg diphenhydramine intravenously. If there is no doubt, add 100 mg of methylprednisolone. Admit the patient for close observation for at least 24 hours.
- If oxygen desaturation occurs, do nothing if there are no other indications of a problem and the desaturation coincides with blue dye injection. This is a false desaturation and is simply a monitoring problem.
- If a blue or hot SLN cannot be identified in a patient with invasive cancer, the axilla must be staged with an axillary lymph node dissection. In a patient with DCIS without known invasive cancer, do nothing further. If the patient has a very aggressive DCIS, consider performing a level I axillary lymph node dissection (simple extended mastectomy; see Chapter 16).
- Perform an axillary lymph node dissection when you cannot localize an SLN in the axilla, even if one was located outside the axilla.
- Postsurgical hemorrhage can occur immediately and up to 10 days after surgery. Hemolysis of clots in the wound can occur during this time and bleeding may be exacerbated by exercise. Only immediate, large postoperative hematomas need reexploration. Smaller hematomas should be followed and, if progressing, should be reexplored.
- Sensory deficit of some type can occur early on (first few weeks) and resolves on its own. Reassure the patient. Observe any motor deficit of the long thoracic or thoracodorsal nerve for up to 6 weeks because such a presentation most likely represents a neuropraxia rather than a severed nerve. If the deficit persists after 6 weeks, reexplore the wound for potential reanastomosis.

- If nerve damage is recognized during surgery, repair with 6.0 absorbable suture.
- For a frozen shoulder, consult occupational or physical therapy for range-of-motion exercises. Water aerobics are also helpful.
- If a lymphocele develops, use a 20-gauge syringe to aspirate it, similar to the procedure used for a simple cyst aspiration. See the patient every 3 to 4 days until the lymphocele is resolved.
- On intraoperative pathology, a false-positive result is rare, but a false-negative is not. Therefore, rely on the final formalin-fixed results for treatment.
- Treat the patient based on the results of the final H&E stain. If intraoperative pathology gave a false-negative reading of the SLN and the SLN turns out to be positive, take the patient back to the operating room for an axillary lymph node dissection, or arrange for randomization on an available clinical trial.

Bibliography

American Society of Breast Surgeons: Statement on Sentinel Lymph Node Biopsy. Available at: www.breastsurgeons.org.

Harlow SP, Krag DN: Sentinel lymph node—why study it: Implications of the B-32 study. Semin Surg Oncol 2001;20:224-229.

Grube BJ, Giuliano AE: Observation of the breast cancer patient with a tumor-positive sentinel node: Implications of the ACOSOG Z0011 trial. Semin Surg Oncol 2001;20:230-237.

Orr RK: The impact of prophylactic axillary node dissection on breast cancer survival: A bayesian meta-analysis. Ann Surg Oncol 1999;6:109-116.

Schwartz GF, Giuliano AE, Veronesi U: Proceeding of the consensus conference of the role of sentinel lymph node biopsy in carcinoma or the breast April 19-22, 2001, Philadelphia, PA, USA. Breast J 2002;8:124-138.

Tuttle TM, Zogakis TG, Dunst CM, et al: A review of technical aspects of sentinel lymph node identification for breast cancer. J Am Coll Surg 2002;195:261-268.

CHAPTER 12

MEDIASTINAL SENTINEL LYMPH NODE BIOPSY

Virgilio Sacchini and Alice Chung

Step 1. Surgical Anatomy

- The internal mammary (IM) lymph node chain is confined in the anterior extrapleural chest space, leaning on the so-called transverse thoracic muscle, which is often involuted to a thin aponeurotic fascia. The fusion between the visceral and parietal pleura usually begins 2.5 to 3 cm from the lateral sternal border (Fig. 12-1).
- The internal mammary artery (IMA) runs through this space along the lateral sternal border, with its distance from the border increasing from 10 mm at the first intercostal space to 20 mm at the sixth space.
- At the third intercostal space, the IMA is usually 12 to 13 mm from the sternal border.
- From the IMA originate the anterior intercostal arteries, two for each intercostal space, running between the two intercostal muscles, one inferior and the other superior, both anastomosed with the posterior intercostal artery (see Fig. 12-1). Other minor collateral veins go to the transverse thoracic muscle.
- The IM lymph nodes are usually located in the same plane as the IM vessels or in an anterior plane, within the fatty tissue surrounding the artery and veins. There are usually four to six nodes per site, with different distribution in the intercostal spaces (Fig. 12-2).
- Usually there is one node in each intercostal space. In the first and second spaces, the lymph node is usually medial to the IM vessels, whereas in the inferior spaces they are lateral to the vessels (see Fig. 12-2). Usually no lymph nodes are found below the heads of the ribs.
- Two IM veins run along the artery, one medially and the other laterally. The medial vein is usually the smaller of the two (see Fig. 12-1). These two veins have collaterals similar to those of the IMA.
- The lymphatic vessels of the medial portion of the breast, and especially those located in the deep portion of the breast, lead to the IM chain. These lymphatics cross the major pectoral muscle in its medial aspect and traverse the subsequent intercostal muscles. A small number of nodes are occasionally found in the thin lymphatic net located between the external and the internal intercostal muscles. The lymphatics that cross the internal intercostal muscle go to the IM nodes.

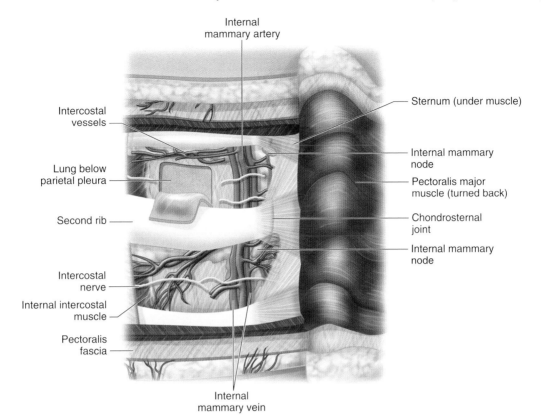

Figure 12-1

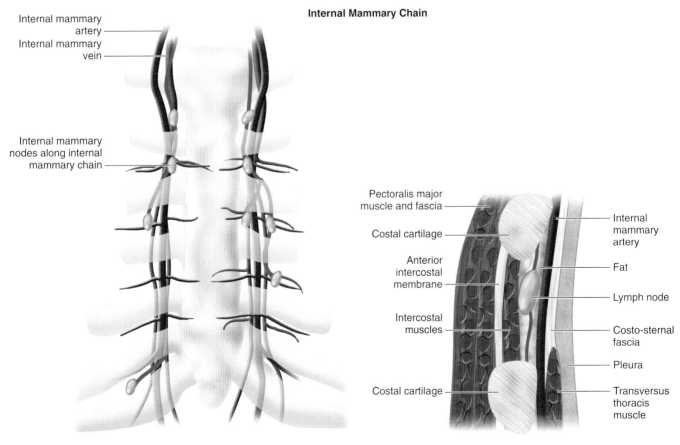

A

B

Figure 12-2

1. Indications for Procedure

- Complete removal of the IM chain *en bloc* with the parietal pleura, transected IM vessels, rib, and intercostal muscle, as well as the major pectoral muscle and the breast, has been described extensively by several authors. These authors completed subset studies or clinical trials comparing the standard Halsted mastectomy with this extended procedure. In all cases, the authors reported no benefit in survival and an increased morbidity and mortality with the extended procedure.
- The introduction of the sentinel node technique in breast cancer has led to the detection of sentinel nodes outside of the axilla.
- Some believe that mediastinal sentinel lymph node biopsy (MSLNB) leads to more accurate staging and contributes to the overall management of the patient with breast cancer.
- MSLNB is a feasible, low-risk operation when directed by radio-guided lymph node mapping.
- Maximally accurate staging should improve the "individualization" of treatment, contributing to reduced incidence of overtreatment or undertreatment. The American Joint Committee on Cancer has included the status of the IM lymph node biopsy in defining the stage of breast cancer.
- Differences in survival according to degree of axillary or IM involvement were well reported in studies with long-term follow-up of extended radical mastectomies.
- Migration of the staging based on information obtained from IM biopsy has been reported in 10% of cases.
- Others claim that migration of the stage may not dramatically influence the choice of adjuvant therapy.
- MSLNB should be considered:
  - ▲ When the node is visible on lymphoscintigraphy.
  - ▲ When a positive IM node may change the systemic treatment, in particular when the change is from a hormonal adjuvant treatment to chemotherapy (e.g., negative axillary sentinel node biopsy, small cancers, hormonal receptor positive).
- Patients with enlarged mediastinal or IM lymph nodes demonstrated on preoperative computed tomography or magnetic resonance imaging scans may also be considered appropriate candidates for this operation.
- Because the overall survival benefits of IM lymph node biopsy remain unconfirmed, the technique of IM sentinel node biopsy should be as nonaggressive as possible to minimize potential complications or cosmetic sequelae.

Step 2. Preoperative Considerations

- Preoperative lymphoscintigraphy with peritumoral injection of radioisotope is performed (Fig. 12-3). This will guide the dissection to the appropriate interspace. Lymphazurin blue dye may be injected intradermally or intraparenchymally before the start of the procedure. However, the value of blue dye mapping in IM node biopsy is limited. The superficial lymphatics that take up the blue dye will not likely drain to the deep IM nodes, and use of a peritumoral injection will require blind dissection of the IM basin without knowing to which interspace the dissection should be directed.
- The normal rate of identification of IM lymph nodes as sentinel nodes ranges between 0% and 4%, with some authors reporting 60% when the isotope injection was performed deeply in the breast, close to the fascia of the pectoralis major.

Right oblique anterior

Anterior

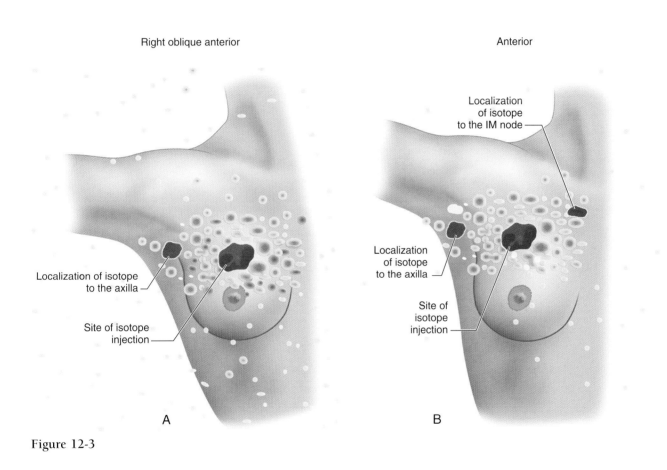

Localization
of isotope
to the IM node

Localization
of isotope
to the axilla

Localization
of isotope
to the axilla

Site of
isotope
injection

Site of isotope
injection

A

B

Figure 12-3

Step 3. Operative Steps

1. Incision

- This procedure is usually performed under general anesthesia, although there have been reports of cases performed under local anesthesia with sedation. Therefore, preoperative assessment for patients undergoing IM node biopsy is no different than for any patient undergoing standard axillary sentinel node biopsy with possible axillary lymph node dissection.
- Access to the IM node is usually obtained through a wide excision or mastectomy incision. Only occasionally is a new skin incision required. In these cases, we recommended a 3-cm curvilinear incision 3 to 4 cm from the lateral sternal margin, for cosmetic purposes (Fig. 12-4).
- The pectoral major muscle is exposed for 2 to 3 cm linearly from the nipple to the lateral sternal border. In the case of breast conservation surgery, the breast parenchyma should be detached from the major pectoral fascia to achieve this exposure (Fig. 12-5).

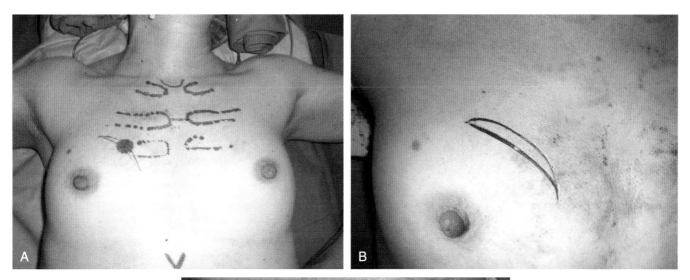

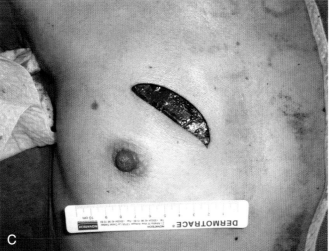

Figure 12-4

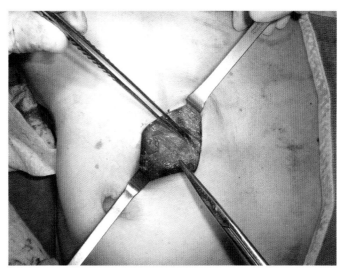

Figure 12-5

- The muscle is then split to expose the superior intercostal space (Fig. 12-6). Some vessels may run along the fibers of the pectoralis major, requiring coagulation or ligation.
- The external and internal intercostal muscles are cut transversely from the sternal border in a lateral direction for 3 to 4 cm (Fig. 12-7). The division should be done in the middle, between the two ribs or along the superior costal border, to avoid injury of the anterior intercostal vessels. In cutting the internal intercostal muscle, particular care must be taken to avoid injury to the inferior parietal pleura.

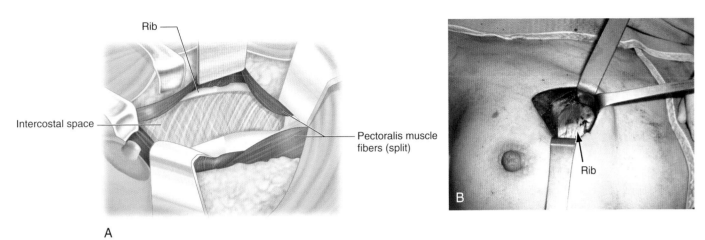

Figure 12-6

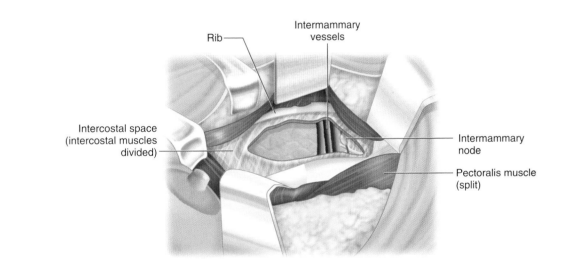

A

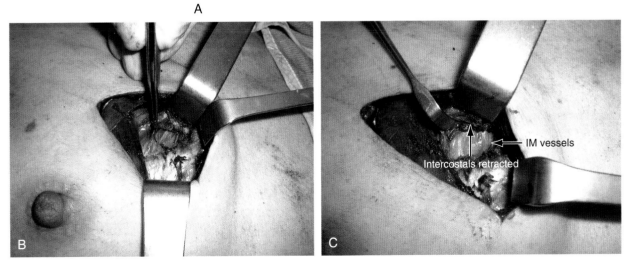

Figure 12-7

- The IM vessels are surrounded by adipose and lymphatic tissue. They are situated in an extra-pleural space starting 2.5 to 3 cm from the medial border of the lung (see Fig. 12-7). Confining the dissection to this space helps to prevent injury of the pleura. The artery and veins are usually covered by fibrous fatty tissue, which is separated, and the small vessels are coagulated. The artery is usually found 10 to 15 mm from the lateral sternal border.
- Figure 12-8 shows the MSLN at the angle of the intercostal vessels and the IM vessels.
- A vessel loop is placed to encircle the IM artery (Fig. 12-10). This prevents major bleeding in the case of inadvertent injury. The vessel loop may also prevent retraction of the artery in case of transection. If transection does occur, prompt disarticulation or transection of the rib should be done to clamp the open artery. The largest IM vein, usually lateral to the artery, may also be encircled. During this maneuver, some small venous collaterals may bleed, requiring coagu-lation or ligature. If bleeding occurs, the vein may be ligated or clipped. Particular attention should be paid to preserving the IMA because it is a major resource in the event of coronary reperfusion surgery.
- The perivasal adipose tissue is then divided with the scissors, and the gamma probe is used to locate the node. In the case of a hot node, the probe indicates its precise position. The node may be medial or lateral to the vessels. Once identified, the node should be handled with care to avoid coagulation or disruption of the capsule, where micrometastases are most frequently found. Small vessels around the node may be coagulated or clipped (Fig. 12-9).

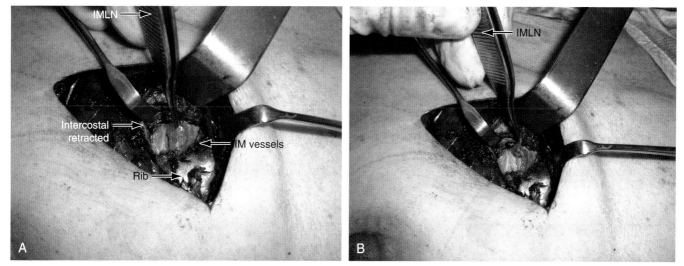

Figure 12-8

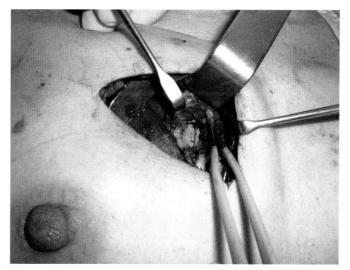

Figure 12-9

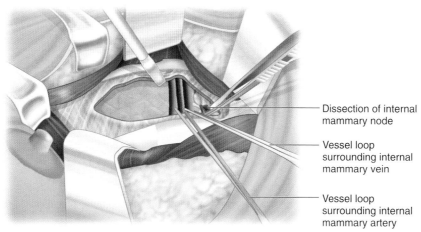

Figure 12-10

2. Closing

* Once the node is removed, the surgical field may be irrigated and examined for abnormal bubbles to confirm the integrity of the pleura (Fig. 12-11, *A*), and the split intercostal and pectoral muscle is then sutured using 2-0 polyglactin, avoiding excessive traction that may transect the muscular fibers (Fig. 12-11, *B*). The breast parenchyma may be reapproximated to restore the shape of the breast in case of conservative surgery, and the skin closed (Fig. 12-12).

Step 4. Postoperative Care

* The average time of the procedure is 18 minutes; there is no additional postoperative care required.
* Routine chest radiography is not required unless a pneumothorax is suspected.
* In the event of a pneumothorax, a chest tube is not necessary unless the lung itself has been injured.
* Postoperative antibiotics are not indicated unless required for other conditions.

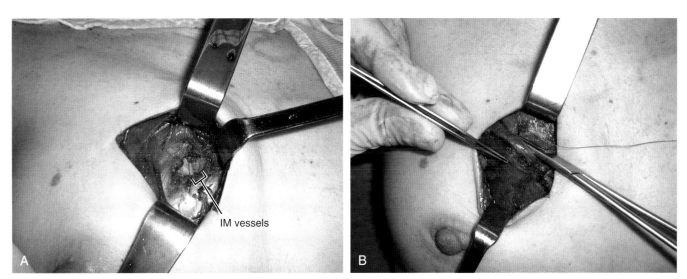

Figure 12-11

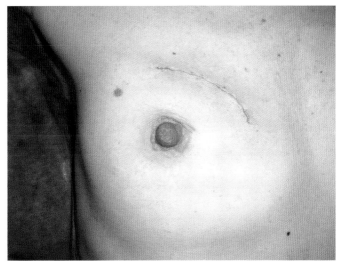

Figure 12-12

Step 5. Pearls and Pitfalls

- ◆ Preoperative lymphoscintigraphy is the essential tool in the preoperative and intraoperative planning of IM node biopsy. In the equivocal case, intraoperative ultrasonography may be used to identify whether an IM lymph node is of sufficient size to warrant dissection.
- ◆ During division of the intercostal muscles to gain access to the IM nodes, the interspace may be very narrow. In this case, removal of the panel of intercostal muscles between the appropriate ribs may provide better exposure.
- ◆ Injury to the underlying pleura may occur during division of the internal intercostal muscle. If an injury is recognized intraoperatively, it can easily be repaired with fine absorbable suture.
- ◆ The placement of vessel loops around the IM vessels aids in preventing major bleeding in the case of iatrogenic injury to the artery or vein. The vessel loop can prevent retraction of the vessel in the case of arterial or venous transection and allow for prompt repair or ligation. In such a case, disarticulation or transection of the rib should be performed to allow control of the artery. Care must be taken to preserve the IMA as it may become necessary as a conduit for coronary reperfusion or pedicled transverse rectus abdominis muscle reconstruction.
- ◆ If an injury involves pneumothorax, the pleura may be sutured with 3-0 polyglactin. A red rubber catheter is used to evacuate air from the pleural space.
- ◆ Special consideration should be given to patients who have had previous median sternotomy with bypass using the IMA as a conduit to the coronary vessels. The plane of the IM nodes has been disturbed by prior dissection of the IMA and the procedure carries more risk in this case.
- ◆ Patients with breast implants may also pose a challenge in gaining adequate exposure of the IM nodes. IM node biopsy is still feasible in these patients, but dissection of the implant away from the biopsy field should be performed outside of the capsule, with care taken to avoid puncturing the implant.

Bibliography

Benti R, Bruno A, Glacomelli M, et al: Internal mammary chain lymphoscintigraphy (IML) and IML-guided internal mammary chain biopsy (GIMB) in breast cancer. Tumori 1997;83:533-536.

Jansen L, Doting MH, Rutgers EJ, et al: Clinical relevance of sentinel lymph nodes outside the axilla in patients with breast cancer. Br J Surg 2000;87:920-925.

Johnson N, Soot L, Nelson J, et al: Sentinel node biopsy and internal mammary lymphatic mapping in breast cancer. Am J Surg 2000;179:386-388.

Lacour J, Le M, Caceres E, et al: Radical mastectomy versus radical mastectomy plus internal mammary dissection: Ten year results of an international cooperative trial in breast cancer. Cancer 1983;51:1941-1943.

Meier P, Ferguson DJ, Karrison T: A controlled trial of extended radical versus radical mastectomy: Ten-year results. Cancer 1989;63:188-195.

Sugg SL, Ferguson DJ, Posner MC, Heimann R: Should internal mammary nodes be sampled in the sentinel lymph node era? Ann Surg Oncol 2000;7:188-192.

Stibbe PE: The internal mammary lymphatic glands. J Anat 1918;70:257-264.

Testut L, Jacob O: Traité d'Aanatomie Topographique avec Applications Médico-Chirurgicales. Paris, O. Doin, 1905.

Urban JA: Clinical experience and results of excision of the internal mammary lymph node chain in the primary operable breast cancer. Cancer 1959;12:14-22.

Valdes-Olmos RA, Jansen L, Hoefnagel CA, et al: Evaluation of mammary lymphoscintigraphy by a single intratumoral injection for sentinel node identification. J Nucl Med 2000;41:1500-1506.

Veronesi U, Marubini E, Mariani L, et al: The dissection of internal mammary nodes does not improve the survival of breast cancer patients: 30-Year results of a randomized trial. Eur J Cancer 1999;35:1320-1325.

CHAPTER 13

AXILLARY LYMPH NODE DISSECTION

V. Suzanne Klimberg

- Figure 13-1 demonstrates the surgical anatomy of the axilla from the axillary view.

Step 2. Preoperative Considerations

- The indications for axillary lymph node dissection (ALND) include the following:
  ▲ Positive sentinel lymph
  ▲ Contraindication to sentinel lymph node detection (e.g., pregnancy)
  ▲ Clinically palpable nodes
  ▲ Inflammatory breast cancer

Step 3. Operative Steps

1. Setup

- Drape the arm into the field using a stockinette so that it can be freely mobilized (Fig. 13-2).
- Make sure general anesthesia does not include a muscle relaxant so that the nerves can easily be identified during the dissection.

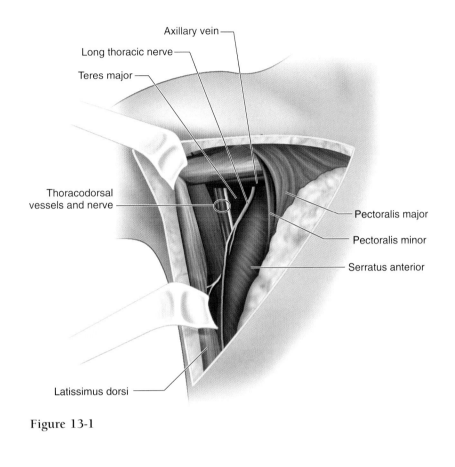

Figure 13-1

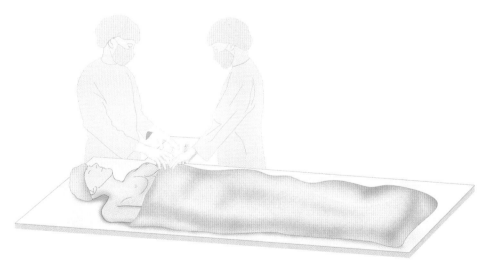

Figure 13-2

2. Incision

◆ The incision is made below the hair line in the horizontal Langer line from the palpable border of the pectoralis major (PM) to the palpable border of the latissimus dorsi (LD), (demonstrated by ink in Fig. 13-3). A longer incision does not provide better exposure because these muscles define the medial and lateral borders of the axilla, respectively.

◆ The incision also can be made along and just lateral to the border of the PM (Fig. 13-4).

◆ Alternatively, the incision of an outer quadrant lesion can be extended to the axilla. In an extreme upper outer lesion, the dissection can be performed through the lumpectomy scar.

◆ Take skin directly over a palpable node or one that has eroded the skin.

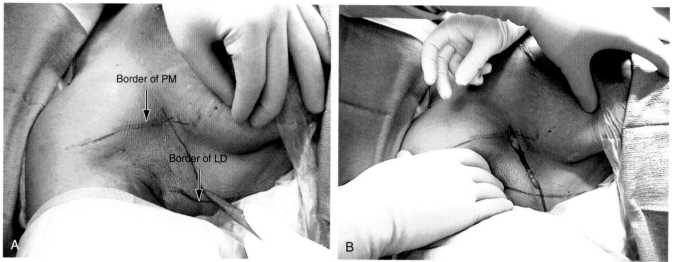

Figure 13-3

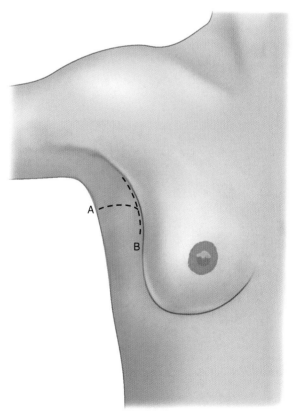

Figure 13-4

3. **Dissection**

Superior Skin Flap Dissection

- ◆ Develop the superior flap in the approximate 7-mm plane of relatively avascular fat between the skin and the glandular tissue (Figs. 13-5 and 13-6).
- ◆ The skin flaps in the axilla are usually thicker than those from the skin overlying the breast proper. There seldom is need to take the subcutaneous fat above the axillary fascia because all axillary lymph nodes are below this plane.
- ◆ Avoid making the flap too thin because it may cause more seroma formation.
- ◆ The flap extends to the fascia of the PM medially and the LD laterally (Fig. 13-7).

Inferior Skin Flap Dissection

- ◆ The inferior flap is developed similarly to the superior flap to the PM medially and the LD laterally, but the plane tends to be less well defined and almost straight down to the chest wall.

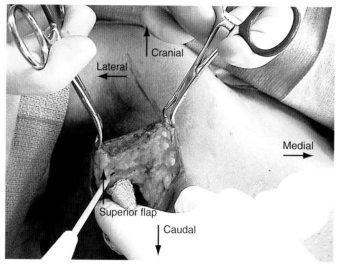
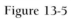

Figure 13-5

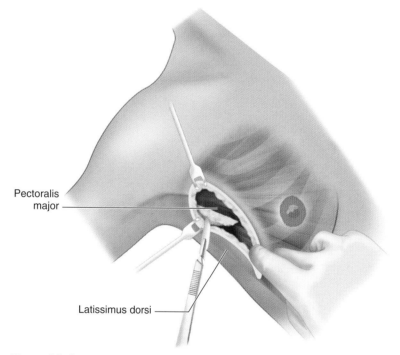

Figure 13-6

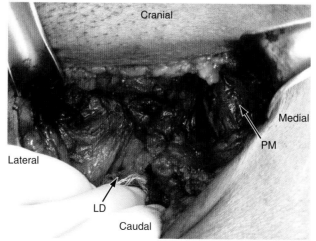

Figure 13-7

Lateral Flap Dissection

◆ Make this flap slightly thicker (~1 cm or more with increasing body mass index). Take the flap down to the LD (Fig. 13-8).
◆ Start inferiorly for the fastest way to find the LD and to avoid injury to any nerves or vessels. If the LD cannot be readily palpated, use the electrocautery to stimulate the muscle to indicate its location and where to start.
◆ Stay right on the anteromedial border of the muscle. Drifting medially may cause thermal injury or transect the thoracodorsal nerve or vessels.
◆ Dissecting lateral to the LD will make the flap unnecessarily thin while retrieving no additional lymph nodes. A thin flap increases the risk of seroma.
◆ Incise the fascia of the anteromedial border of the LD from inferior to superior to free the axillary contents from the LD.
◆ Continue superiorly to the level of the white tendon of the LD, which is usually found where the PM crosses over the LD anteriorly. This is the area where the axillary vein rests, and continuing too far superiorly may cause injury to the axillary vein (Fig. 13-9).

Medial Flap Dissection

◆ Develop the medial skin flap in the same plane, connecting the superior and inferior flaps. Open the PM fascia from the superior flap above to the inferior flap below to open up the axillary contents (Fig. 13-10).

Pectoralis Minor Dissection

◆ Use the electrocautery to free the edge of the PM; the lateral border of the pectoralis minor (PMi) will then be visible under a filmy layer of tissue (Fig. 13-11).
◆ Similarly dissect out the lateral border of the PMi. Stay off the muscle itself. There is no need to take further fascia. Avoid going too superior on the PMi to prevent thermal injury to the axillary vein or brachial plexus.

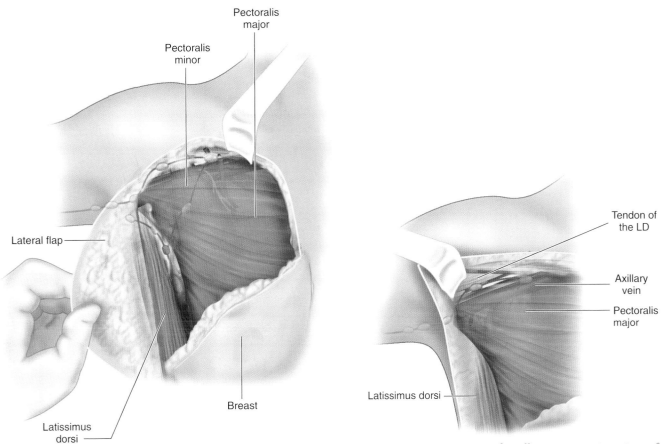

Figure 13-8 Latissimus dorsi muscle with breast removed for demonstration.

Figure 13-9 Location of axillary vein at junction of white tendon of LD and PM with breast removed for demonstration.

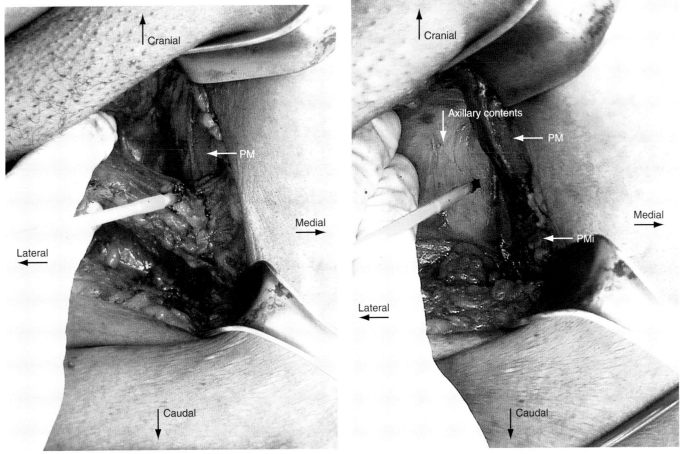

Figure 13-10 Making medial flap.

Figure 13-11

- Identify the medial pectoral bundle (Fig. 13-12) coming around the upper third of the lateral border of the PMi and stop the dissection not more than a few centimeters above that.
- Use an appendiceal retractor to lift up the PMi medially. If the medial extent of the axillary vein cannot be easily visualized, take the medial pectoral bundle with a tie.
- Avoid clips here because the rest of the dissection requires considerable retraction, which could dislodge clips.
- Palpate between the PM and PMi and resect any suspect palpable nodes. If lymph nodes are involved in this area, resect the head of the PMi for full visualization of the axillary lymph node bed.

Identification of the Axillary Vein

- Flex the arm medially and anteriorly to relax the PMi (see Fig. 13-13).
- Retract the PM and PMi medially with an appendiceal retractor.
- Using your nondominant hand, retract the level II lymph nodes (those immediately behind the PMi) caudally and laterally. Make a crescent-shaped incision in the fascia. Retraction then frees the axillary vein at the medial extent of the dissection (Fig. 13-14). This is the easiest place to identify the vein.
- Although a level I and II dissection properly stages the axilla, feel the level III lymph nodes (posteromedial to the PMi). If these are suspect, bluntly dissect the nodes, freeing them to the clavipectoral fascia medially, the so-called Halsted ligament.
- Avoid taking the level III lymph nodes because this increases the risk of lymphedema. The venous plexus just below the medial extent of the axillary vein is often the site of unrecognized bleeding. Double-check this area before closing and use clip and tie for hemostasis.

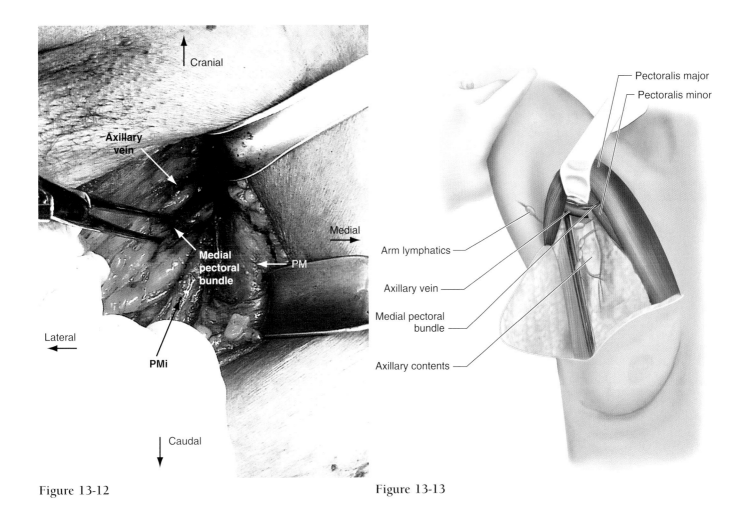

Figure 13-12

Figure 13-13

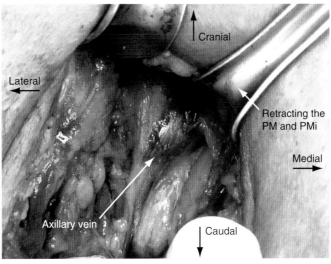

Figure 13-14

Superior Vein Dissection

- Lift the PMi medially and retract the axillary contents inferiorly and laterally (Fig. 13-15).
- Make an incision just below the axillary vein, taking care not to skeletonize the vein (Fig. 13-16). Clean the axillary vein medial to lateral with a knife to avoid thermal injury to the vein.
- Take superficial vessels with clip and tie. Clip occasional lymphatics coming over the vein. It is important to avoid skeletonizing the vein.
- Take care to stay 1 cm below the vein to avoid injury to the vein as well as the main lymphatic trunk of the arm, that sometimes can be identified running parallel just beneath the axillary vein (Fig. 13-17).
- A new technique that can be added to the ALND to help identify and thus allow protection of the lymphatics draining the arm is called *axillary reverse mapping* (see Chapter 14).
- Using a claw-like motion of the nondominant hand, retract inferiorly and perpendicular to the teres major to identify the thoracodorsal nerve, which sits deep just anterior to the teres major muscle in the medial angle created by the meeting of the thoracodorsal vessels with the axillary vein (see Figs. 13-15 and 13-16).
- Gentle pinching of the nerve ensures identification by activation of the LD.
- Use retraction and blunt dissection to reflect tumorous lymph nodes off the vein and avoid injury to the nerve.
- If possible, resect tumorous involvement of the vein by resecting part of the vein. Use a 6.0 polypropylene Halsted stitch followed by a whip stitch to repair the vein.
- Alternatively, resect as much tumor off of the vein as possible and leave multiple clips on the vein to identify landmarks for later radiation therapy.
- If necessary, all of the vein may be resected, but this significantly increases the risk of subsequent lymphedema.

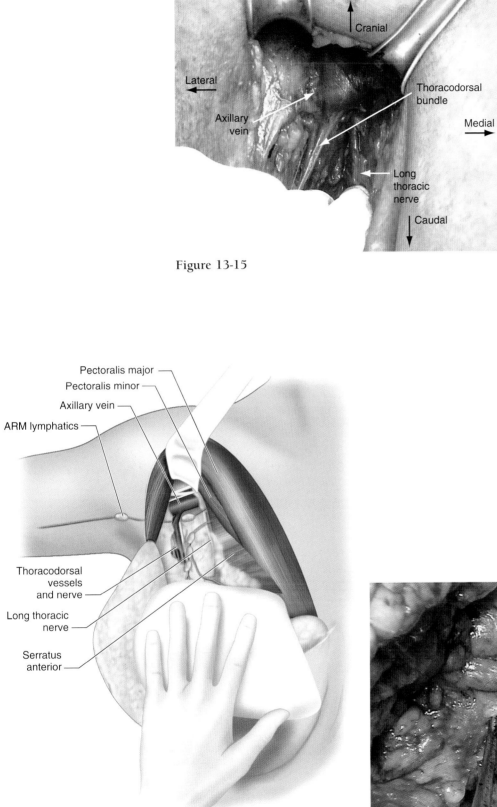

Figure 13-15

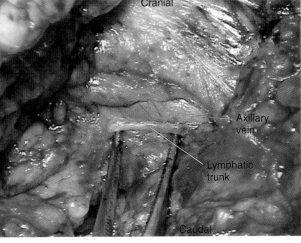

Figure 13-16

Figure 13-17

Posterior-Lateral Dissection

- Free the thoracodorsal nerve from superior to inferior by blunt dissection with a long, fine tonsil clamp (Fig. 13-18).
- Retract the axillary contents laterally and dissect medially, hugging the serratus. The thoracodorsal nerve should be very deep, almost to the level of the teres (Fig. 13-19). Take care not to retract too hard to avoid pulling the nerve out laterally, causing misidentification. Gentle pinching of the nerve ensures identification by activation of the serratus muscle.
- Similarly, use a long, fine tonsil clamp to free the nerve from superior to inferior. Avoid severing the nerve by keeping the plain of dissection parallel to the course of the nerve.
- Retract the axillary contents inferiorly, freeing them from the teres major posteriorly.
- Control troublesome bleeding from the venous plexus that overlies the teres using cautery, harmonic, or clip and tie.
- There are usually three to five intercostobrachial nerves that supply sensation to the medial-posterior aspect of the arm. These are the only nerves that run medial-to-lateral in this dissection. They should be spared if they do not directly interfere with the dissection.
- Take care to protect the thoracodorsal nerve and long thoracic nerve and vessels.

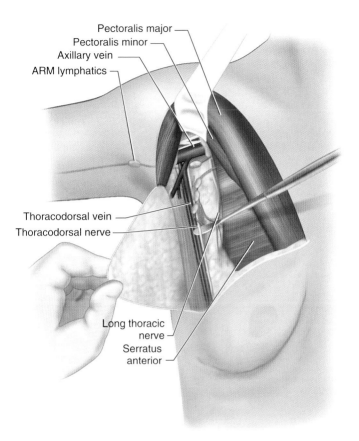

Pectoralis major
Pectoralis minor
Axillary vein
ARM lymphatics

Thoracodorsal vein
Thoracodorsal nerve

Long thoracic nerve
Serratus anterior

Figure 13-18

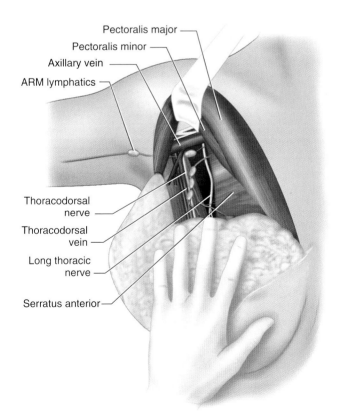

Pectoralis major
Pectoralis minor
Axillary vein
ARM lymphatics

Thoracodorsal nerve
Thoracodorsal vein
Long thoracic nerve

Serratus anterior

Figure 13-19

Medial Chest Wall Dissection

♦ Reflect and retract the axillary contents medially.
♦ First, identify the thoracodorsal nerve superiorly; then, using a knife (heat may damage the nerve), cut just anterior to the nerve from known to unknown. Take care to cut in the long axis so that if the nerve is cut, it will merely be a slice and not a transection (Figs. 13-20 [TD, thoracodorsal] and 13-21).
♦ As the axillary contents are freed from the thoracodorsal nerve, identify the more medial long thoracic nerve, and similarly free it (see Fig. 13-19).

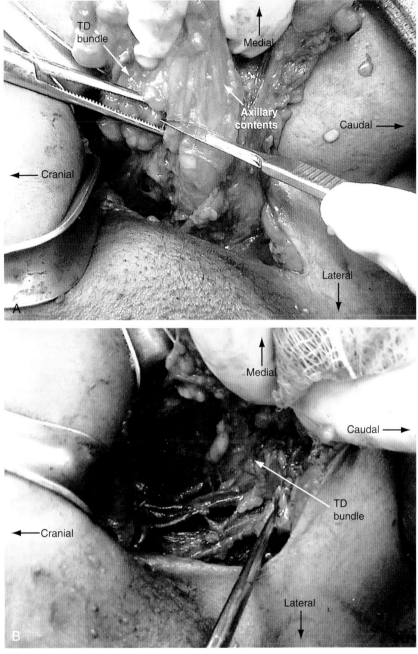

Figure 13-20

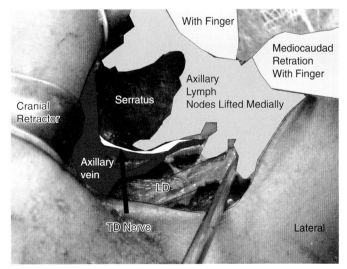

Figure 13-21

- Reflect the axillary contents laterally over your hand and use electrocautery to complete the dissection from the serratus (Fig. 13-22).
- Deliver the axillary contents en bloc from the wound to complete the ALND (Fig. 13-23).

4. Irrigation and Packing of the Wound

- The wound is thoroughly irrigated with hot water to remove devascularized fatty tissue. Water is used for irrigation because tumor cells, if present, will be removed or osmotically lysed. The wound is then packed with hot lap pads. It is also thought that heat drives the clotting reaction forward, improving hemostasis. However, irrigation that is too hot can result in a burn.

5. Clean Field

- Gloves and instruments are changed and the field redraped. It is thought that blood-soaked towels or instruments might seed tumor cells.

6. Hemostasis

- Examine the field thoroughly for torn vessels that are not necessarily bleeding and ligate them with clip or tie. Avoid electrocautery near the larger veins or nerves to prevent thermal injury. Avoid using clips near the nerves because of the possibility of later nerve impingement or fibrosis.

7. Drain Placement

- A single, large (~19 Fr) drain is placed in the anterior axillary line, above or below the bra line. A round Blake drain allows for easiest removal. Two drains are unnecessary. This placement keeps it within the patient's sight. Because the drain is the last thing to be removed and leaves an open wound, placing it in the bra line causes undue and prolonged pain (Fig. 13-24).

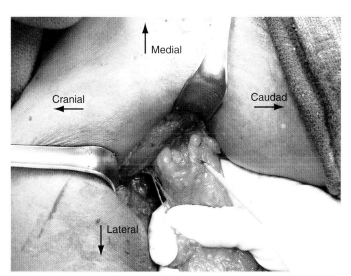

Figure 13-22

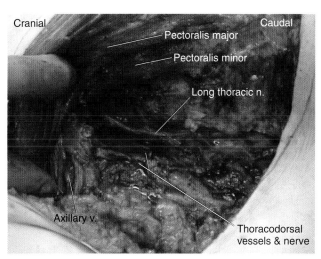

Figure 13-23

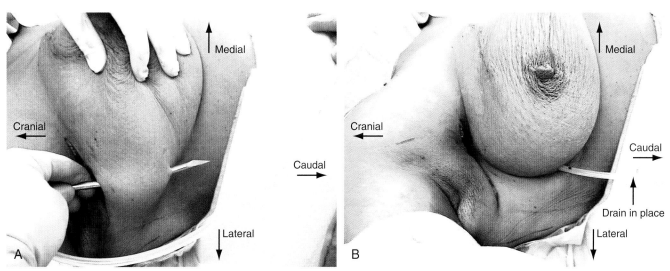

Figure 13-24

8. Closure

- A variety of different closures are adequate, as long as a seal is maintained so that the drain works. A 3.0 running polydioxanone (PDS) suture with a 4.0 subcuticular stitch is the fastest to place.

9. Dressing

- Simple Steri-Strips placed horizontally on the wound or external glue are all that are necessary. Pressure dressings do not prevent seromas.

Step 4. Postoperative Care

- The patient usually requires an overnight hospital stay because she must (1) be able to take pain-relieving and other medications, (2) be able to eat and maintain hydration, and (3) learn how to take care of the drain. Patients with comorbid conditions may require longer stays.
- The patient should be instructed to keep her elbow at her side to lessen fluid production and give the flaps a chance to heal down to the chest wall to prevent seroma formation once the drain has been removed. The drain should be removed after 7 days if the drainage is less than 30 mL and should be left in no longer than 10 days to prevent infection. Although the practice is somewhat controversial, some practitioners elect to cover drains with antibiotics. If drain prophylaxis is chosen, consult with the hospital for the antibiotic that best covers staphylococcal infection.
- Hematomas occur in less than 1% of cases. A small, stable, next-day hematoma can simply be watched. An enlarging or large hematoma should be opened through the incision, bleeders ligated, and closed. Most of the time, a specific origin of bleeding cannot be located.

Step 5. Pearls and Pitfalls

- Seromas occur in about 30% of cases.
  - ▲ Drain the patient percutaneously with a 20-gauge syringe every 2 to 4 days until the flap is healed down and there is no more ballotable fluid.
  - ▲ If the fluid continues to accumulate after 3 weeks, palpate the most inferior extent of the fluid and make a 3-cm incision in the inferior portion of the palpable seroma. Alternatively, ultrasound can be used.

- ▲ Instruct the patient to manually drain the wound three times a day with a cotton swab inserted into the wound to act as a wick.
- ▲ If the wound still does not heal after 2 weeks, take the patient back to the operating room and remove or scarify the capsule that has formed and close with multiple 3.0 absorbable stick ties.
- ▲ Replace the drain if necessary.
- ◆ Injury to the thoracodorsal or long thoracic nerve, if recognized during surgery, can be repaired primarily using simple interrupted 9.0 nylon sutures.
- ◆ Numbness or dysesthesia in the posterior medial arm results from destruction of one or more of the intercostobrachial nerves, which is more often than not unavoidable.
  - ▲ Numbness may improve over time because there are multiple intercostobrachial nerves. Offer reassurance.
  - ▲ Amitriptyline or similar neurogenic drugs may be useful for dysesthesias of the arm or chest wall, sometimes referred to as *phantom pain*.
- ◆ In case of injury to the thoracodorsal vessels, clip or tie the vessels. Repair is not necessary because of the dual blood supply to the LD.
- ◆ Injury to the lymphatics cannot usually be repaired, and the surgeon usually is not aware of the injury. The axillary reverse mapping procedure can be used to avoid such injury (see Chapter 14).
- ◆ Nerve injuries often are identified postoperatively.
  - ▲ A long thoracic nerve injury presents with a winged scapula. A thoracodorsal nerve injury presents with weakness of internal rotation and extension or the inability to hold a book under the arm.
  - ▲ Do not reoperate immediately. These presentations may be due to neurapraxia because of intraoperative tension. Wait at least 3 months before reoperation to identify and anastomose the nerves.
- ◆ Some patients experience postoperative chronic shoulder bursitis after laying supine on the operative table with the arm immobilized.
  - ▲ Find the trigger point, which is usually located on the middle to lower medial border of the scapula.
  - ▲ Inject the trigger point with a mixture of 0.5% short-acting anesthetic with epinephrine, 0.5% long-acting anesthetic, and 30 mg methylprednisolone. The patient should experience immediate relief from the anesthetic and long-term relief from the steroid.
  - ▲ A total of two or three injections may be necessary if symptoms recur. Oral analgesics and aquatic aerobics may provide additional relief.
- ◆ If the patient experiences frozen shoulder, consult occupational or physical therapy for range-of-motion exercises. If the condition is due to pain, a trigger point injection is often helpful. If the range of motion fails to improve or the condition is not associated with pain, consider an injection of botulinum toxin (Botox; Allergan, Inc., Irvine, CA).

Bibliography

Kass K, Henry-Tillman RS, Mancino AT, Klimberg VS. Lymphedema review. Womens Oncol Rev 2002;2:240-252.

CHAPTER 14

AXILLARY REVERSE MAPPING

V. Suzanne Klimberg

Step 1. Surgical Anatomy

* The anatomy of the axillary lymphatic system has been well described (Fig. 14-1); however, the areas from which these lymphatics derive have not. Only recently has there been a delineation between the axillary lymph nodes draining the breast and those draining the arm (Fig. 14-2; SLN, sentinel lymph node). Axillary reverse mapping (ARM) is a method of separating nodes draining the breast from those draining the arm so that the arm lymphatics can be preserved and lymphedema prevented. Five variations have been identified of ARM lymphatics including 1) above or below the axillary vein; 2) a sling pattern that may come as much as 4 cm below the axillary vein; 3) a lateral apron; 4) a medial apron; and 5) a twine or cord like pattern of multiple small nodes. All of these usually emanate from the arm just lateral to the thoracodorsal vessels just under the axillary vein—the so-called "axillary ring". Often there is a large node that sits in this area from which the variations spring.

Step 2. Preoperative Considerations

* Variations in arm lymphatic drainage put the arm lymphatics at risk for disruption during an axillary or SLN dissection. Therefore, ARM, or mapping the drainage of the arm with blue dye (BD), decreases the likelihood of inadvertent disruption of the lymphatics.
* ARM may be used for lesions of any size and for those with lymph node involvement.
* Significant disturbance of the breast (e.g., previous axillary surgery) may have already disrupted the arm lymphatics such that ARM may not be efficacious in this group of patients.

Step 3. Operative Steps

1. Setup

* Available materials for localization and biopsy of the SLN include technetium-99m (Tc-99m) sulfur colloid (filtered or unfiltered) and Tc-99m albumin (see Chapter 11).
* Two to 5 mL of 1% isosulfan BD (1% isosulfan blue) is reserved for injection into the arm. Methylene blue has been demonstrated to cause necrosis of the skin when injected intradermally

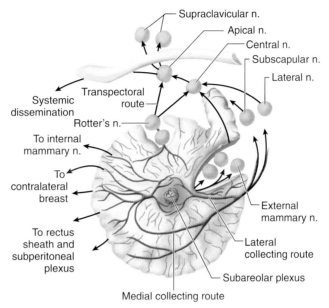

Figure 14-1

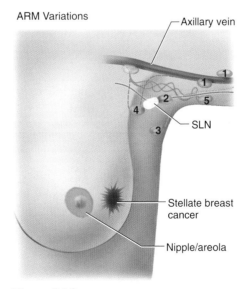

Figure 14-2

or subcutaneously, and therefore its use should be avoided if possible. When using methylene blue, it is necessary to dilute it by at least half.

◆ The patient is placed supine with the arm extended at a right angle.

2. Injection of Radiopharmaceutical

◆ If an SLN biopsy is to be performed, the radioactive tracer may be injected into the breast as instructed in Chapter 11.

3. Injection of Blue Dye

◆ Inject 2 to 5 mL of BD subcutaneously in the ipsilateral upper inner arm along the medial intramuscular groove of the arm to locate the lymphatics draining from the arm (Fig. 14-3).
◆ This location has the most rapid drainage and it will hide the tattoo from the BD.
◆ After injection, massage the site and then elevate the arm for 5 minutes to enhance arm lymphatic drainage.
◆ Inform the anesthesiologist when the BD is injected because a drop may be seen on the oxygen saturation monitor.

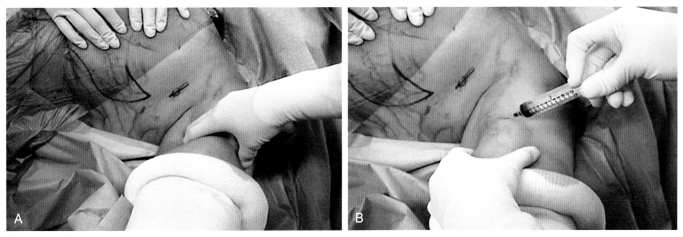

Figure 14-3

4. Excision of Sentinel Lymph Nodes

◆ Once the axillary fascia has been incised, care should be taken not to disturb any blue lymphatics (Fig. 14-4, *A* and *B*). The gamma probe should be used to locate the radioactive nodes. Blue
lymphatics should be identified, followed to their destination, and separated from the SLN.
One should dissect down to but not lift up the SLN to avoid misidentification of the SLN. Blue
lymphatics can been seen from the SLN incision in approximately one third of cases, and may
be juxtaposed to the SLN in approximately 5%.

5. Axillary Lymph Node Dissection

◆ The incision is made in the usual fashion (see Chapter 13, Fig. 13-3) unless a mastectomy is
being done at the same time, in which case the axillary lymph node dissection (ALND) is performed through the mastectomy incision (see Chapters 15 and 16).
◆ Once the axillary fascia has been breached, protect all blue nodes and lymphatics seen during
dissection (see Chapter 16). This sometimes can be difficult because the blue arm lymphatics
can present as a large apron lying over the breast axillary contents (see Fig. 14-2). This apron
can lie medially or, more commonly, laterally. The blue ARM node may be attached to a large
lymphatic (as large as 6 mm) that may not appear blue itself. The lymphatic may present as a
sling lying 3 to 4 mm below the vein that needs to be dissected free (Fig. 14-5).

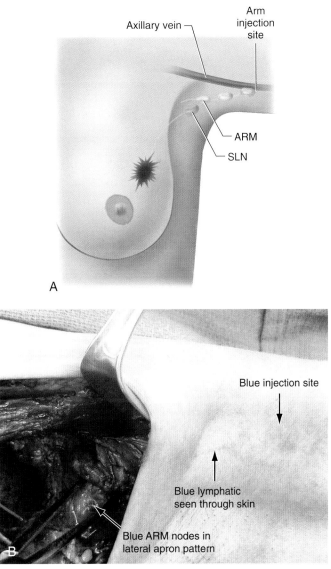

Figure 14-4

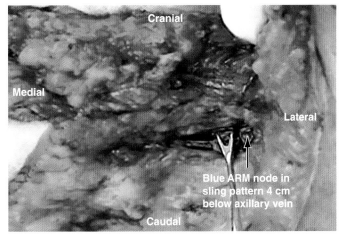

Figure 14-5

6. Intraoperative Assessment of Blue Nodes

- Palpate the blue ARM nodes. In theory, lymph nodes blocked by tumor could divert the tracer to an alternate node, and there is a potential for crossover to the ARM node. If there is concern that the ARM node is involved, it should be excised or biopsied.
- Assess the blue ARM nodes for radioactivity. If the blue ARM node shows a level of radioactivity greater than 10% of that the "hottest" SLN, it should be taken and sent for pathology because it is also an SLN. This happens in 2% to 3% of patients.

7. Hemostasis

- Obtain hemostasis with clip, tie, or electrocautery, but take care when deep in the axilla to avoid the blue lymphatics and nodes.

8. Closure

- Close the axillary or other fascia in layers with 3-0 absorbable sutures, as described in Chapter 13.

9. Dressing

- Steri-Strips parallel to the incision or wound glue are sufficient. Such a dressing allows the patient to shower immediately after surgery. There is no need for a pressure dressing.

Step 4. Postoperative Care

- Caution the patient against significant arm movement or any exercise that would jostle the breast and axilla.
- As soon as the wound is healed (average <1 week), mobilize the patient's arm to regain range of motion.

Step 5. Pearls and Pitfalls

- Lymphedema has not been reported after successful preservation of the lymphatics identified by ARM when coupled with either SLN biopsy or ALND; however, follow-up has been short. Lymphedema may occur if the ARM lymphatics are entrapped in matted involved nodes, in which case the ARM lymphatic may need to be sacrificed. Lymphedema can occur anytime after surgery, even years later, but is rare without axillary intervention or adjuvant irradiation. The best protection for the patient is still to avoid infection and to treat any arm infection early and aggressively.
- Most patients have a blue tattoo at the injection site, which may last anywhere from a few days to 6 months. If a dermal injection is avoided, tattooing is minimized. BD may be injected in the hand, but when injected under the arm it identifies the blue ARM nodes more quickly and has the distinct advantage of being hidden.
- If you suspect a blue dye reaction, give the patient 50 mg diphenhydramine intravenously. If there is no doubt, add 100 mg methylprednisolone. Admit the patient for close observation for at least 24 hours.
- If oxygen desaturation occurs, do nothing if there are no other indications of a problem and the desaturation coincides with BD injection. This is a false desaturation and is simply a monitoring problem.

Bibliography

Boneti C, Korourian S, Bland K, et al: Axillary reverse mapping: Mapping and preserving arm lymphatics may be important in preventing lymphoedema during sentinel lymph node biopsy. J Am Coll Surg 2008;206:1038-1042.

Klimberg VS: A new concept toward the prevention of lymphedema: Axillary reverse mapping. J Surg Oncol 2008;97:563-564.

Mansel R, Fallowfield L, Kissin M, et al: Randomized multicenter trial of sentinel node biopsy versus standard axillary treatment in operable breast cancer: The ALMANAC Trial. J Natl Cancer Inst 2006;98:599-609.

Sakorafas G, Peros G, Cataliotti L: Sequelae following axillary lymph node dissection for breast cancer. Expert Rev Anticancer Ther 2006;6:1629-1638.

Thompson M, Korourian S, Henry-Tillman R, et al: Axillary reverse mapping (ARM): A new concept to identify and enhance lymphatic preservation. Ann Surg Oncol 2007;14:1890-1895.

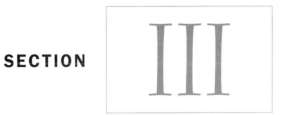

Mastectomy

15

SIMPLE MASTECTOMY

V. Suzanne Klimberg

Step 1. Surgical Anatomy

- ◆ Figure 15-1 shows the borders of the simple mastectomy (SM).
  - ▲ Superiorly—1st and 2nd rib
  - ▲ Inferiorly—the rectus
  - ▲ Medially—the sternum
  - ▲ Laterally—the ill-defined border of the breast approximately the mid axillary line

Step 2. Preoperative Considerations

- ◆ The indications for SM include the following:
  - ▲ First and most important, review the diagnostic biopsy results (either from your institution or elsewhere) with the pathologist. A cytologic diagnosis is not adequate evidence to remove a breast.
  - ▲ Prophylactic contralateral SM is indicated in those patients with a high risk of bilaterality (lobular pathology, locally advanced, inflammatory invasive breast cancer [IBC], multicentricity with a family history) or who cannot reliably be screened (difficult mammography or examination).
  - ▲ For either a primary or contralateral mastectomy, decide ahead of time whether there is a risk of undetected or underestimated IBC. If the risk is sufficiently high, consider a sentinel lymph node biopsy before removal of the breast. If IBC is found in the final pathologic examination and the axilla was not staged before removal of the breast, the patient will need a level I and II axillary lymph node dissection.
  - ▲ Other common uses of SM are in patients who have just undergone a lumpectomy and axillary staging and final pathology has revealed positive margins, patients who later develop a local recurrence, and those who simply desire a mastectomy.
  - ▲ In men, it is not uncommon to perform an SM for refractory gynecomastia.

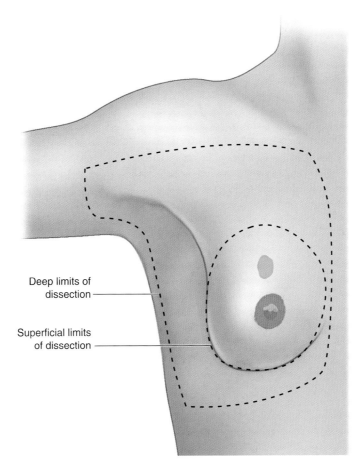

Deep limits of
dissection

Superficial limits
of dissection

Figure 15-1

Step 3. Operative Steps

1. **Anesthesia**

  ◆ General anesthesia is best and safe for most patients. Spinal or epidural anesthesia or local blocks can be used alone or in combination to avoid general anesthesia, or with general anesthesia to reduce postoperative pain. SM can be performed using local anesthesia alone with a mixture of short- and long-acting anesthetics injected in the fat plane between the skin and the glandular tissue of the breast. Others have reported using the instillation of a local anesthetic to facilitate the dissection.

2. **Position**

  ◆ The patient is positioned at the edge of the table with the arm abducted at 90 degrees (Fig. 15-2). This positioning provides the best exposure to the patient and avoids the need for constant leaning over that could lead to back strain.
  ◆ Padding on the arm board should be adjusted so that the arm is level with the body. Too much or too little padding may cause a brachial nerve neuropraxia. For SM, there is no need to drape the lower arm into the field because the arm will remain stationary. Padding should be placed under the wrist to avoid radial nerve neuropraxia.

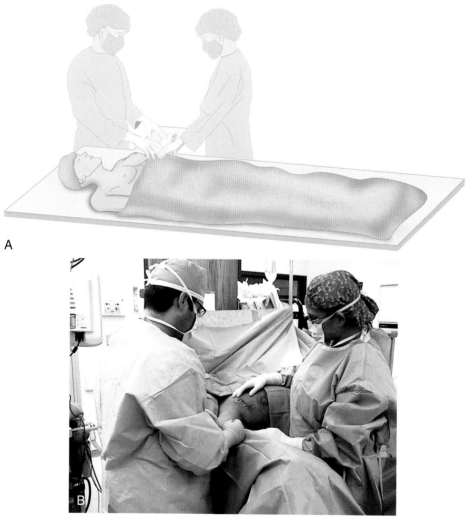

A

B

Figure 15-2

3. Incision

- The standard incision is an ellipse in the plane of the tumor and the nipple-areolar complex, and can be done in virtually any orientation (Fig. 15-3). Ideally, if the tumor is at the 3 o'clock position, the incision will be horizontal, and if at the 12 o'clock position, it will be vertical. In practice, most incisions are horizontal or diagonal. The medial border will be 2 or 3 cm from the sternal edge and the lateral border should extend only to the lateral border of the pectoralis major or edge of the latissimus.
- Skin directly over a tumor, especially a superficial one (<1 cm from skin), should be taken.
- Avoid taking too big an ellipse, or closure will be difficult.
- The tendency to extend the lateral border of the incision posteriorly to incorporate redundant skin and fat underneath the arm increases the risk of lymphedema and should be avoided.
- If immediate reconstruction is contemplated, a "skin-sparing" incision is used. This can simply consist of a much smaller ellipse around the nipple–areolar complex when using implants, or a circular incision encompassing or just inside the nipple–areolar complex when bringing tissue and skin for a tissue reconstruction (Fig. 15-4).
- When the areolar requires removal, a lollipop incision—making a radial incision (laterally or infraareolar) in the inframammary fold—can give better exposure and projection to the reconstructed breast.
- Some have begun to use a total skin-sparing or nipple-sparing procedure using an inframammary fold incision or a vertical radial incision from the limbus to the inframammary fold.

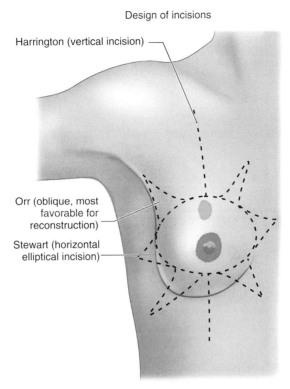

Design of incisions

Harrington (vertical incision)

Orr (oblique, most favorable for reconstruction)

Stewart (horizontal elliptical incision)

Figure 15-3

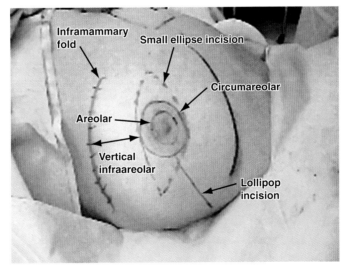

Inframammary fold

Small ellipse incision

Circumareolar

Areolar

Vertical infraareolar

Lollipop incision

Figure 15-4

4. Dissection

Superior Skin Flap Dissection

- In the average patient there is an approximately 7-mm plane of relatively avascular fat between the skin and the glandular tissue; this is the plane that should be used to develop the flap (Fig. 15-5). The thickness of the plane varies with the habitus of the patient.
- Too thin or too thick a flap results in greater than ordinary bleeding, and you may end up leaving more breast tissue behind than intended. If the flap is too thick, simply take a little more tissue, usually with a knife or curved Mayo scissors. If the flap is too thin, especially at the base, necrosis might result. Therefore, as you approach the chest wall, purposefully make the flap thicker to avoid severing feeder vessels, but not so thick as to produce a ridge of tissue on closure. Using a dilator can help define the plan of the flap (Fig. 15-6).
- The flap should be taken superiorly to the level of the first or second rib and the fascia of the pectoralis major incised (Fig. 15-7) medially to the edge of the sternum, taking care to preserve the internal mammary perforators, and laterally to the edge of the pectoralis major. Because the fascia of the breast melds with the fascia of the pectoralis, the latter is incised in preparation for the anterior dissection.
- A lap is left in place to deter oozing while the other flaps are developed.

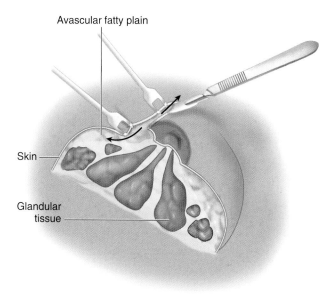

Avascular fatty plain

Skin

Glandular tissue

Figure 15-5

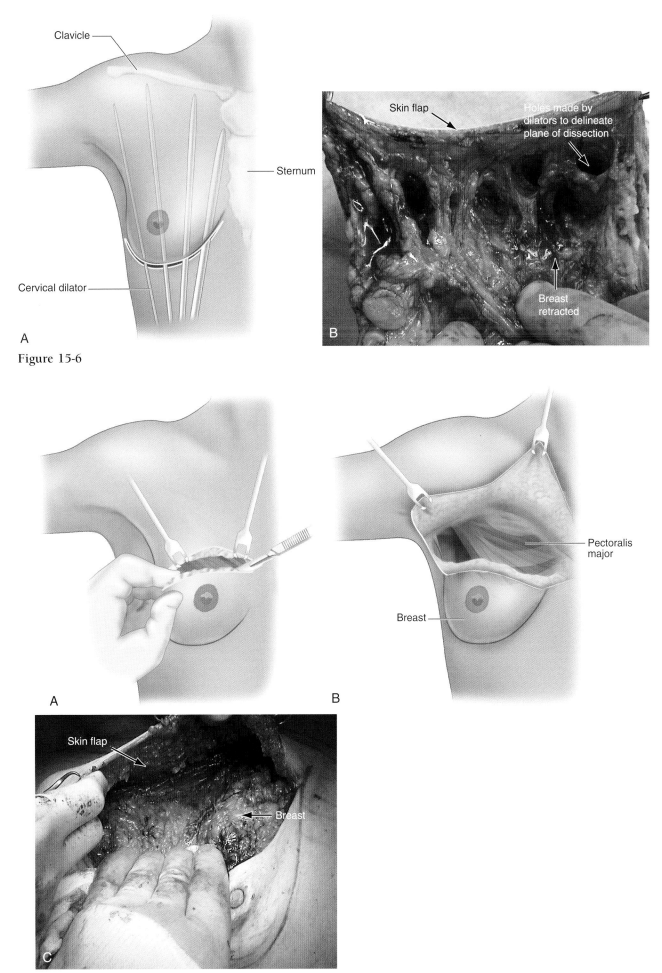

Clavicle

Sternum

Cervical dilator

A

Figure 15-6

Skin flap

Holes made by dilators to delineate plane of dissection

Breast retracted

B

Pectoralis major

Breast

A

B

Skin flap

Breast

C

Figure 15-7

Inferior Skin Flap Dissection

- The inferior flap is developed similarly to the superior flap, using the dilator (Fig. 15-8) or hot or cold cutting dissection, but the plane tends to be less well defined.
- The breast tissue extends to the rectus inferiorly, just at or below the inframammary fold. The fascia of the pectoralis major is incised with electrocautery.
- The pectoralis major and rectus muscles can be easily torn in the medial part of this dissection, so care must be taken not to retract too vigorously in this area. If either muscle is torn the surgeon can elect to sew it back into place.

Medial Skin Flap Dissection

- The medial flap is developed in the same plane connecting the superior and inferior flaps. The opening in the pectoralis flap is connected from above to below along the sternal border. Note that the dissection is directly on top of the chest wall and that past-pointing with the electrocautery or knife can lead to a pneumothorax.
- As you develop the medial flap, identify and avoid the perforators (Fig. 15-9). Clips should not be used here because they can leave palpable scars later in this thin area. These vessels tend to retract. A stick tie should be used to quell bleeding.

Lateral Skin Flap Dissection

- The lateral dissection is slightly thicker than the other flaps and less well defined.
- The flap is taken down to about the level of the pectoralis muscles and then diagonally into the chest wall (serratus), taking the breast tissue but staying out of the axilla and well away from the nerves.
- Take care not to past-point because the serratus is all that separates you from the chest wall and a pneumothorax.

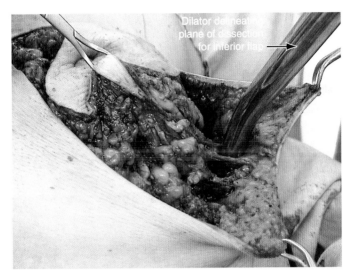

Figure 15-8

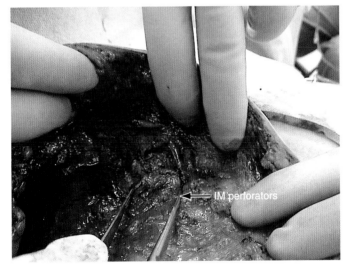

Figure 15-9

Anterior Chest Wall Dissection

- With the surgeon standing below the arm, the breast is retracted down and electrocautery is used in the plane of the muscle fibers to remove the breast en bloc with the fascia of the pectoralis major (see Fig. 15-7).
- Especially in cases of ductal carcinoma in situ or cancer with multiple calcifications, radiographs can be obtained of the ex vivo breast to determine if and where calcifications are left behind, and that area intraoperatively reexcised. Figure 15-13 shows the completed dissection.

Total Skin-Sparing Mastectomy

- When a total skin-sparing mastectomy is performed (see Fig. 15-4, *B*), a cervical dilator can be used to develop the flap from any incision (Fig. 15-10). See Chapter 16 for greater detail.
- Once the flap is developed, the anterior dissection is completed first. A C-Strang retractor is very helpful to lift the breast off the chest wall (Fig. 15-11). The skin flap is then taken superiorly, using the cautery to cut between and connect the cervical dilator holes, which serve as a guide to the correct plane.
- When the nipple–areolar complex is reached, it is dissected sharply from the skin with care taken to remove all of it (Fig. 15-12). A separate core biopsy should be taken and sent to pathology to ensure negative margins during surgery.

5. Irrigation and Packing of the Wound

- The wound is thoroughly irrigated with hot water to remove devascularized fatty tissue. Water is used for irrigation because tumor cells, if present, will be removed or osmotically lysed. The wound is then packed with hot lap pads. It is also thought that heat drives the clotting reaction forward, improving hemostasis.

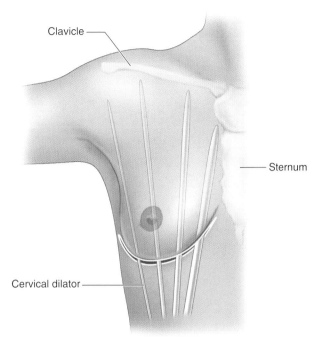

Figure 15-10

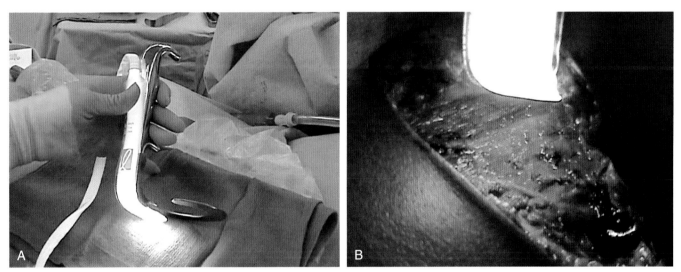

Figure 15-11

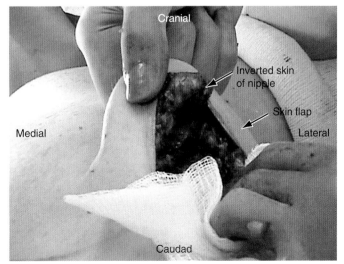

Figure 15-12

6. Clean Field

- Gloves and instruments are changed and the field redraped. It is thought that blood-soaked towels or instruments might seed tumor cells.

7. Hemostasis

- The flaps and chest wall are thoroughly inspected for signs of bleeding or for cut vessels that are not bleeding. A stick suture is needed in the area of the perforators because they tend to retract. Avoid using clips near the nerves because of the possibility of later nerve impingement.

8. Drain Placement

- A single large drain is placed in the anterior axillary line, either above or below the bra line. The drain should drape into the axilla and rest in the inframammary sulcus (Fig. 15-13). Two drains are unnecessary. Because the drain is the last thing to be removed and leaves an open wound, placing it in the bra line causes undue and prolonged pain for the patient.

9. Closure

- A variety of different closures are adequate, as long as a seal is maintained so that the drain works. A 3.0 running polydioxanone suture (PDS) with a 4.0 subcuticular stitch is the fastest to place (Fig. 15-14).

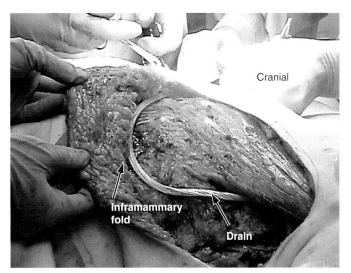

Figure 15-13

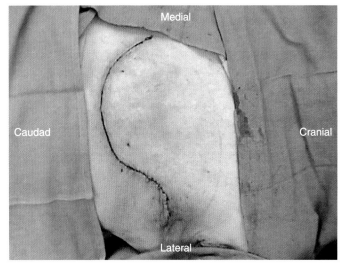

Figure 15-14

10. **Dressing**

   ◆ Simple Steri-Strips placed horizontally on the wound (to avoid blisters seen with perpendicu-larly placed Steri-Strips) or external glue are all that is necessary. The pressure dressings used in the past do not prevent seromas.

Step 4. Postoperative Care

   ◆ The patient usually requires an overnight hospital stay because she must (1) be able to take pain-relieving and other medications, (2) be able to eat and maintain hydration, and (3) learn how to take care of the drain. Patients with comorbid conditions may require longer stays.
   ◆ Patients undergoing accompanying bilateral implant reconstruction (usually not unilateral) and tissue reconstruction may need a longer time to recover.
   ◆ The patient should be instructed to keep her elbow at the side to lessen fluid production and give the flaps a chance to heal down to the chest wall, thus preventing seroma formation after the drain has been removed. The drain should be removed after 7 days if the drainage is less than 30 mL and should be left in no longer than 10 days to prevent infection. Although the practice is somewhat controversial, some practitioners elect to cover drains with antibiotics specific for staphylococci.
   ◆ Hematomas occur in less than 1% of cases. A small, stable, next-day hematoma can simply be watched. An enlarging or large hematoma (one that encompasses more than one fourth of the chest wall) should be opened through the incision, bleeders ligated, and closed. Most of the time, a specific origin of bleeding cannot be located.

Step 5. Pearls and Pitfalls

- Closure is insufficient.
  - With large tumors, a significant amount of skin may be taken (to encompass the tumor), making a simple closure impossible.
  - Once the wound has been thoroughly irrigated, the inferior flap can be extended below the inframammary fold to easily bring the skin edges together. Failing that, the surgeon can swing a local flap.
- The flap is too thin.
  - If the dermis has been back-walled in one or several areas, it may affect flap viability.
  - Flap viability can be checked intraoperatively by administering one or two vials of fluorescein (after giving a test dose to check for allergic reaction). Under a Wood's lamp, necrotic areas will be dark, in sharp contrast to viable areas that fluoresce green, thus outlining the areas that need to be resected.
- Pneumothorax is a rare complication.
  - If it is recognized intraoperatively, it requires only evacuation with a red rubber catheter under positive-pressure ventilation and closure of the opening with a previously placed pursestring suture.
  - If it is recognized after surgery, a small chest tube left in place less than 24 hours will suffice.
- If margins are positive on pathologic examination, and you believe you have done a good anatomic dissection and no further areas can be dissected, then postoperative irradiation is required for local control.
- The drain is leaking.
  - This may be a sign of a nonfunctioning drain.
  - First, strip the drain to make sure it is working. If it is not working, pull it. The patient will need to be seen every few days to check for and drain the accumulating seroma percutaneously with a 20-gauge syringe.
- If the drain is removed prematurely, it is not necessary to replace it, but the patient does need to be followed every few days to check for and drain any fluid accumulation.

- Seroma feels like ballotable fluid and occurs in approximately 30% of patients.
  - ▲ A 20-gauge butterfly on a 30- to 50-mL syringe is used to drain the seroma. The needle is placed at an angle and preferably over a rib (to avoid pneumothorax) in the most dependent portion of the wound. The patient should be seen every few days to check and drain reaccumulation. An unattended seroma can cause flap necrosis.
  - ▲ If a seroma persists beyond 3 to 4 weeks after surgery, an incision (~3 cm) is made in the most dependent portion of the wound and dressed with gauze. This should close within 2 weeks.
  - ▲ It is rare for a seroma to last more than 3 months. If it does, surgical removal of the capsule is required (Fig. 15-15).
- Uninfected flap necrosis can be watched, with the patient taking showers and the eschar removed as necessary. If it is infected, the patient should go back to the operating room and the necrotic area resected. If implants have been placed, they should be removed.
- Cellulitis occurs in less than 5% of the patients and can be treated with antibiotics. Intravenous antibiotics are required for up to 6 weeks in those with previous irradiation. Formation of an abscess, either with the drain in place or associated with a seroma, requires evacuation and packing.
- Neuropraxia can occur from local anesthesia used for postoperative pain or from malpositioning of the arm. Reassure the patient that function will return, although it may take as long as 6 weeks.
- Lymphedema is a late complication and can occur any time after surgery, even years later, but is rare without axillary intervention or adjuvant irradiation. The best protection for the patient is to avoid infection and to treat any arm infection early and aggressively (see Chapter 14 for a discussion of axillary reverse mapping).

Bibliography

Bland KI, Chang HR, Copeland EM: Modified radical mastectomy and total (simple) mastectomy. In Bland KI and Copeland EM (eds): The Breast: Comprehensive Management of Benign and Malignant Diseases, 2nd ed. Philadelphia, WB Saunders, 1998, pp 881-912.

Fisher B, Anderson S, Bryant J, et al: Twenty-year follow-up of a randomized trial comparing total mastectomy, lumpectomy, and lumpectomy plus irradiation for the treatment of invasive breast cancer. N Engl J Med 2002;347:1233-1241.

Rohrich RJ, Ha RY, Kenkel JM, Adams WP Jr: Classification and management of gynecomastia: Defining the role of ultrasound-assisted liposuction. Plast Reconstr Surg 2003;111:909-923.

Society of Surgical Oncology: Statement on Prophylactic Mastectomy [updated March 2007]. Available at www.surgonc.org/default. aspx?id=47.

Vicini FA, Recht A: Age at diagnosis and outcome for women with ductal carcinoma-in-situ of the breast: A critical review of the literature. J Clin Oncol 2002;20:2736-2744. Review.

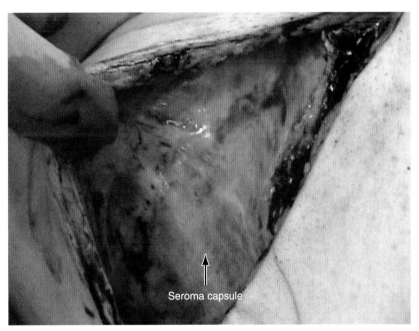

Figure 15-15

CHAPTER 16

SIMPLE EXTENDED AND MODIFIED RADICAL MASTECTOMY

V. Suzanne Klimberg

Step 1. Surgical Anatomy

- Figure 16-1 demonstrates the extent of dissection of the chest wall. The dissection extends from the 1st or 2nd rib superiorly, to the rectus inferiorly, to the sternum medially, and to the latissimus laterally. The classic anatomy of the lymph nodes is demonstrated in Figure 16-2.
- Figure 16-3 shows the en bloc anatomy of the chest wall.
- Figure 16-4 shows a transverse view of the anatomy and the positioning of nerves and vessels, demonstrating the positions of the thoracodorsal bundle and the long thoracic nerve relative to the axillary musculature.

Step 2. Preoperative Considerations

- The primary indication for a simple extended mastectomy (SEM) is for a ductal carcinoma in situ larger than 4 cm (because of risk of recurrence and unidentified invasive cancer), when a sentinel lymph node (SLN) is not identified or SLN biopsy cannot be performed. The procedure is rarely performed today.
- The indications for a modified radical mastectomy (MRM) include the following:
  - ▲ Negative margins for the primary tumor cannot be achieved, and the SLN is positive.
  - ▲ The tumor is larger than 5 cm.
  - ▲ Nodes are clinically palpable.
  - ▲ Inflammatory breast cancer is present.
  - ▲ Multiple tumors are present (although recent data indicate that SLN biopsy is feasible in such patients).

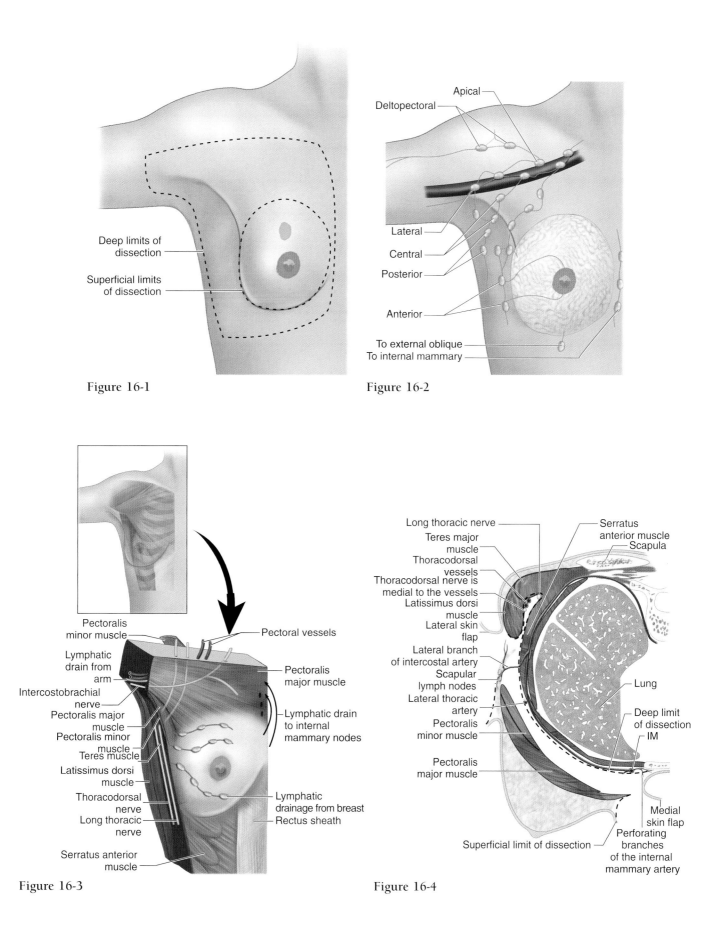

Deep limits of
dissection

Superficial limits
of dissection

Figure 16-1

Apical

Deltopectoral

Lateral

Central

Posterior

Anterior

To external oblique
To internal mammary

Figure 16-2

Pectoralis
minor muscle

Lymphatic
drain from
arm

Intercostobrachial
nerve

Pectoralis major
muscle

Pectoralis minor
muscle

Teres muscle

Latissimus dorsi
muscle

Thoracodorsal
nerve

Long thoracic
nerve

Serratus anterior
muscle

Pectoral vessels

Pectoralis
major muscle

Lymphatic drain
to internal
mammary nodes

Lymphatic
drainage from breast

Rectus sheath

Figure 16-3

Long thoracic nerve

Teres major
muscle

Thoracodorsal
vessels

Thoracodorsal nerve is
medial to the vessels

Latissimus dorsi
muscle

Lateral skin
flap

Lateral branch
of intercostal artery

Scapular
lymph nodes

Lateral thoracic
artery

Pectoralis
minor muscle

Pectoralis
major muscle

Superficial limit of dissection

Serratus
anterior muscle

Scapula

Lung

Deep limit
of dissection

IM

Medial
skin flap

Perforating
branches
of the internal
mammary artery

Figure 16-4

Step 3. Operative Steps

1. Setup

- Patient setup and positioning are the same as for simple mastectomy, except that in MRM the arm is prepped and draped into the field using a stockinette so that it can be freely mobilized (Fig. 16-5).
- Make sure the general anesthetic does not include a muscle relaxant so that the nerves can be easily identified during the procedure.

2. Incision

- Encompass the mass or scar by making an ellipse in the plane of a line drawn between the tumor and the nipple–areolar complex (Fig. 16-6).
- The ellipse will be horizontal if the lesion is at 3 o'clock in the left breast and vertical if the lesion is at 12 o'clock. In practice, most incisions are either horizontal or diagonal.
- Make the medial border of the incision 2 or 3 cm from the sternal edge and the lateral border coinciding with the lateral border of the pectoralis major (PM; when the breast is retracted medially).
- Take skin from directly over a tumor, especially a superficial one (<1 cm from skin).
- Avoid taking too large an ellipse or closure will be difficult.
- Avoid extending the lateral border of the incision posteriorly to incorporate redundant skin and fat underneath the arm; this increases the risk of lymphedema.
- Begin with the superior incision (Fig. 16-7).
- If you plan on immediately reconstructing the patient, use a "skin-sparing" incision (Fig. 16-8). Use a much smaller ellipse around the nipple–areolar complex when placing implants, or a circumareolar incision encompassing the nipple–areolar complex when bringing tissue and skin from a tissue reconstruction. Use a lollipop incision—a radial incision off the circumareolar incision—when exposure is inadequate.
- In benign disease, perform an areolar or nipple skin-sparing procedure through an inframammary fold incision or infra-areolar vertical incision; in cancer, do this cautiously and only when the tumor is deep to the skin, away from and not involving the nipple–areolar complex.

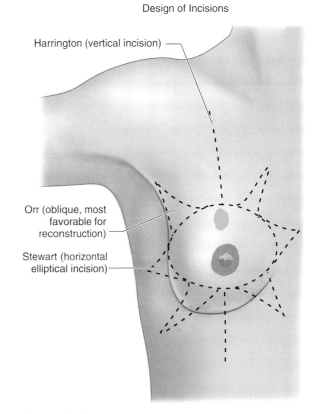

Design of Incisions

Harrington (vertical incision)

Orr (oblique, most
favorable for
reconstruction)

Stewart (horizontal
elliptical incision)

Figure 16-6

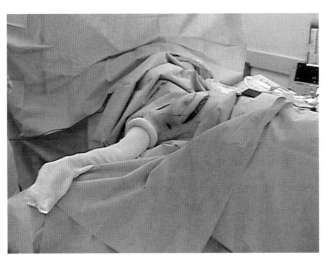

Figure 16-5 Arm mobile in stockinette.

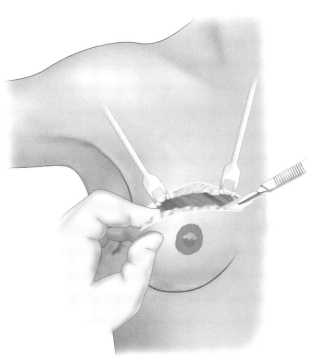

Figure 16-7

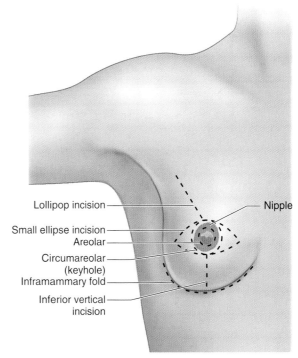

Lollipop incision

Small ellipse incision

Areolar

Circumareolar
(keyhole)

Inframammary fold

Inferior vertical
incision

Nipple

Figure 16-8

3. Dissection

Superior Skin Flap Dissection

♦ Develop the superior flap at an approximately 7-mm-deep plane in the relatively avascular fat between the skin and the glandular tissue (Figs. 16-9 and 16-10).
♦ Whether performing a traditional incision, a skin-sparing incision, or a total skin-sparing incision, Pratt cervical dilators may be used (Fig. 16-11) to develop the flap from the lower incisions over the extent of the flap (Fig. 16-12). The dilator tracks also serve as a guide to the plane of dissection leaving holes to guide the proper plane of dissection (Fig. 16-13).
♦ If the amount of bleeding seems greater than ordinary or expected, the flap may be too thin or too thick.
   ▲ If the flap is too thick, simply take a little more tissue using a knife or curved heavy scissors.
   ▲ Avoid making the flap too thin, especially at the base of the flap, which may jeopardize the vascular supply and cause necrosis. Therefore, as you approach the chest wall, deliberately make the flap thicker to avoid feeder vessels, but not so thick as to produce a ridge on closure.
♦ Make the flap and incise the fascia of the pectoralis major (PM) medially from the edge of the sternum and laterally to the edge of the PM (see Fig. 15-7).
♦ Leave a lap pad packed in the flap to deter unnecessary oozing while the other skin flaps are developed.

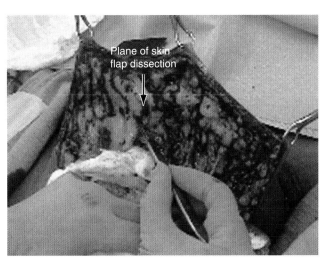

Figure 16-9

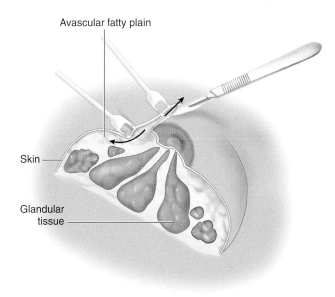

Figure 16-10

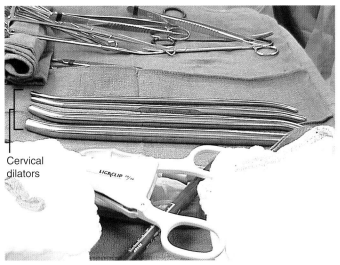

Figure 16-11

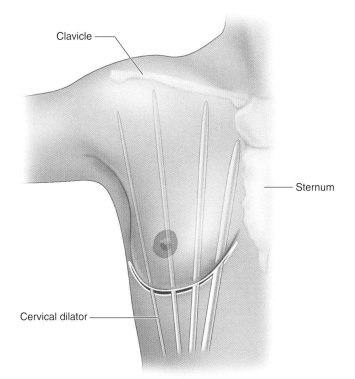

Figure 16-12

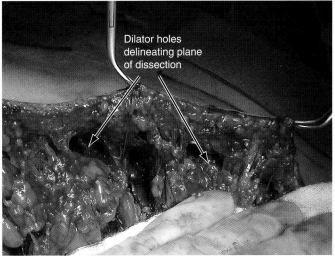

Figure 16-13

Inferior Skin Flap Dissection

◆ The inferior flap is developed similar to the superior flap, but the plane tends to be less well defined.
◆ The breast tissue extends to the inferior border of the PM, adjoining the rectus inferiorly just at or below the inframammary fold (Fig. 16-14). The fascia of the PM is incised with electrocautery.
◆ The PM and rectus can be easily torn in the medial part of this dissection. Less retraction in this part of the dissection is advisable.

Medial Skin Flap Dissection

◆ Develop the medial skin flap in the same plane as the superior and inferior flaps, thus connecting them. Open the PM fascia from the superior flap above to the inferior flap below and just lateral to the sternal border. Note that the dissection is directly on top of the chest wall and that past-pointing with the electrocautery or knife can lead to a pneumothorax.
◆ As you make the medial flap, identify and avoid the perforators (Fig. 16-15). Identify them along the lateral border of the sternum to prevent immediate, as well as delayed postoperative, profuse bleeding.
◆ Clamp or stick-tie perforators only if necessary because they are a major blood supply to the medial skin flap. Avoid the use of clips here because they can produce palpable scars later in this thin area. Perforators tend to retract, so use a 3.0 stick tie for hemostasis.

Lateral Skin Flap Dissection

◆ Make this flap slightly thicker (approximately 1 cm or more, depending on the patient's body habitus). Take the flap down to the latissimus dorsi (LD) muscle (Fig. 16-16).
◆ Start inferiorly to locate the LD most quickly and avoid injury to any nerves or vessels.
◆ Use the electrocautery to test around the area inferiorly where the muscle should be. Visible twitching of the LD indicates where to start the dissection.
◆ Stay directly on the anteromedial border of the muscle. Medial drift may result in thermal injury or transection of the thoracodorsal nerve or vessels. Dissection lateral to the LD makes the flap unnecessarily thin while retrieving no additional lymph nodes. A thin flap increases the risk of seroma.
◆ Follow the anteromedial border of the LD superiorly.
◆ Stop at the level of the LD (the white tendon where the PM crosses over the LD anteriorly may be visible). Going too far superiorly may cause injury to the axillary vein.

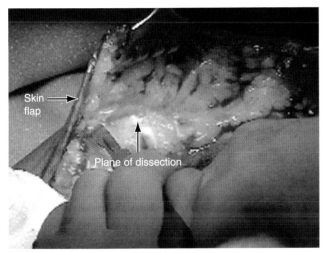

Figure 16-14

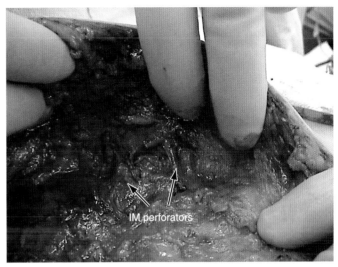

Figure 16-15

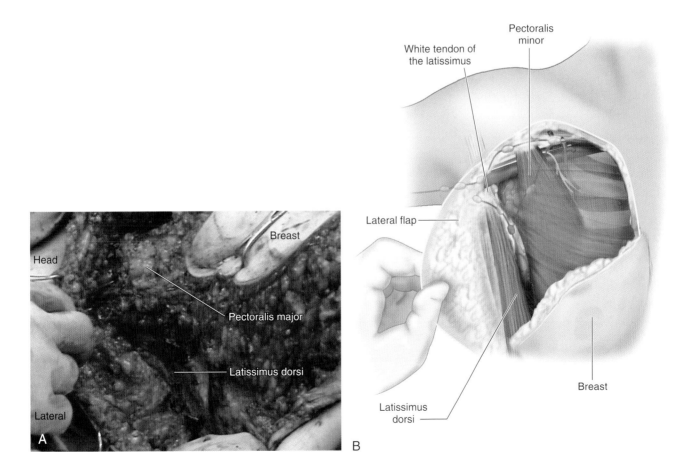

Figure 16-16

Anterior Chest Wall Dissection

▲ The procedure is the same as that in a simple mastectomy. Incise the PM fascia superiorly (Fig. 16-17). Begin to resect fascia from the muscle, carrying it down inferiorly (Fig. 16-18). Alternatively, the dissection can be completed from lateral to medial or inferior to superior depending on incision and exposure.

▲ Examine the radiologic studies and rock the tumor (if palpable) back and forth to determine the likelihood of PM involvement posteriorly. Be mindful of possible muscle involvement in any patient with a posteriorly located lesion.

▲ If the muscle is involved, resect the area around it without disturbing the tumor, using electrocautery.

▲ Bimanually palpate the muscle to rule out unexpected diffuse muscle involvement, which, if present, necessitates resection of the entire PM, as in a radical mastectomy.

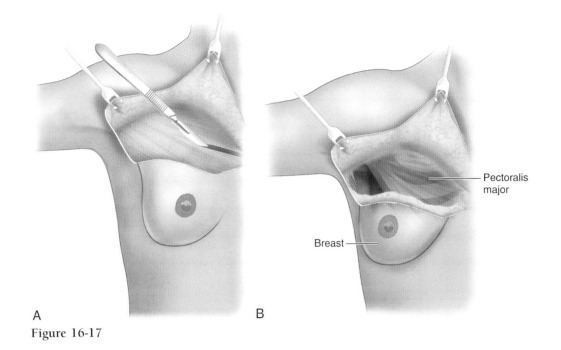

A

B

Pectoralis major

Breast

Figure 16-17

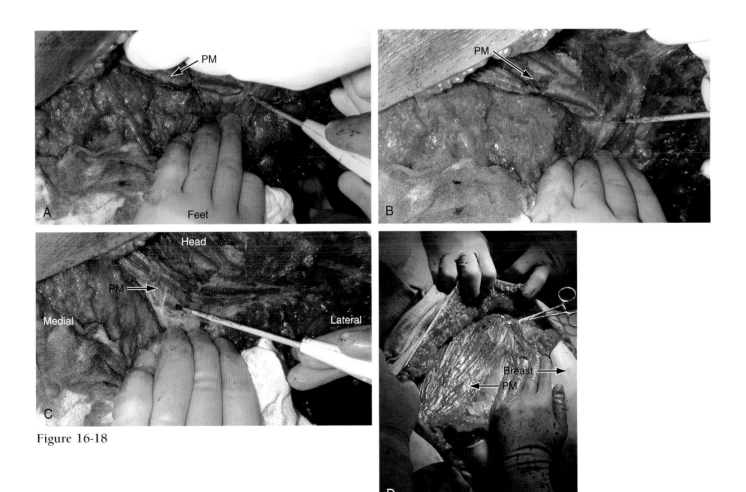

A   PM   Feet

B   PM

C   Head   PM   Medial   Lateral

D   Breast   PM

Figure 16-18

Pectoralis Minor Dissection/Resection

▲ Reflect the breast laterally (Fig. 16-19). The weight of the breast puts tension on the lateral border of the PM.

▲ Use electrocautery to free the edge of the PM. The lateral border of the pectoralis minor (PMi) will then be visible under a filmy layer of tissue (see Fig. 16-19).

▲ Similarly dissect out the lateral border of the PMi (see Fig. 16-19). Stay off the muscle itself. There is no need to take further fascia. Avoid going too superior on the PMi, risking thermal injury to the axillary vein or brachial plexus.

▲ Identify the medial pectoral bundle (Figs. 16-20 and 16-21) coming around the upper third of the lateral border of the PMi, and stop the dissection no more than a few centimeters above the medial pectoral bundle. This is not necessary for an SEM because that procedure takes the level I lymphatics (i.e., those lateral to the PMi).

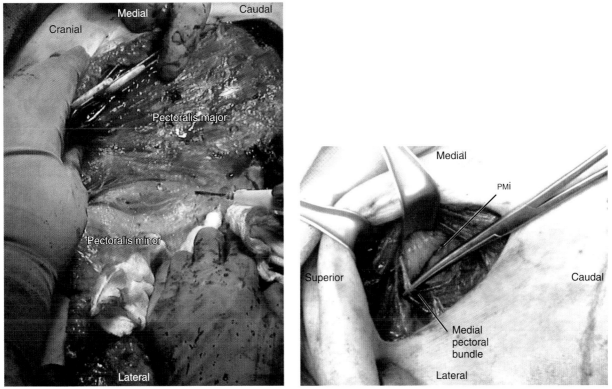

Figure 16-19

Figure 16-20

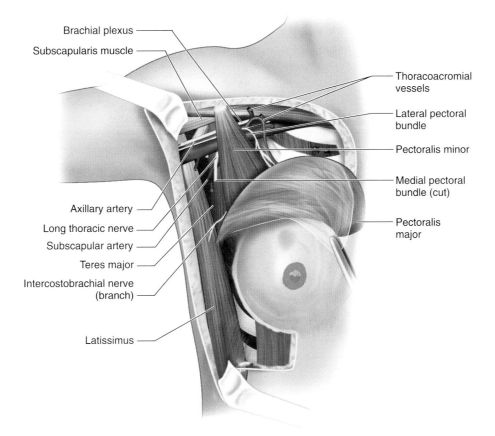

Figure 16-21

▲ Use an appendiceal retractor to lift up the PMi medially (Fig. 16-22). If the medial extent of the axillary vein cannot be easily visualized, take the medial pectoral bundle with clip and tie. Do not use clips alone here because the rest of the dissection requires considerable retraction in this area and clips will be easily dislodged.

▲ Palpate between the muscles and resect any suspect, palpable nodes (Rotter's nodes). If lymph nodes are involved in this area, resect the PMi for full visualization of the axillary lymph node bed.

◆ Resection of the PMi:

▲ This resection is not included in an SEM or necessary for an MRM unless there is involvement of the PMi or inability to access the axillary vein medially. Removal of the PMi is termed a *Patey MRM*. Without resection of the PMi, the operation is referred to interchangeably as the *Auchincloss, Madden,* or *Handley MRM*.

▲ Finger-dissect on the medial side of the PMi near its insertion on the coracoid process (Fig. 16-23).

▲ Put your finger directly behind the tendon that inserts into the coracoid process and transect with the electrocautery.

▲ Retract the cut tendon laterally and use electrocautery to transect the origin of the muscle from the 2nd through 5th ribs.

Identification of the Axillary Vein

◆ When PMi is not resected the assistant will need to flex the patient's arm medially and anteriorly to relax the PMi, resting the patient's arm on yours (Fig. 16-24).

◆ Retract the PM and PMi medially with an appendiceal retractor (see Fig. 16-22).

◆ Using your nondominant hand, retract the level II lymph nodes (those immediately behind the PMi) caudad and laterally. This is not necessary for an SEM.

◆ Make a crescent-shaped incision in the fascia. Retraction then frees the axillary vein at the medial extent of the dissection (see Fig. 16-22). Medially is the easiest place to identify the vein.

◆ Alternatively, retract the level I lymph nodes (those lateral to the PM and PMi) caudad and sharply dissect directly down at the level of the axillary vein, taking care to stay 1 cm below the vein because lymphatics may course just below the vein (Fig. 16-25). This is most commonly done for an SEM.

◆ A level I and II dissection properly stages the axilla. Palpate the level III lymph nodes (medial to the PMi). If they are suspect, bluntly and blindly dissect the nodes free to the clavipectoral fascia, medially.

◆ Avoid taking the level III lymph nodes because this increases the risk of lymphedema on average from approximately 30% with a level I and II lymph node dissection to approximately 50% with a level I to III dissection.

◆ The venous plexus just below the medial extent of the axillary vein is often the site of unrecognized bleeding. Double-check this area before closing.

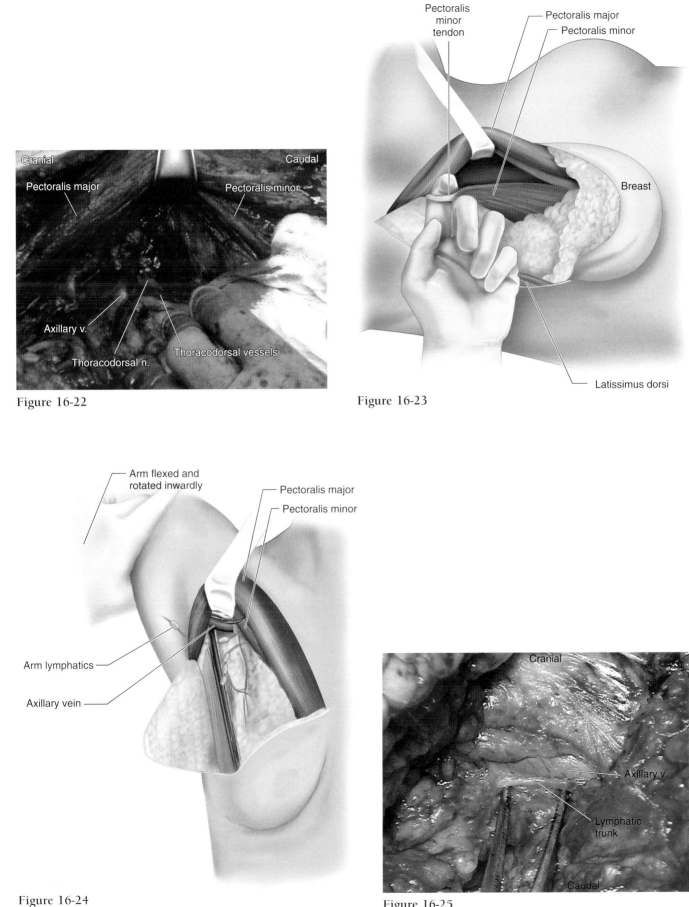

Figure 16-22

Figure 16-23

Figure 16-24

Figure 16-25

Superior Vein Dissection

- See Figure 16-22 for anatomic landmarks.
- Lift the PMi and retract medially and axillary tissue inferiorly.
- Incise the fascia lying just below the axillary vein. If there is a venous plexus here, use multiple clips. This is the most common site of residual bleeding.
- Clean the axillary vein from medial to lateral with a knife to avoid thermal injury to the vein.
- Take superficial vessels with clip and tie. Clip occasional lymphatics coming over the vein. It is important not to skeletonize the vein.
- Take care to stay 1 cm below the vein to avoid injury to the vein as well as the main lymphatics from the arm that can often be identified running parallel to and just beneath the axillary vein (see Fig. 16-25). Also see Chapter 14 for Axillary Reverse Mapping that can be added to MRM.
- Retracting inferiorly, identify the thoracodorsal nerves, which sit deep just anterior to the teres major in the medial angle created by the meeting of the thoracodorsal vessels and the axillary vein (Figs. 16-26 and 16-27).
- Gentle pinching of the nerve ensures identification by activation of the LD.
- Use retraction and blunt dissection to reflect tumorous lymph nodes off of the vein and to avoid injury to the nerve.
- Resect tumorous involvement of the vein if possible by resecting part of the vein.
- Alternatively, resect as much tumor off of the vein as possible and leave multiple clips on the vein to identify landmarks for later radiation therapy.
- All of the vein may be resected if necessary, but this will certainly increase the risk of post-operative lymphedema.

Posterolateral Chest Wall Dissection

- See Figures 16-26 and 16-27 for anatomic landmarks.
- Free the thoracodorsal nerve from superior to inferior by blunt dissection with a long, fine tonsil clamp (Fig. 16-28).
- Retract the axillary contents inferiorly and dissect medially, hugging the serratus. The long thoracic nerve should lie very deep, almost to the level of the teres. Do not retract too vigorously to avoid pulling the nerve out laterally, causing misidentification. Gentle pinching of the nerve ensures identification by activation of the serratus muscle.
- Use a long, fine tonsil clamp to free the long thoracic nerve from superior to inferior. Avoid severing nerves by keeping the plain of dissection parallel to the course of the nerves.
- Retract the axillary contents inferiorly, freeing them from the teres major posteriorly.
- Control troublesome bleeding from the venous plexus that overlies the teres with cautery or clip and tie.
- There are usually three to five intercostobrachial nerves that supply sensation to the postero-medial aspect of the arm (Fig. 16-29). These are the only nerves that run medial to lateral in this dissection. Take them with a clip, but spare them if they do not directly interfere with the dissection.
- Take care to protect the thoracodorsal nerve, long thoracic nerve, and associated vessels from injury.

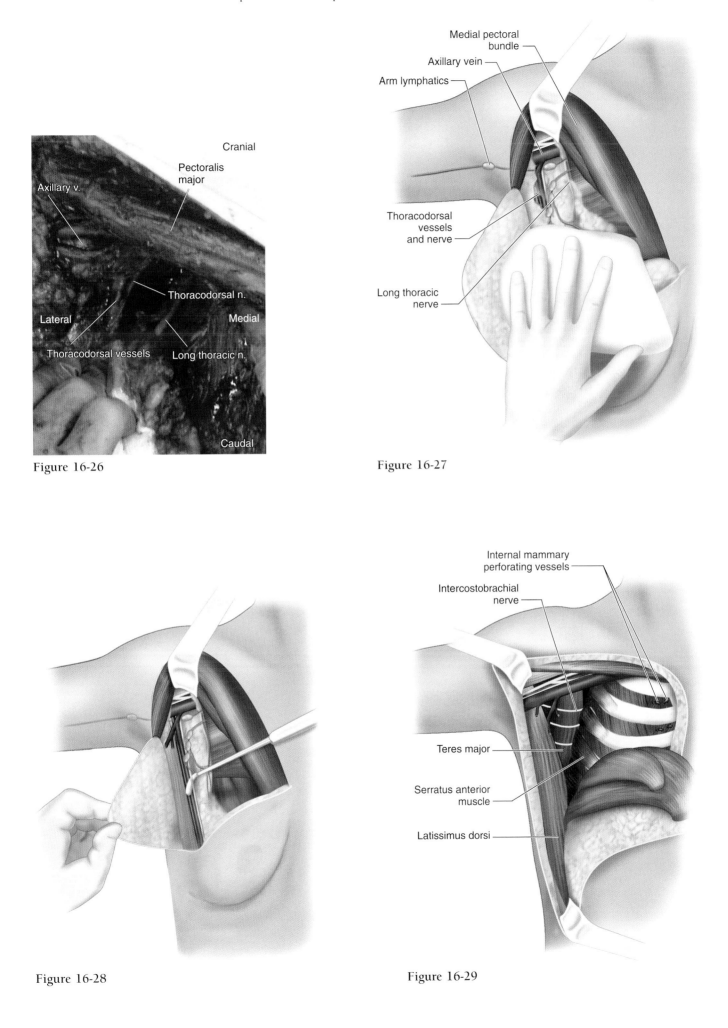

Cranial

Pectoralis major

Axillary v.

Thoracodorsal n.

Lateral

Medial

Thoracodorsal vessels

Long thoracic n.

Caudal

Figure 16-26

Medial pectoral bundle

Axillary vein

Arm lymphatics

Thoracodorsal vessels and nerve

Long thoracic nerve

Figure 16-27

Figure 16-28

Internal mammary perforating vessels

Intercostobrachial nerve

Teres major

Serratus anterior muscle

Latissimus dorsi

Figure 16-29

Medial Chest Wall Dissection

- ◆ Drape a towel over the chest.
- ◆ Reflect and retract the breast and axillary contents medially (Fig. 16-30).
- ◆ First, identify the thoracodorsal nerve lying superiorly and use a knife to cut just anterior to the nerve from known to unknown. Take care to cut along the long axis so that if the nerve is cut, it will merely be a slice and not a transection.
- ◆ As the axillary contents are freed from the thoracodorsal nerve (see Fig. 16-30), identify the long thoracic nerve lying more medially, and similarly free it.
- ◆ Reflect the breast and axillary contents laterally over your hand (Fig. 16-31) and use electrocautery to complete the dissection from the serratus.
- ◆ Deliver the breast and axillary contents en bloc from the wound to complete the MRM (Fig. 16-32).

Pathologic Marking

- ◆ Identify with a clip or stitch the superior and lateral borders of the dissection. The lymph nodes are taken en bloc with the specimen so there is no need to mark them separately.

4. Irrigation and Packing of the Wound

- ◆ The wound is thoroughly irrigated with hot water to remove devascularized fatty tissue. Water is used for irrigation because tumor cells, if present, will be removed or osmotically lysed. The wound is then packed with hot lap pads. It is also thought that heat drives the clotting reaction forward, improving hemostasis. However, irrigation that is too hot can result in a burn.

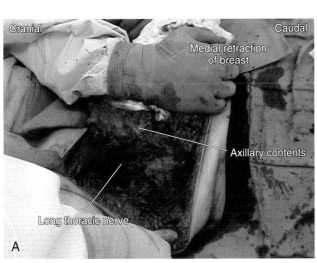

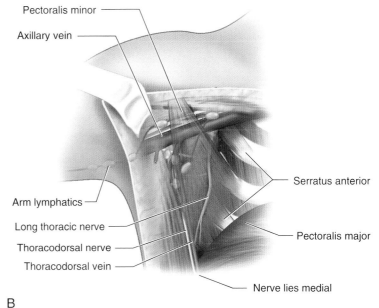

Figure 16-30

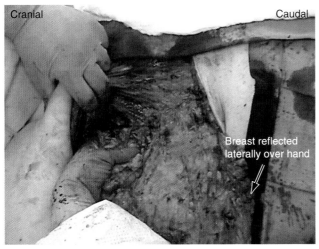

Figure 16-31

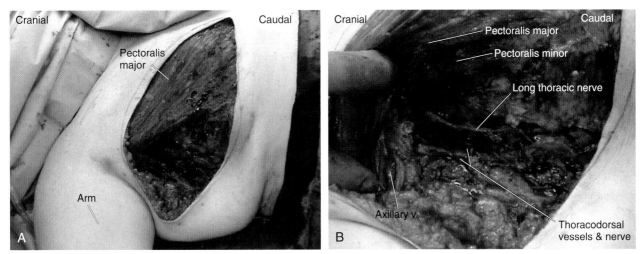

Figure 16-32

5. **Clean Field**

◆ Gloves and instruments are changed and the field re-draped. It is thought that blood-soaked towels or instruments might seed tumor cells.

6. **Hemostasis**

◆ Examine the field thoroughly for torn vessels that are not necessarily bleeding and ligate them with clip or tie. Avoid electrocautery near the larger veins or nerves to prevent thermal injury. Avoid using clips near the nerves because of the possibility of later nerve impingement or fibrosis.

7. **Drain Placement**

◆ A single large drain is placed in the anterior axillary line, either above or below the bra line (Fig. 16-33). Two drains are unnecessary. This placement keeps the drain in the patient's sight. Because the drain is the last thing to be removed and leaves an open wound, placing it in the bra line causes undue and prolonged pain for the patient.

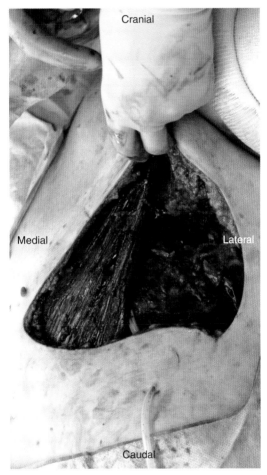

Figure 16-33

8. Closure

◆ A variety of different closures are adequate, as long as a seal is maintained so that the drain works. A 3.0 running polydioxanone suture (PDS) with a 4.0 subcuticular stitch is the fastest to place (Fig. 16-34).

9. Dressing

◆ Simple Steri-Strips placed horizontally on the wound (to avoid blisters seen with perpendicularly placed Steri-Strips) or external glue are all that is necessary. The pressure dressings used in the past do not prevent seromas.

Step 4. Postoperative Care

◆ The patient usually requires an overnight hospital stay because she must (1) be able to take pain-relieving and other medications, (2) be able to eat and maintain hydration, and (3) learn how to take care of the drain. Patients with comorbid conditions may require longer stays.

◆ Patients undergoing accompanying bilateral implant reconstruction (usually not unilateral) and tissue reconstruction may need a longer time to recover. The patient should be instructed to keep her elbow at the side to lessen fluid production and give the flaps a chance to heal down to the chest wall, thus preventing seroma formation after the drain has been removed. The drain should be removed after 7 days if the drainage is less than 30 mL and should be left in no longer than 10 days to prevent infection. Although the practice is somewhat controversial, some practitioners elect to cover drains with antibiotics specific for staphylococci.

◆ Hematomas occur in less than 1% of cases. A small, stable, next-day hematoma can simply be watched. An enlarging or large hematoma (one that encompasses more than one fourth of the chest wall) should be opened through the incision, bleeders ligated, and closed. Most of the time, a specific origin of bleeding cannot be located.

◆ About 60% of patients experience nausea or vomiting secondary to anesthesia. A combination of preoperative dronabinol (Marinol; Solvay Pharmaceuticals, Marietta, GA) and prochlorperazine (Compazine; GlaxoSmithKline, Brentford, United Kingdom) has been shown to drastically reduce the incidence of this complication.

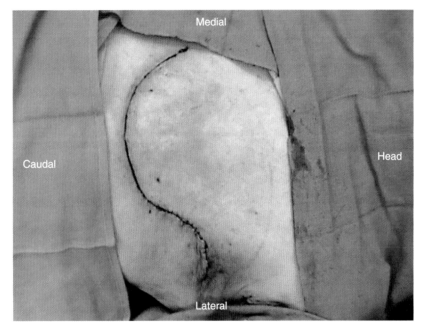

Figure 16-34

Step 5. Pearls and Pitfalls

- ◆ The flap is too thin.
  - ▲ If the dermis has been back-walled in one or several areas, it may affect flap viability.
  - ▲ Flap viability can be checked intraoperatively by administering one or two vials of fluorescein (after giving a test dose to check for allergic reaction). Under a Wood's lamp, necrotic areas will be dark, in sharp contrast to viable areas that fluoresce green, thus outlining the areas that need to be resected.
- ◆ Torn PM or rectus muscles can be sewn back in place with interrupted 3.0 absorbable sutures.
- ◆ Pneumothorax, if recognized intraoperatively, requires only evacuation with a red rubber catheter under positive-pressure ventilation and closure of the opening with a previously placed pursestring suture. If recognized after surgery, a small chest tube left in place less than 24 hours will suffice.
- ◆ Thermal injury to the thoracodorsal nerve is irreparable. To repair a transected nerve, trim the ends and primarily repair with simple 6.0 interrupted absorbable sutures.
- ◆ Resection of the lateral pectoral bundle may cause atrophy of the PM and flattening of the chest wall, affecting mainly cosmesis. Reassurance is all that can be offered.
- ◆ Some patients experience postoperative chronic shoulder bursitis after laying supine on the operative table with the arm immobilized.
  - ▲ Find the trigger point, which is usually located on the middle to lower medial border of the scapula.
  - ▲ Inject the trigger point with a mixture of 0.5% short-acting anesthetic with epinephrine, 0.5% long-acting anesthetic, and 30 mg methylprednisolone. The patient should experience immediate relief from the anesthetic and long-term relief from the steroid.
  - ▲ A total of two or three injections may be necessary if symptoms recur. Oral analgesics and aquatic aerobics may provide additional relief.
- ◆ The axillary vein is injured.
  - ▲ Apply pressure to control hemorrhage until the circulator can get a vascular set on the field and a small, curved vascular clamp can be applied to the site. Do not use regular clamps on the vein or you may tear it further.
  - ▲ Repair the vein using an in-and-out Halsted stitch.
  - ▲ Release the clamp and follow with a running 5.0 polypropylene back stitch.
- ◆ Numbness or dysesthesia in the posterior medial arm results from destruction of one or more of the intercostobrachial nerves, which is usually unavoidable.
  - ▲ Numbness may improve over time because there are multiple intercostobrachial nerves. Offer reassurance.
  - ▲ Amitriptyline or similar neurogenic drugs may be useful for dysesthesias of the arm or chest wall, sometimes referred to as *phantom pain*.
- ◆ Seromas occur in about 30% of cases.
  - ▲ Drain the patient percutaneously with a 20-gauge syringe every 2 to 4 days until the flap is healed down and there is no more ballotable fluid.
  - ▲ If the fluid continues to accumulate after 3 weeks, palpate the most inferior extent of the fluid and make a 3-cm incision directly over the area.
  - ▲ Instruct the patient to manually drain the wound three times a day with a cotton swab inserted into the wound to act as a wick.
  - ▲ If the wound still does not heal after 2 weeks, take the patient back to the operating room and remove or schlerify the capsule that has formed and close with multiple 3.0 absorbable stick ties (Fig. 16-35).
  - ▲ Replace the drain if necessary.

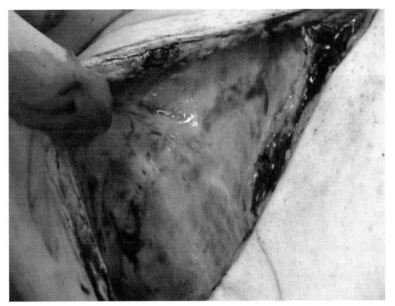

Figure 16-35

- ◆ Injury to the lymphatics cannot usually be repaired, and the surgeon usually is not aware of the injury. If injured lymphatics are identified, clip their ends to avoid the possibility of subsequent seroma.
- ◆ Injury to the thoracodorsal or long thoracic nerve can be repaired primarily using simple interrupted 9.0 sutures.
- ◆ In case of injury to the thoracodorsal vessels, clip or tie the vessels. Repair is not necessary because of the dual blood supply to the LD.
- ◆ If the patient experiences frozen shoulder, consult occupational or physical therapy for range-of-motion exercises. If the condition is due to pain, a trigger point injection is often helpful. If the range of motion fails to improve or the condition is not associated with pain, consider an injection of botulinum toxin (Botox; Allergan, Inc., Irvine, CA).
- ◆ Nerve injuries often are identified postoperatively.
  - ▲ A long thoracic nerve injury presents with a winged scapula. A thoracodorsal nerve injury presents with weakness of internal rotation and extension or the inability to hold a book under the arm.
  - ▲ Do not reoperate immediately. These presentations may be due to neuropraxia because of intraoperative tension. Wait at least 3 months before reoperation to identify and anastomose the nerves.

Bibliography

Bland KI, McCraw JB, Copeland EM: General principles of mastectomy: Evaluation and therapeutic options. In Bland KI, Copeland EM (eds): The Breast: Comprehensive Management of Benign and Malignant Diseases (2nd ed). Philadelphia, WB Saunders, 2004, pp 865-883.

Fisher B, Anderson S, Bryant J, et al: Twenty-year follow-up of a randomized trial comparing total mastectomy, lumpectomy, and lumpectomy plus irradiation for the treatment of invasive breast cancer. N Engl J Med 2002;347:1233-1241.

Fisher B, Jeong JH, Anderson S, et al: Twenty-five year follow-up of a randomized trial comparing radical mastectomy, total mastectomy followed by YRT. N Engl J Med 2002;347:567-575.

Van Dongen JA, Voogd AC, Fentiman IS, et al: Long-term results of a randomized trial comparing breast-conserving therapy with mastectomy: European Organization for Research and Treatment of Cancer 10801 trial. J Natl Cancer Inst 2000;92:1143-1150.

Veronesi U, Cascinelli N, Mariani L, et al: Twenty-year follow-up of a randomized study comparing breast-conserving surgery with radical mastectomy for early breast cancer. N Engl J Med 2002;347:1227-1232.

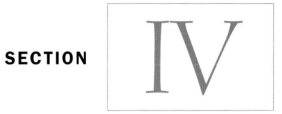

Breast Reconstruction

Oncoplastic Approaches to the Partial Mastectomy for Breast Conservation Therapy

Chin-Yau Chen, Kristine E. Calhoun, and Benjamin O. Anderson

Step 1. Surgical Anatomy

- A comprehensive understanding of normal ductal anatomy, as well as its influence on the distribution of cancer in the breast, is critical to planning an oncoplastic partial mastectomy.[1,2] An understanding of this anatomy has not been widely discussed in the context of breast surgery, despite the fact that the concept of segmental ductal anatomy was thoroughly described in 1840 by Sir Astley Cooper in his classic two-volume atlas of comparative mammary anatomy.[3]

- At present, it is uncertain whether the segmental anatomy of the breast is relatively constant, like the segmental anatomy of the liver, or if the ductal segmental anatomy varies from individual to individual or breast to breast. A fundamental challenge for the oncoplastic surgeon is to determine how each individual cancer is distributed within the breast and to assess whether the lesion can be resected as a single en bloc fibroglandular resection, as is recommended by the National Comprehensive Cancer Network (NCCN).[4]

- The modern anatomic analysis of ductal anatomy reported by Love and Barsky suggests that the number of major ductal systems is probably fewer than 10 (Fig. 17-1, A). The size of ductal segments is variable: in some cases, a segment can be a narrow "pie slice" of tissue; in other cases, one ductal segment can occupy up to 25% of the total breast volume[5] (Fig. 17-1, B).

- Not all ducts pass radially from the nipple to the periphery of the breast; rather, some travel directly back from the nipple toward the chest wall. According to Cooper, single ductal segments radiate to the margin of the sternal (medial) and clavicular (superior) aspects of the breast, with two or three ductal branches layered on each other, thus creating a fuller pad of fibroglandular tissue in the axillary (lateral) and abdominal (inferior) aspects of the breast.[3] Although the ductal branches appear to interdigitate with each other within the breast parenchyma, the segments do not communicate with each other through ductal anastomoses.

- In contrast to the ductal anatomy, the fibroglandular tissue of the breast has a rich anastomotic circulatory bed, thereby allowing oncoplastic resection and mastopexy advancement of the parenchyma to be safely performed. The well-collateralized vasculature of the breast makes it possible to move and remodel fibroglandular tissue within the skin envelope without major

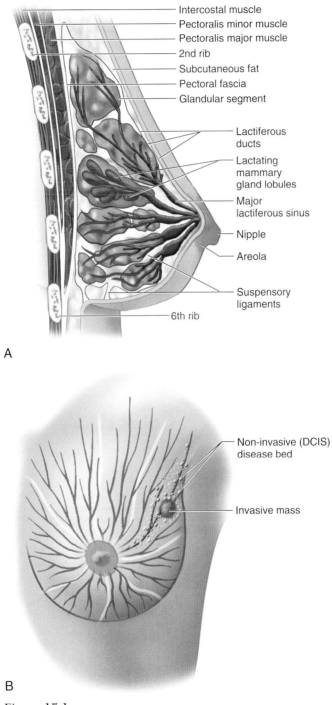

Intercostal muscle
Pectoralis minor muscle
Pectoralis major muscle
2nd rib
Subcutaneous fat
Pectoral fascia
Glandular segment

Lactiferous ducts

Lactating mammary gland lobules

Major lactiferous sinus

Nipple

Areola

Suspensory ligaments

6th rib

A

Non-invasive (DCIS) disease bed

Invasive mass

B

Figure 17-1

risk of breast devascularization and necrosis. The most common source of arterial blood supply in the human breast arises from the axillary and internal mammary arteries. By maintaining communication with one of these two arterial connections, and by limiting the degree of dissection between the fibroglandular tissue and skin, an adequate blood supply for the breast parenchyma is maintained during tissue advancement and mastopexy closure.

◆ Using magnetic resonance imaging, the distribution of a breast cancer can be classified into three patterns: (1) localized, (2) segmentally extended, or (3) irregularly extended.[6] Ductal carcinoma in situ (DCIS) is often multifocal but unicentric in nature, that is, spreading as many small, noninvasive tumor foci that can appear discontinuous on histologic analysis but which are actually intraductally connected within a single major ductal segment.[7] When invasive carcinoma arises in a segmental bed of DCIS, it commonly arises at the periphery rather than the center of the DCIS.[8] For this reason, the oncoplastic surgeon needs to be thoughtful in designing a tissue resection that encompasses both the noninvasive and invasive components of disease. Cancer resection intending to remove only a palpable invasive carcinoma will often produce inadequate surgical margins for its nonpalpable, noninvasive portion. Furthermore, the oncoplastic surgeon should not assume that the invasive cancer is centrally located within a segment of noninvasive disease (see Fig. 17-1, B). Instead, mammographic images should be scrutinized for the presence of microcalcifications that may suggest an eccentric distribution of disease that follows the natural ductal segmental anatomy of the breast.

◆ Using oncoplastic surgical techniques for breast preservation, breast surgeons can achieve wide surgical margins while preserving the shape and appearance of the breast[9] (Table 17-1). Although oncoplastic techniques vary in type and approach, the general principle of fashioning the tissue resection to the anatomic shape of the cancer minimizes the removal of uninvolved breast tissue while ensuring that wide margins, ideally more that 1 cm, are achieved in an optimal number of patients.[1,2]

Step 2. Preoperative Considerations

◆ To plan an optimal oncoplastic surgical resection, the surgeon should recognize the limited degree to which imaging may accurately predict the true histologic extent and orientation of disease, especially its noninvasive component.

◆ A combination of imaging modalities (diagnostic mammography with magnification views, ultrasonography, and magnetic resonance imaging when indicated) may yield the best estimates of tumor size.[10]

◆ Multiple localization wires can help define the radiographic extent of the nonpalpable calcified lesions[11] (Fig. 17-2).

◆ Consultation with plastic surgery colleagues may be warranted for surgeons without formal plastic surgery training for the more complex oncoplastic procedures.

TABLE 17-1	Oncoplastic Approaches for Partial Mastectomy	
TYPE OF ONCOPLASTIC LUMPECTOMY	CANCER LOCATION	CANCER DISTRIBUTION
Parallelogram mastopexy lumpectomy	Peripheral, except the upper inner quadrant*	Localized or small, segmentally extended
Batwing mastopexy lumpectomy	Central breast	Centrally distributed, without involvement of nipple
Reduction mastopexy lumpectomy	Lower breast, 4 to 8 o'clock position	Localized or small, segmentally extended
Donut mastopexy lumpectomy	Upper or lateral	Segmentally extended

*For lumpectomy in the upper inner quadrant of the breast, it is better not to remove a skin island to avoid nipple–areolar deviation upward and medially.

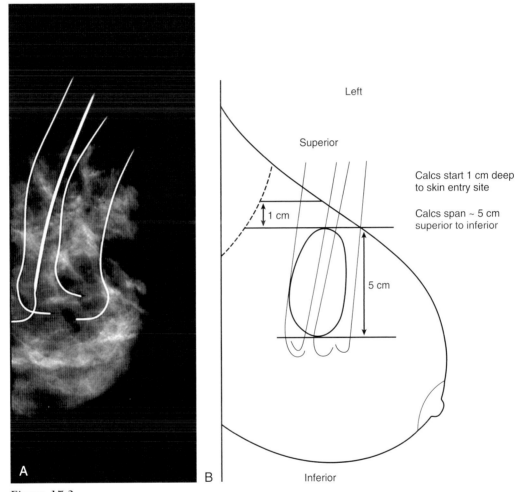

Figure 17-2
A and B courtesy of Dr. Kate Dee, Seattle, Wash.

- Although surgical margins should ideally exceed 10 mm, this width is often incompatible with an acceptable cosmetic outcome. The general principle of "wider is better" for surgical margins needs to be tempered by a realistic understanding of breast cosmesis. Low local recurrence rates after breast conservation therapy, especially in the era of postlumpectomy irradiation, can be achieved with intermediate surgical margin widths between 1 and 10 mm.[4]
- Before the procedure, the patient's skin landmarks should be marked with the patient in the upright position for the purpose of planning the skin incision(s). Relevant skin landmarks include the inframammary crease, the anterior axillary fold at the pectoralis major muscle, the posterior axillary fold of the latissimus dorsi muscle, the sternal border of the breast, and the periareolar circle (Fig. 17-3).
- Identifying these landmarks with the patient in the upright position is very important to the final cosmetic outcome because these anatomic sites may be difficult to locate accurately once the patient is anesthetized and lying supine on the operating room table. During surgery, the boundaries of the target lesion can be marked sonographically for tumors visible by ultrasound. The location of the skin incision(s) can be adjusted as needed to ensure that the skin island to be resected is located directly above the target lesion.

Step 3. Operative Steps

1. Parallelogram Lumpectomy with Mastopexy Closure

- This procedure is a full-thickness excision best used for localized or small, segmental cancers located peripherally in the breast with respect to the nipple–areolar complex (NAC). The purpose of removing a skin island is to provide adequate access for wide excision of the target lesion while setting the stage for mastopexy closure of the resulting intraparenchymal, full-thickness defect (Fig. 17-4). The size of the resected skin island is limited by the degree to which it shifts the NAC on the breast in relation to the chest wall and anatomic boundaries.
- Mild to moderate elevation of the NAC can create a pleasing lift effect (Fig. 17-5). Excessive lifting is not desirable, particularly with resections involving the upper inner quadrant of the breast. In the upper inner quadrant, skin island excisions should be small, or the resection and closure should be performed using a simple reapproximation of breast tissue and skin without removal of any skin island.[12]

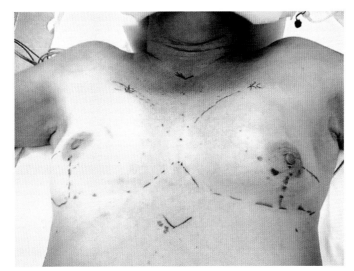

Figure 17-3

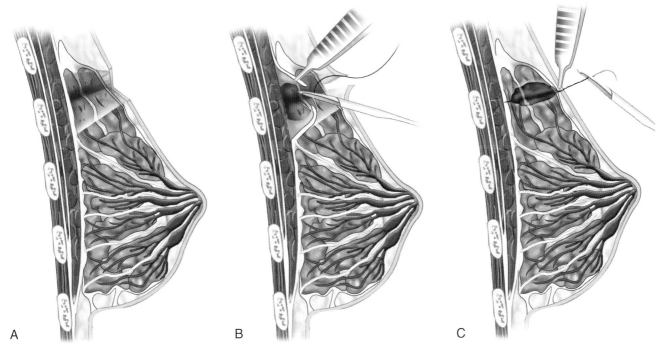

A

B

C

Figure 17-4

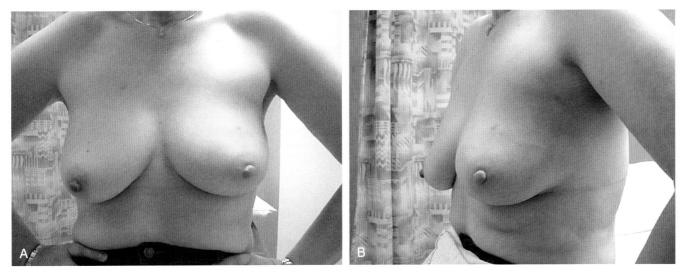

A

B

Figure 17-5

Incision

- A rounded parallelogram with two equal-length lines is drawn, thus marking the skin island to be excised in conjunction with the underlying target lesion and surrounding tissues. The width of the skin parallelogram can be used to estimate the distance by which the NAC becomes shifted toward the resection after skin closure. Before making the incision, the surgeon needs to consider how much the NAC will be deviated and balance this effect with the width of the anticipated surgical margins. For lesions in the upper breast, incisions should be curvilinear, following Kraissl's lines[13] (Fig. 17-6). Instead of a circumareolar pattern, Kraissl noted that the skin tension lines run transversely owing to gravity's effect on the breasts.
- For lesions in the lower breast, including the 3 o'clock and 9 o'clock positions, the parallelogram is placed radially (Fig. 17-7). At the corner of the parallelogram that comes closest to the nipple, the design can be positioned such that the closed incision after resection approaches the NAC tangential to the periareolar line (see Fig. 17-7, *A*). This reduces deviation of the NAC toward the lesion, a condition that can result from scar contraction. In the standing position, radial scars at 3 o'clock or 9 o'clock generally follow Kraissl's lines and rarely become hypertrophic. This radial approach gives more projection to the nipple (see Fig. 17-7, *B* and *C*), avoiding the downward displacement that can be caused by a purely horizontal scar.

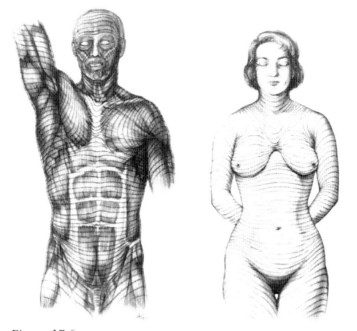

Figure 17-6
From Kraissl CJ: The selection of appropriate lines for elective
surgical incisions. Plast Reconstr Surg 1951;8:1-28.

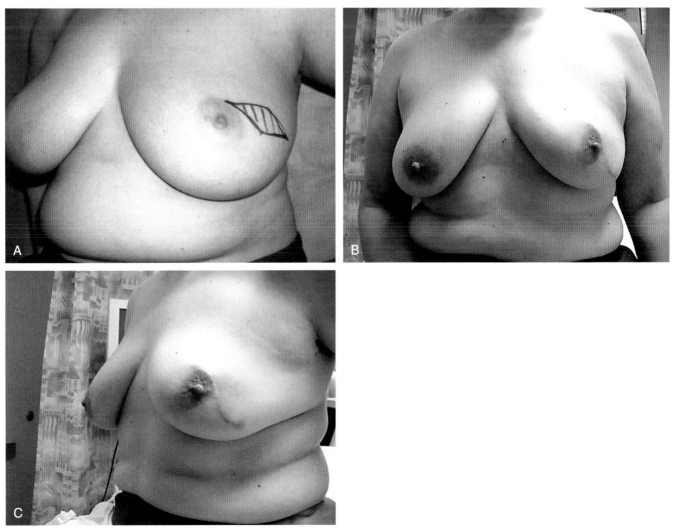

Figure 17-7

◆ In the patient example shown in figure 17-8, the parallelogram has been marked in the upper breast (see figure 17-8, *A-C*) in preparation for incision.

Dissection

◆ After excision of the skin island, short-distance skin flaps are raised along both sides of the wound. Dissection is then carried down to the chest wall and the breast gland is lifted off the pectoralis muscle (Fig. 17-8, *D-F*). An advantage of this maneuver is that it allows bimanual palpation of the target lesion to identify where the breast tissue should be divided.

◆ After full-thickness excision of the tumor, and before mastopexy closure, four to six marking clips are placed at the base of the defect in the surrounding fibroglandular tissue. These radiopaque markers help the radiation oncologist target the tumor bed. Those open faces of tissue created for mastopexy closure are not actually adjacent to cancer and do not need be marked.

◆ For adequate evaluation of margin status by the pathologist, sharp rather than cautery dissection should be considered. The advantage of sharp dissection is that it will not alter the histologic margins of the resected tissues. Larger intraparenchymal vessels can be ligated or coagulated during the dissection and cautery can then be used on the exposed fibroglandular tissue faces to control bleeding.

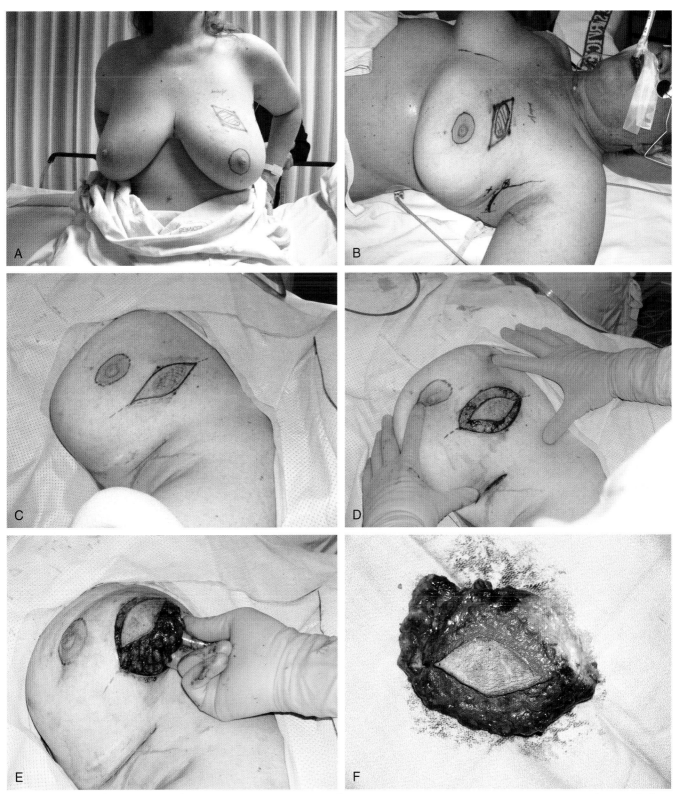

Figure 17-8. Parallelogram partial mastectomy, preoperative and intraoperative images. **A.** Preoperative target marking and placement of parallelogram. **B.** Intraoperative marking with patient in supine position. **C.** Rounding of parallelogram incision corners. **D.** Initial skin incision revealing wide exposure over target lesion. **E.** Full thickness dissection back to chest wall to facilitate delivery of target lesion. **F.** Inked resected specimen.

Mastopexy Closure

◆ The fibroglandular tissue at the level of the pectoralis fascia is sufficiently undermined so that breast tissue advancement can be performed over the muscle, without being too extensive to threaten the blood supply to the residual breast tissue (see Fig. 17-4, *A* and *B*). Once the fibroglandular tissues are mobilized and hemostasis is obtained, the margins of the residual cavity are shifted together by the advancement of breast tissue over muscle, and the defect is sutured at the deepest edges using 3-0 absorbable suture (Fig. 17-8, *G*; see Fig. 17-4, *C*).

◆ The direction of tissue advancement can be adjusted depending on the locations of the fibroglandular defect and the excess tissue that can be shifted to close it. In some cases, fatty tissue from the lateral breast can be shifted medially with relatively little tissue loss being notable after surgery. In a pendulous breast with a low-riding NAC, upward shifting can be desirable to restore a more youthful appearance.

◆ The superficial layer is then closed by interrupted subdermal 3-0 absorbable sutures. Skin is closed by 4-0 absorbable subcuticular sutures in routine fashion (Fig. 17-8, *H*). The cavity between the deep and superficial layer will be filled by seroma, which will reabsorb during radiation therapy (see Fig. 17-5).

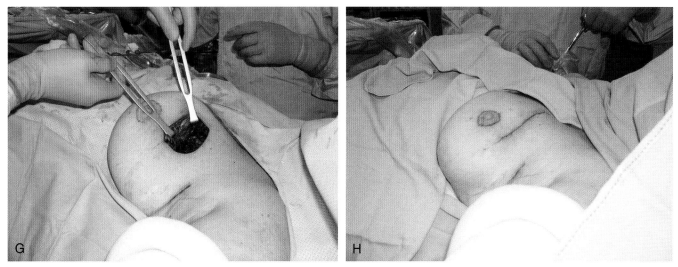

Figure 17-8, cont'd. G. Deep fibroglandular closure using mastopexy advancement technique to close breast tissue over exposed muscle. **H.** Final skin closure after completion of mastopexy advancement.

2. Batwing Lumpectomy with or without Mastopexy Closure

◆ This approach is particularly useful for the resection of cancers that are located deep to or in close proximity to the NAC. The batwing approach can be performed full thickness from skin to chest wall, but in cases where the breast is moderately large and the cancer is superficial, a full-thickness resection back to the chest wall may be unnecessary.

Incision

◆ Two similar semicircle incisions are made with angled "wings" on each side of the areola (Fig. 17-9, *A* and *B*). The two half-circles are positioned to allow them to be approximated to each other at closure. Removal of the skin wings allows the two semicircles to be shifted together without creating redundant skin folds at closure.

Dissection

◆ Dissection is carried deep to the known cancer, although in some cases a partial-thickness dissection is adequate. In most situations, the dissection is carried down to the chest wall and the breast gland is lifted off the pectoralis muscle in a fashion similar to that for the parallelogram lumpectomy (Fig. 17-9, *C* and *D*).
◆ The principle of sharp dissection and the placement of marking clips are the same as for the parallelogram mastopexy lumpectomy.

Mastopexy Closure

◆ After full-thickness resection, some mobilization of the fibroglandular tissue for mastopexy closure may be required. The tissue is elevated off of the chest wall at the plane between the pectoralis muscle and breast gland. There are relatively few major perforators in this plane, so tissue elevation and advancement can be performed with little difficulty, often by sweeping the index finger behind the breast in this natural anatomic plane. The fibroglandular tissue is advanced to close the resulting defect. The deepest parts are approximated by interrupted sutures (Fig. 17-9, *E*). We typically secure the fibroglandular tissue to itself and do not place anchoring stitches into the chest wall. This allows the approximated breast tissues to move on the chest wall and adjust to find their most natural way to settle in for final healing. The superficial layer is then closed in the same fashion as the parallelogram mastopexy lumpectomy (Fig. 17-9, *F*).
◆ This procedure can cause some lifting of the nipple, which in some cases can create asymmetry relative to the noncancerous breast. If desired, a contralateral lift can be performed afterward to achieve symmetry.

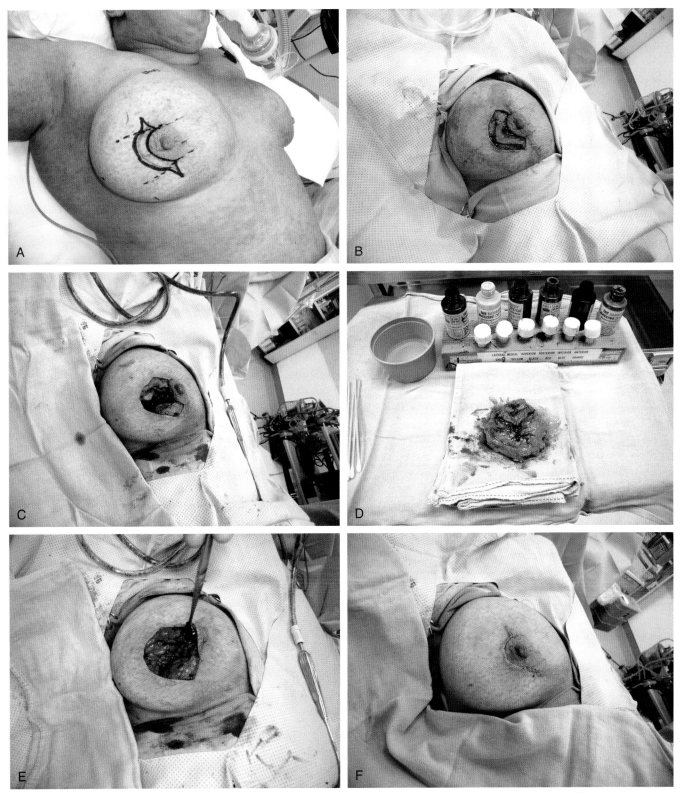

Figure 17-9. Batwing mastopexy lumpectomy. **A.** Skin incision design. **B.** Skin incision exposing underlying fibroglandular tissue containing target lesion. **C.** Full thickness tissue resection following the segmental anatomy of the underlying ductal tree. **D.** Excised specimen. **E.** Deep closure of fibroglandular tissue over exposed chest wall muscle. **F.** Final skin closure.

3. Reduction Mastopexy Lumpectomy

♦ This procedure is used for lesions located in the lower hemisphere of the breast, from the 4 o'clock to 8 o'clock positions. Lower pole cancers that are localized or segmentally distributed are excellent candidates for this procedure, depending in part on the size of the tumor in relation to the breast.

Incision

♦ A reduction mammoplasty keyhole pattern incision is made (Fig. 17-10, *A-C*). The skin above the areola is de-epithelialized in preparation for skin closure (Fig. 17-10, *D*).

Dissection

♦ A superior pedicle flap is created by inframammary incision and undermining of the breast tissue off the pectoral fascia to mobilize the NAC and underlying tissues (see Fig. 17-10, *D*). Mobilization of the breast tissue allows palpation of both deep and superficial surfaces of the tumor, which can aid the surgeon in determining the lateral margins of excision around the target lesion (Fig. 17-10, *E*).
♦ For cancers located in the inferolateral or inferomedial quadrant, the keyhole pattern can be rotated slightly to allow for a more lateral or medial excision, and the NAC is moved in a direction opposite to that of the surgical defect.[14]
♦ Commencing inferiorly and proceeding superiorly beneath the tumor, full-thickness excision of the lesion is completed (Fig. 17-10, *F*). The excision is performed with the intent of performing an en bloc resection that includes the tumor, at least a 1-cm macroscopic margin of normal tissue, and the skin overlying the lesion.
♦ The principle of sharp dissection and the placement of marking clips are the same as for the parallelogram mastopexy lumpectomy.

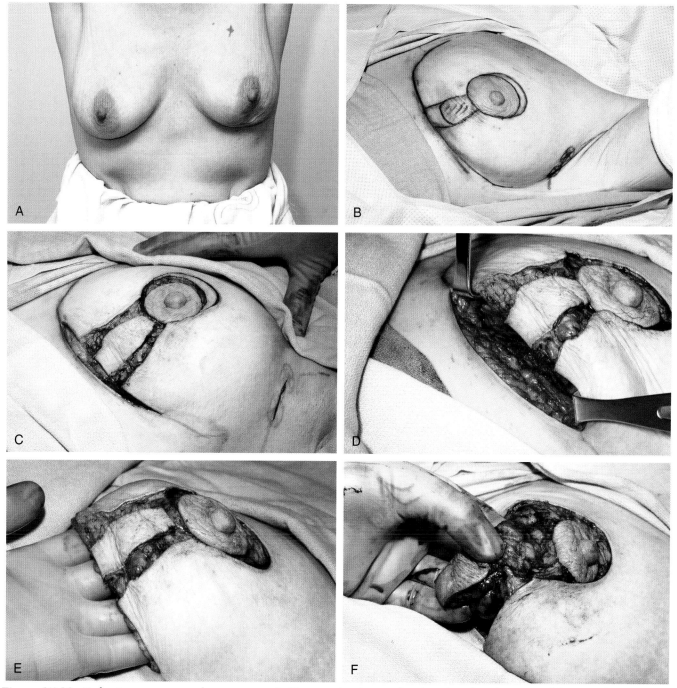

Figure 17-10. Reduction mastopexy lumpectomy. **A.** Preoperative image showing skin dimpling caused by spiculated mass at 6:00. **B.** Skin incision design showing keyhole incision pattern. **C.** Initial skin incision. **D.** Posterior dissection behind lesion at level of chest wall muscle. **E.** Manual examination of dissected tissues facilitating excision of specimen. **F.** Specimen excision. A, B, and E from Anderson BO, Masetti R, Silverstein MJ: Oncoplastic approaches to partial mastectomy: An overview of volume-displacement techniques. Lancet Oncol 2005;6:145-147.

Mastopexy Closure

◆ The NAC is recentralized to recreate a harmonious breast size and shape. The medial and lateral flaps are undermined and sutured together to fill the excision defect, leaving a typical inverted-"T" scar (Fig. 17-10, *G-K*). Uplifting of the NAC by virtue of removal of the skin island superior to it helps restore a youthful appearance of the breast, but can create mild asymmetry relative to the contralateral breast (Fig. 17-10, *L*). If desired, a contralateral lift can be performed afterward to achieve symmetry.

◆ For patients with macromastia, consistent positioning of the breast for radiation therapy may be difficult, resulting in dosing inhomogeneity and suboptimal treatment.[14] These patients can benefit from reduction mastopexy lumpectomy using a unilateral or bilateral approach.

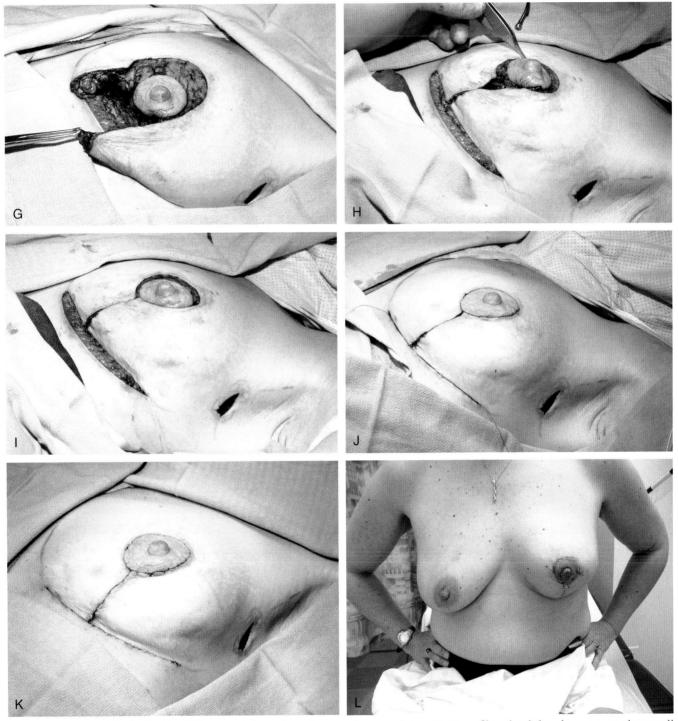

Figure 17-10, cont'd. G. Residual fibroglandular defect after specimen excision. **H.** Deep fibroglandular closure over chest wall. **I.** Deep fibroglandular closure. **J.** Superficial fibroglandular closure. **K.** Final skin closure. **L.** Postoperative result.
K from Anderson BO, Masetti R, Silverstein MJ: Oncoplastic approaches to partial mastectomy: An overview of volume-displacement techniques. Lancet Oncol 2005;6:145-147.

4. Donut Mastopexy Lumpectomy

* This procedure is best chosen for segmentally distributed cancers located in the upper or lateral breast.

Incision

* Two concentric lines are placed around the areola and a "donut" skin island is excised (Fig. 17-11, *A*). De-epithelialization by separating this skin island from the underlying tissues should be done carefully to avoid devascularization of the areolar skin (Fig. 17-11, *B*).
* The width of the donut skin island should be approximately 1 cm, but depends somewhat on the size of areola and expected extent of excision. Removal of this tissue ring is needed to allow both adequate access to the breast tissue and closure of the skin envelope around the remaining fibroglandular tissue that will reduce tissue volume overall.

Dissection

* A skin envelope is created in all directions around the NAC. The quadrant of breast tissue including the target lesion is fully exposed using the same dissection used for a skin-sparing mastectomy (Fig. 17-11, *C*). The full-thickness breast gland is peeled off of the underlying pectoralis muscle and delivered through the circumareolar incision (Fig. 17-11, *D*).
* The segment of breast tissue containing the tumor is resected in a wedge-shaped fashion (Fig. 17-11, *E* and *F*). The width of tissue excision required to achieve adequate surgical margins must be weighed against the difficulty that will be created by an oversized segmental defect. When performing this full-thickness segmental excision, the large face of a no. 10 blade can help make the dissection planes straight.

Mastopexy Closure

* The remaining fibroglandular tissue is returned to the skin envelope. The peripheral apical corners of the fibroglandular tissue are secured to each other and also anchored to the chest wall (Fig. 17-11, *G*). This maintains the proper orientation of the mobilized fibroglandular tissue in the skin envelope during the initial phases of healing. This securing of the peripheral apical corners of fibroglandular tissue to the chest wall is a notable exception to the general approach to mastopexy closure where we approximate fibroglandular tissues to each other, but not to the chest wall, to allow the tissues to shift on the chest wall during the healing phase and find the most natural location for optimal healing and preservation of breast shape. With the donut mastopexy, the degree of separation of fibroglandular tissue from both skin and chest wall could allow the breast gland to "fall" within the breast skin envelope rather than filling it in a uniform fashion.

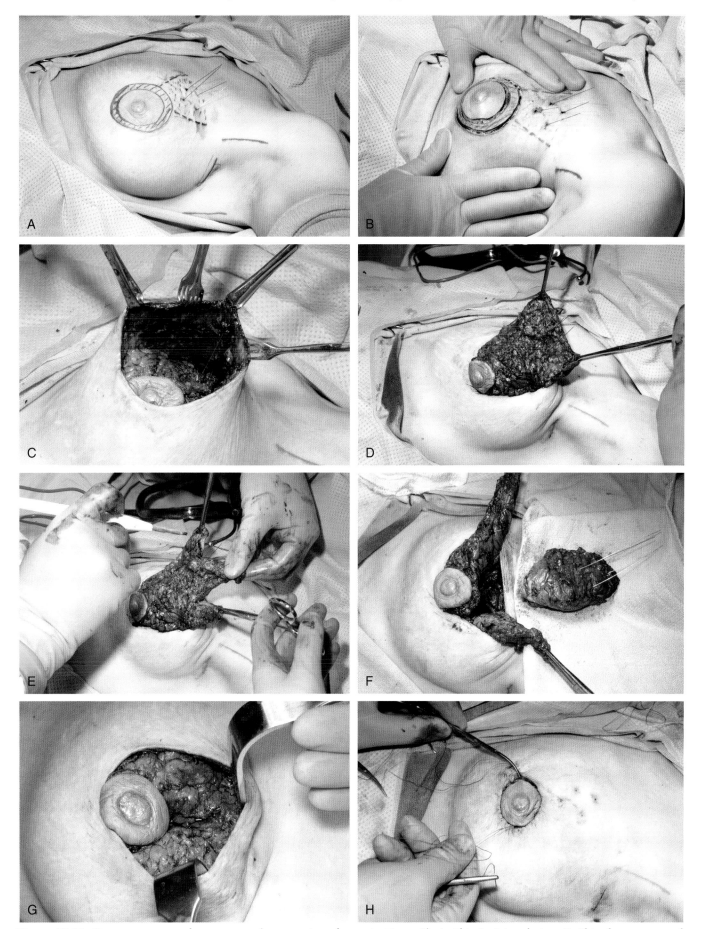

Figure 17-11. Donut mastopexy lumpectomy (same patient shown in Figure 2). **A.** Skin incision design. **B.** Skin donut removed. **C.** Skin flaps raised using same technique as in skin-sparing mastectomy, but centered over the target area to be resected. **D.** Delivery of fibroglandular tissue through skin incision. **E.** Dissection of breast segment including target lesion. **F.** Specimen excised. **G.** Deep closure and flap advancement over exposed chest wall muscle. **H.** Pursestring periarolar closure.

- A pursestring 3-0 absorbable suture is placed around the areola opening (Fig. 17-11, *H*). This pursestring suture is clamped, but not tied, at a size that reapproximates the original NAC. Interrupted inverted 3-0 absorbable sutures are placed subdermally around the NAC. The pursestring suture is tied and then 4-0 subcuticular sutures are used to close the wound (Fig. 17-11, *I*).
- Uplifting of the NAC can create mild asymmetry relative to the unoperated breast (Fig. 17-11, *J*). If desired, a contralateral lift can be performed to achieve symmetry.

Step 4. Postoperative Care

- Drain use is a controversial area. We have found that drains generally are not required in partial mastectomy cases because seroma fluid usually is reabsorbed. However, with more extensive dissections like the donut mastopexy lumpectomy, fluid accumulation can become more pronounced and potentially can distort the orientation of the shifted breast planes during healing. In recent years, we have started to place small closed drains in the partial mastectomy cavity and leave them overnight to avoid excessive fluid accumulation in the dissected breast that might distort the oncoplastic closure.

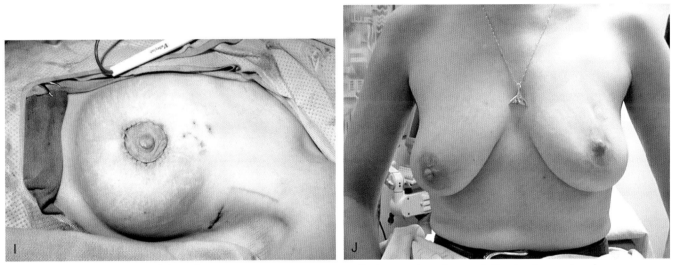

Figure 17-11, cont'd. I. Final skin closure. **J.** Postoperative, postradiation result at 2 years following locoregional treatment.

Step 5. Pearls and Pitfalls

- Complete excision of calcified lesions and masses should be confirmed with specimen radiography during surgery. Specimen radiograms can be very useful to assess the location of the target lesion in the resected tissues and thereby determine if any of the surgical margins appear to be too close.
- Multicolored inking can help orient the specimen and is best performed by the operating surgeon. Multicolored inking kits are now available with six colors (red, blue, yellow, orange, green, and black). They are very useful for labeling all of the surgical margins (superior, inferior, medial, lateral, superficial, and deep).
- In oncoplastic surgery, the surgeon can undermine a very large area of the breast between the pectoralis muscle and breast gland. This plane is generally avascular, with few perforators. If the breast is attached at the skin level, adequate blood flow will be preserved.

References

1. Anderson BO, Masetti R, Silverstein MJ: Oncoplastic approaches to partial mastectomy: An overview of volume-displacement techniques. Lancet Oncol 2005;6:145-157.
2. Chen CY, Calhoun KE, Masetti R, Anderson BO: Oncoplastic breast conserving surgery: A renaissance of anatomically-based surgical technique. Minerva Chir 2006;61:421-434.
3. Cooper AP: On the Anatomy of the Breast. London, Longman, Orme, Green, Brown, and Longmans, 1840. Special Collections, Scott Memorial Library, Thomas Jefferson University, Philadelphia. Available at http://jdc.jefferson.edu/cooper/.
4. National Comprehensive Cancer Network: The NCCN Breast Cancer Treatment Guidelines. The Complete Library of NCCN Clinical Practice Guidelines in Oncology [CD-ROM] Version 1.2007. Jenkintown, Pa, National Comprehensive Cancer Network, 2007.
5. Love SM, Barsky SH: Anatomy of the nipple and breast ducts revisited. Cancer 2004;101:1947-1957.
6. Amano G, Ohuchi N, Ishibashi T, et al: Correlation of three-dimensional magnetic resonance imaging with precise histopathological map concerning carcinoma extension in the breast. Breast Cancer Res Treat 2000;60:43-55.
7. Holland R, Hendriks JH, Vebeek AL, et al: Extent, distribution, and mammographic/histological correlations of breast ductal carcinoma in situ. Lancet 1990;335:519-522.
8. Mai KT, Perkins DG, Mirsky D: Location and extent of positive resection margins and ductal carcinoma in situ in lumpectomy specimens of ductal breast carcinoma examined with a microscopic three-dimensional view. Breast J 2003;9:33-38.
9. Silverstein MJ: An argument against routine use of radiotherapy for ductal carcinoma in situ. Oncology (Huntingt) 2003;17:1511-1533; discussion 1533-1534, 1539, 1542 passim.
10. Silverstein MJ, Lagios MD, Recht A, et al: Image-detected breast cancer: State of the art diagnosis and treatment. J Am Coll Surg 2005;201:586-597.
11. Liberman L, Kaplan J, Van Zee KJ, et al: Bracketing wires for preoperative breast needle localization. AJR Am J Roentgenol 2001;177:565-572.
12. Grisotti A, Calabrese C: Conservation treatment of breast cancer: Reconstructive problems. In Spear SL (ed): Surgery of the Breast: Principles and Art, 2nd ed. Philadelphia, Lippincott Williams & Wilkins, 2006, pp 147-178.
13. Kraissl CJ: The selection of appropriate lines for elective surgical incisions. Plast Reconstr Surg 1951;8:1-28.
14. Masetti R, Di Leone A, Franceschini G, et al: Oncoplastic techniques in the conservative surgical treatment of breast cancer: An overview. Breast J 2006;12(5 Suppl 2):S174-S180.

CHAPTER 18

BREAST RECONSTRUCTION POSTMASTECTOMY WITH TISSUE EXPANDERS AND ALLODERM

Julio Hochberg and James C. Yuen

Step 1. Surgical Anatomy

- Figure 18-1 demonstrates the key anatomic structures that must be considered with breast reconstruction.
- Figure 18-2 shows the relationship of the breast to the pectoralis major muscle (PM) and the chest wall.

Step 2. Preoperative Considerations

- The following issues must be taken into consideration in planning postmastectomy breast reconstruction using tissue expanders and Alloderm:
  - ▲ Size of the breasts and patient's breast size expectation
  - ▲ Scars from previous biopsies, lumpectomies, or mastectomies (Fig. 18-3)
  - ▲ Presence of skin striae

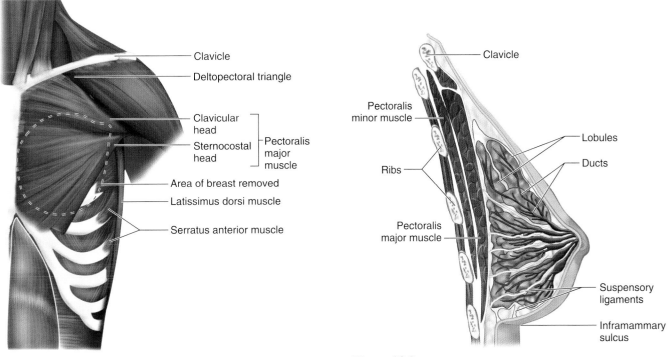

Clavicle

Deltopectoral triangle

Clavicular head

Sternocostal head — Pectoralis major muscle

Area of breast removed

Latissimus dorsi muscle

Serratus anterior muscle

Clavicle

Pectoralis minor muscle

Ribs

Pectoralis major muscle

Lobules

Ducts

Suspensory ligaments

Inframammary sulcus

Figure 18-1

Figure 18-2

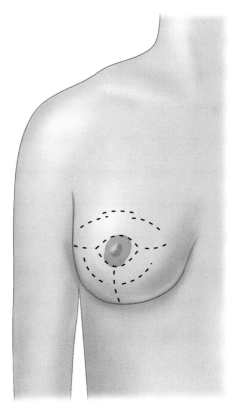

Figure 18-3

▲ Mastectomy types: modified radical (Fig. 18-4, *A*), skin-sparing mastectomy (Fig. 18-4, *B*), total skin-sparing mastectomy (Fig. 18-4, *C*)
▲ Unilateral or bilateral mastectomies; in unilateral mastectomies, the patient is informed about the need for future surgery to the contralateral breast, such as reduction and mastopexy, to improve symmetry
▲ Breast cleavage and tendency for synmastia (Fig. 18-5)

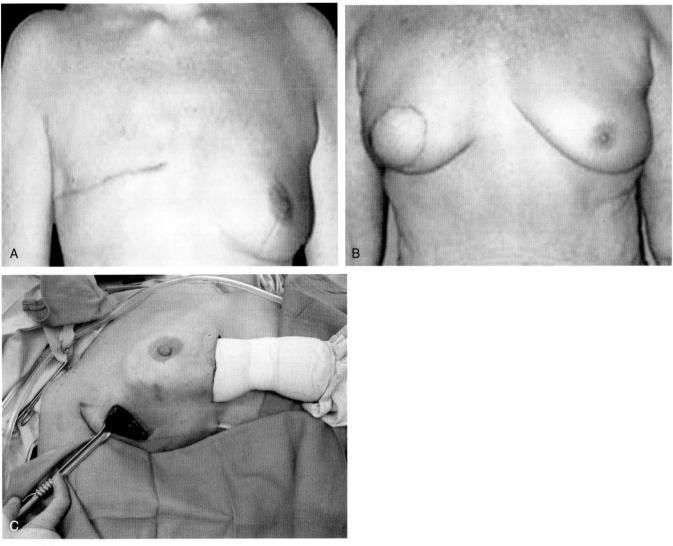

Figure 18-4

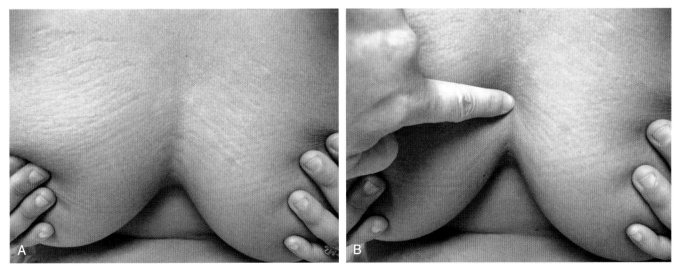

Figure 18-5

▲ History of smoking and previous radiation therapy and the high risk of complications
▲ Choice of tissue expanders: round (Fig. 18-6, *A*) or anatomic shape (Fig. 18-6, *B*), textured surface (Fig. 18-6, *C*), with magnetic integrated injection ports
▲ Size of tissue expander: length, width, projection, volume
▲ Preoperative marking of the breast inframammary sulcus, anterior axillary line, mid-sternum line, and medial edge of the breast with patient in the upright position (Fig. 18-7)

Step 3. Operative Steps

◆ On completion of the mastectomy, meticulous attention is paid to hemostasis using electrocautery. The PM is evaluated for its integrity. Portions of muscle removed during the tumor resection may require reconstruction. Position of the inferior muscle border in relation to the inframammary crease (marked by a stitch before mastectomy) is determined (Fig. 18-8). The skin is evaluated for its circulatory status and thickness.

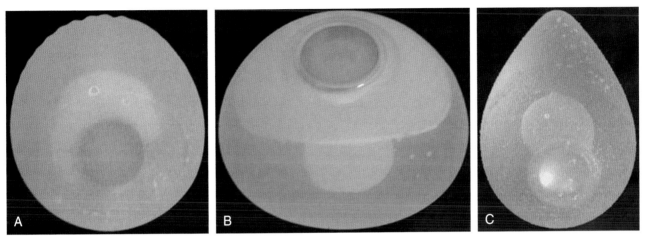

Figure 18-6

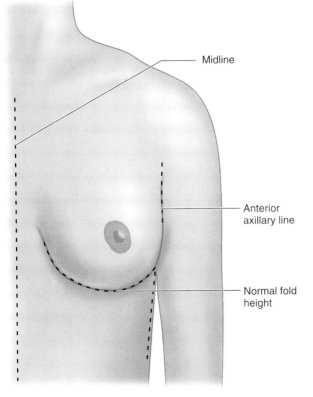

Figure 18-7

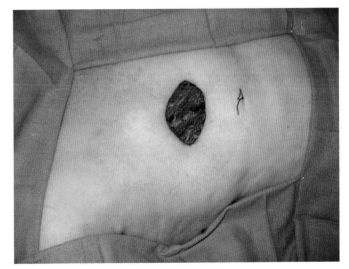

Figure 18-8

- Botox (botulinum toxin type A; Allergan, Irvine, CA) 100 IU diluted in 60 mL of injectable normal saline is injected in the PM using a 21-gauge spinal needle in a fan shape (Fig. 18-9). The objective is to diminish muscle spasm, and thus pain, immediately after surgery and during expansion over the next several months.
- Bupivacaine HCl (0.25%) without epinephrine (Hospira Inc., Lake Forest, IL) is injected in the chest wall muscles to diminish immediate postoperative pain. A 21-gauge spinal needle is used and the injection proceeds in a fan shape, as in Figure 18-9, B. The serratus, teres, and latissimus dorsi are also injected.
- To dissect the expander pocket, the PM is dissected from the chest wall, starting from its lateral edge using the electrocautery (Figs. 18-10, A and B); then, by digital dissection, the muscle is easily detached from the chest wall in its upper two thirds (Fig. 18-10, C and D). In the inferior aspect the muscle is firmly attached to the chest wall and the dissection requires electrocautery (Fig. 18-10, E). Dissection of the PM from the pectoralis minor (PMi) proceeds in the upper lateral aspect of the pocket.

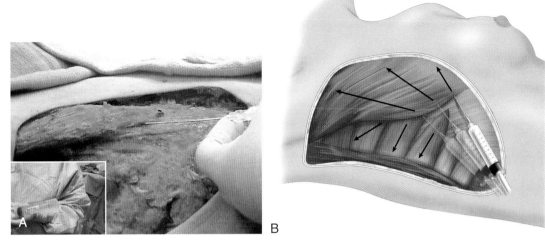

Figure 18-9

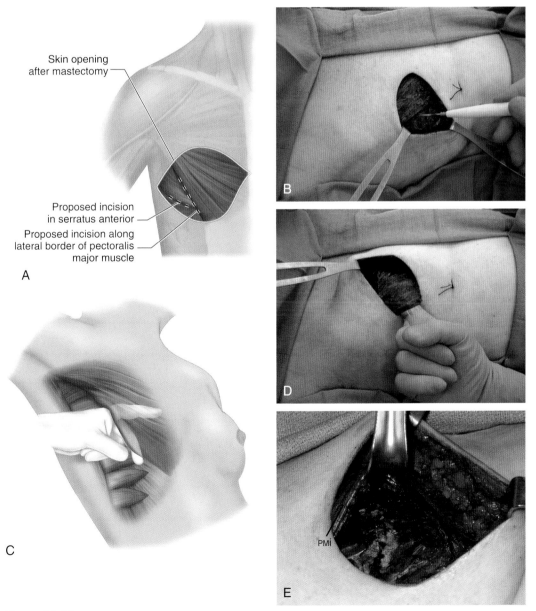

Skin opening after mastectomy

Proposed incision in serratus anterior

Proposed incision along lateral border of pectoralis major muscle

PMi

Figure 18-10

◆ The tissue expander is carefully inspected for leaks or nicks before use. A 21-gauge butterfly needle is inserted in the magnetic port, air is removed from the tissue expander (Fig. 18-11, *A*), and 5 mL of methylene blue is injected (Fig. 18-11, *B*) to serve as a monitor for leaks during the case. The expander is immersed in saline to check for leaks before implantation (Fig. 18-11, *C*). A new pair of gloves is worn before touching and handling the tissue expander.
◆ The tissue expander is positioned in the submuscular pocket (Fig. 18-12). Any muscular bands that may distort the expander must be transected with electrocautery. If the pocket is too small, the expander may not have adequate room to unfold, increasing the risk of tissue erosion. If the pocket is too large, the expander may not remain in proper position for filling and expansion. Extreme care should be taken to avoid damage to the expander during surgery.

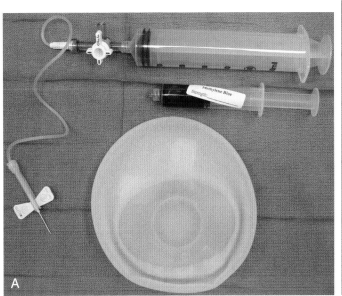

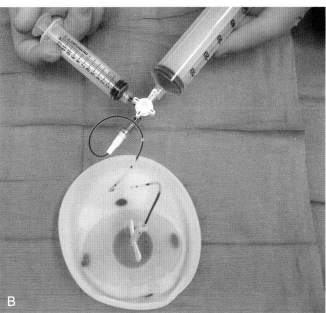

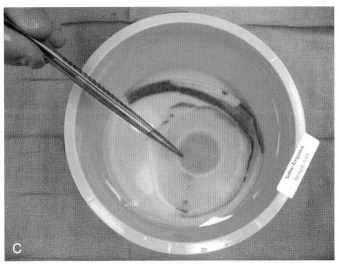

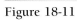

Figure 18-11

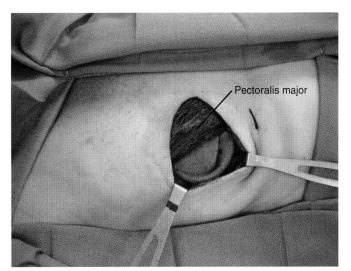

Figure 18-12

- Alloderm (Lifecell, Brauchberg, NJ), a regenerative tissue matrix allograft, is used to close the lateral aspect of the muscular pocket. A 12 × 4-cm, medium-thickness, previously hydrated Alloderm (Fig. 18-13, *A*) is applied to the lateral edge of the PM and sutured with a continuous running 3-0 polyglactin 910 (Vicryl; Ethicon, Somerville, NJ; Fig. 18-13, *B*). The lateral edge of the Alloderm is cut to fit the defect and sutured in the same fashion to the serratus anterior muscle (Fig. 18-13, *C*). Separate, simple interrupted sutures of 3-0 Vicryl are applied every 2 cm for reinforcement of the suture line.
- Muscle defects can also be reconstructed with Alloderm.
- When the PM origin is too high in relation to the inframammary sulcus (Fig. 18-14), the inferior muscle edge is detached from the chest wall and an inferolateral sling of Alloderm is constructed and sewn in similarly to accommodate the expander (Fig. 18-15). Two pieces of 12 × 4-cm of Alloderm may be required.
- If the incision is remote from the site of expansion, the expander may be filled to tissue tolerance at the time of surgery. If wound stability or skin viability is a concern, inflate only slightly to fill the pocket space without applying undue tension to the overlying tissues (see Fig. 18-15).
- A closed drain system is applied, using a 15-Fr Blake drain (Bard, Covington, GA), brought out through a separated stab wound in the medial axillary line at the level of the inferior mammary sulcus. It is secured with a 2-0 nylon suture. The drain is connected to a closed wound suction evacuation bulb reservoir (ReliaVac; Bard).
- The wound is closed with simple interrupted 3-0 Vicryl at the subcutaneous level, a continuous running 5-0 poliglecaprone 25 (Monocryl; Ethicon) suture at the skin level, and two layers of Dermabond (Ethicon).

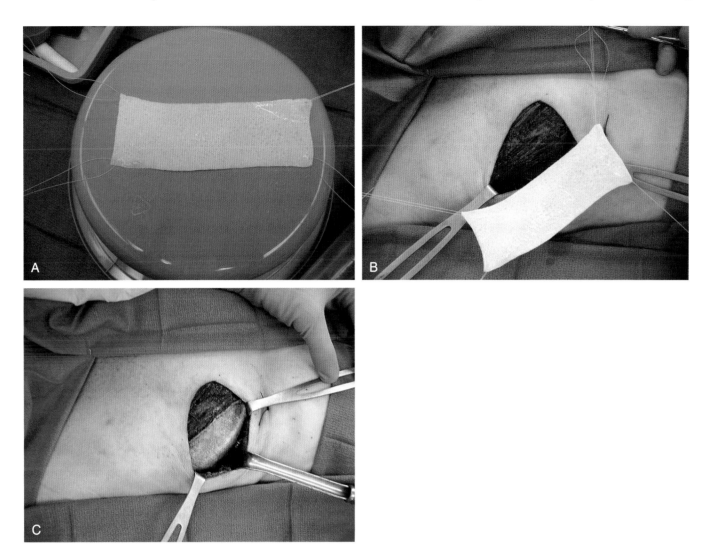

Figure 18-13

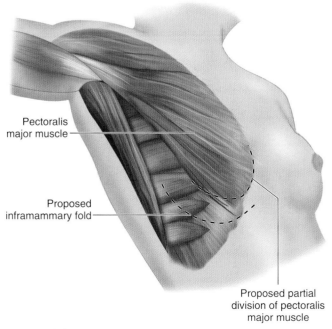

Pectoralis
major muscle

Proposed
inframammary fold

Proposed partial
division of pectoralis
major muscle

Figure 18-14

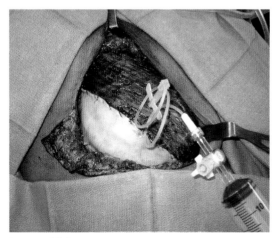

Figure 18-15

Step 4. Postoperative Care

- A liquid skin adhesive (Dermabond; Ethicon) is applied to the incisions.
- No dressing is applied over the reconstructed breast to avoid undue pressure over the skin flaps.
- Dressings are applied only to the drain.
- Antibiotics and analgesics are administered.
- Exercises using the upper extremities are avoided in the first 2 weeks, including driving.
- A petroleum-based ointment is applied after the ninth postoperative day. The dry Dermabond will peel with ease, and the sutures can then be removed.

1. Tissue Expander Filling

- The wound should be stable before tissue expansion begins.
- Although the injection port usually can be identified by palpation, a port locator should always be used to verify its location and orientation. There are a variety of port locators, instruments that correspond to the different brands of tissue expanders.
- The PMT Integra tissue expander (PMT, Chanhassen, MN) has a locator that produces light when in contact with the metal port. Its circular periphery is determined, and the center is localized (Fig. 18-16, *A*). The PSS H Umbrella tissue expander (SSP, Victor, MO) magnetic injection port locator determines the center of the port in an absolutely perpendicular manner (Fig. 18-16, *B*). The Mentor tissue expander (Mentor, Irving, TX) port locator has a small magnetic pendulum that straightens over the center of the port (Fig. 18-16, *C*).
- Inflation is typically performed in sessions spaced at weekly intervals. Unnecessary delays may produce a resistant capsule.
- To avoid contamination, each inflation session is performed using sterile draping and a closed filling system.
- Fill volumes during each session depend on the patient and tissue tolerance. The initial volume is usually between 100 and 150 mL of sterile injectable saline and is delivered using a 21-gauge needle. The needle should enter perpendicular to the top of the injection port. Expansion should proceed in moderate increments of approximately 50 mL per session. A patient fill volume record is maintained.
- A certain amount of clear drainage normally accumulates around the expander and will appear at the site of the injection.
- The expansion ideally continues until the desired volume chosen by the patient is exceeded by 10% to 20%. This will help overcome the normal retraction of the skin.

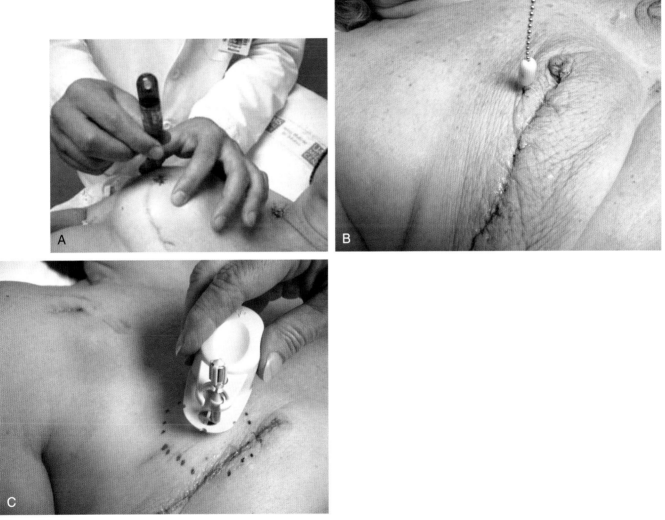

Figure 18-16

2. Exchange of Tissue Expander for Saline Implant

- ◆ A second-stage surgery to exchange the tissue expander for permanent saline implants is scheduled when the expansion is completed.
- ◆ Skin is marked to determine the areas that will require capsulotomies (C), capsuloplasties (CA), liposuction (L), or lipectomies (LI). Capsular contractures, displacements of the expander, and irregularities of the subcutaneous tissue or axillary skinfold are the indications for these procedures (Fig. 18-17).
- ◆ A 5-cm incision is made in the lateral aspect of the original mastectomy scar (Fig. 18-18, A). The capsule is incised with the electrocautery.
- ◆ The expander is deflated using an 18-gauge needle attached to a tuberculin syringe modified to serve as an adaptor to the suction tubing.
- ◆ The expander is removed with a Kelly clamp, avoiding damage to the capsule (Fig. 18-18, B).
- ◆ The capsular pocket is examined for possible band formations, deformities, contractures, or tumor.
- ◆ Capsulotomies under direct visualization (see Fig. 18-17) are performed usually in the medial and inferior sites of the capsule, if indicated.

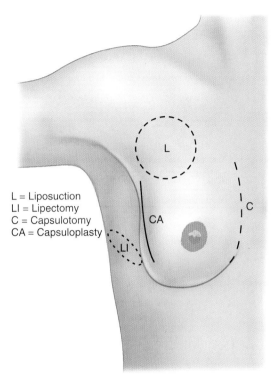

L = Liposuction
LI = Lipectomy
C = Capsulotomy
CA = Capsuloplasty

Figure 18-17

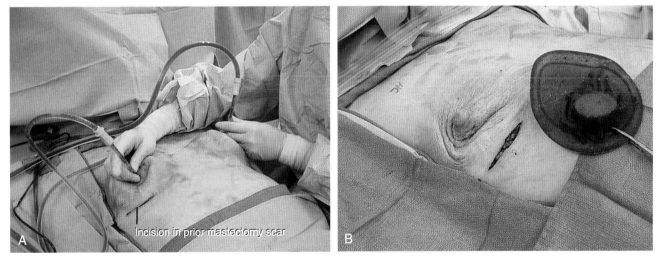

Incision in prior mastectomy scar

Figure 18-18

- Capsulorrhaphies using 3-0 Vicryl sutures are performed in the lateral or inferior sites of the capsule under direct visualization, in cases of lateral or inferior displacement of the expander (Fig. 18-19).
- Axillary lipectomies are performed when excess subcutaneous tissue and skin form extra folds of skin in the axilla, causing discomfort (see Fig. 18-17).
- Liposuction of localized areas of excess subcutaneous tissue (see Fig. 18-17) can be performed to optimize cosmesis. The demarcated areas are infiltrated with epinephrine 1:200,000 to diminish bleeding. Then excess fat is removed through a 2-mm incision using a 2-mm cannula.
- A saline implant, smooth round high or medium profile, of the chosen volume, is connected to special tubing (Fig. 18-20, *A*).
- Simple interrupted 3-0 Vicryl sutures are applied to the capsular opening and left untied, tagged with hemostats.
- The implant is deflated and introduced into the submuscular capsular pocket (Fig. 18-20, *B*).

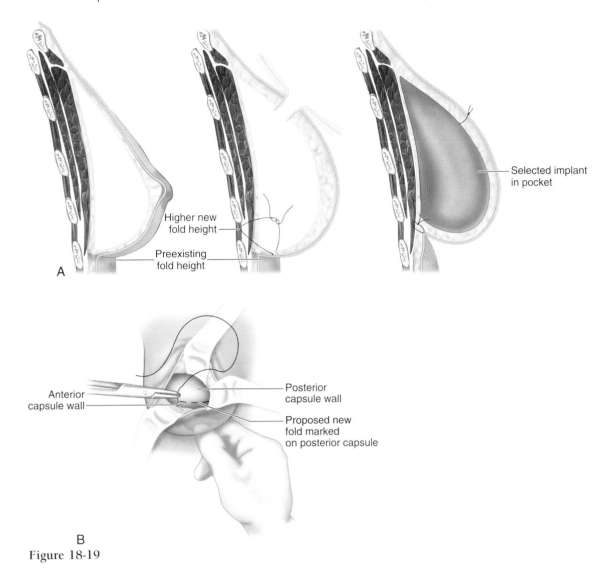

A

Higher new fold height

Preexisting fold height

Selected implant in pocket

Anterior capsule wall

Posterior capsule wall

Proposed new fold marked on posterior capsule

B

Figure 18-19

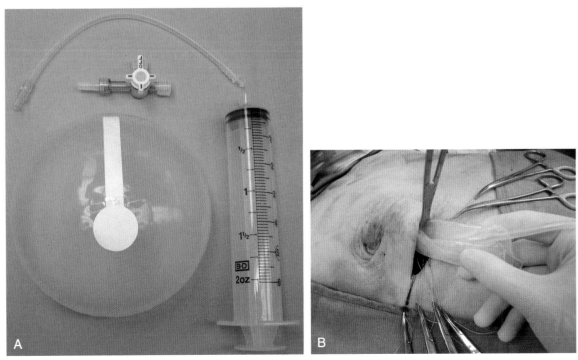

A

B

Figure 18-20

* The saline implant is inflated with sterile injectable saline to the desired volume using a closed filling system (Fig. 18-21). When the desired result is achieved, the tubing is removed and the valve is closed. The sutures are then tied. Closure is completed with Vicryl 3-0 simple interrupted subcutaneous sutures and, in the skin, a 5-0 Monocryl continuous running suture. Dermabond is applied in two layers.
* A sports bra may be applied loosely.
* The patient is given analgesics and kept on a postoperative course of oral antibiotics until the drains are removed.

3. Nipple–Areolar Complex Reconstruction

* Patients who have had a modified radical mastectomy (see Fig. 18-4, *A*) or skin-sparing mastectomy (see Fig. 18-4, *B*) may desire reconstruction of the nipple-areolar complex (NAC).
* Mark the NAC site with the patient in a sitting position. The NAC is located approximately at 18 to 19 cm from the suprasternal notch (Fig. 18-22).

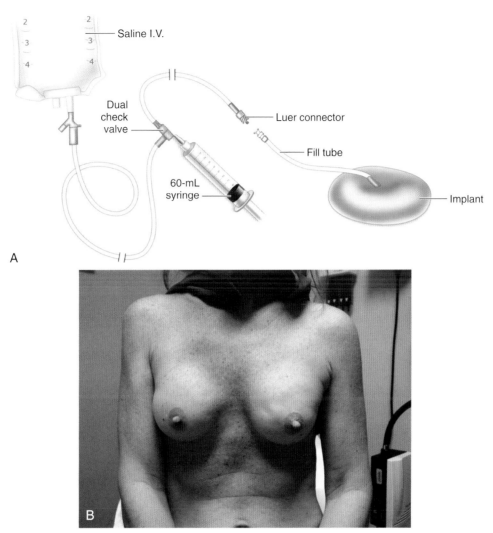

Figure 18-21

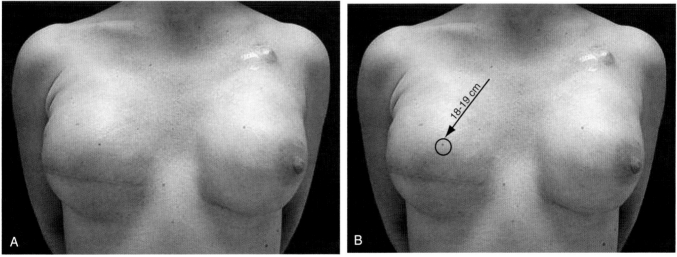

Figure 18-22

- The site of the new areola disk is de-epithelialized using a no. 15 blade, taking care to remove only the epidermis and leaving the dermis viable to accept the skin graft (Fig. 18-23).
- Hemostasis is achieved with electrocautery.
- A 1-mm circular skin frame is left intact surrounding the de-epithelialized new nipple site.
- A small pocket is dissected under the nipple site. A 3-mm incision is done in the lower aspect of the skin frame and a tenotomy scissors is used to undermine the pocket. Three layers of thick Alloderm, previously hydrated, are placed in the pocket for greater nipple projection. The pocket is closed with Monocryl 5-0 simple interrupted sutures.
- A circular, full-thickness skin graft is harvested from the elbow skin and is sutured to the skin frame using 6-0 Monocryl. The donor site at the elbow is closed with Vicryl 3-0, Monocryl 5-0, and Dermabond.
- When possible, nipple sharing from the opposite breast is used instead of the elbow graft.

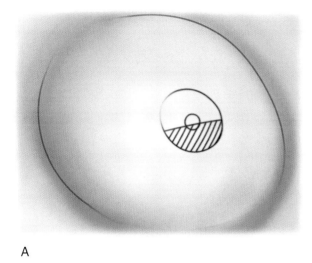

A

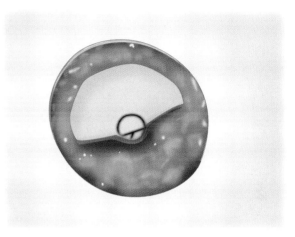

B

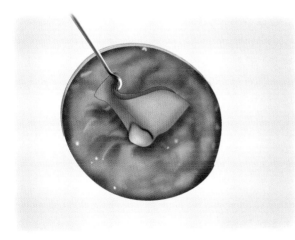

C

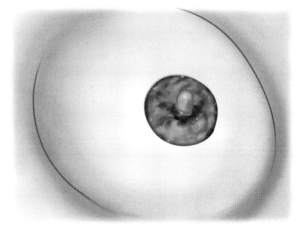

D

Figure 18-23

◆ To reconstruct the areola, a full-thickness skin graft is harvested from the medial aspect of the upper thigh and defatted. The graft is sutured to the reconstructed breast using nylon 5-0 bolster sutures. In the center of the areola graft, a 7-mm diameter disk of the skin graft is excised to expose the new nipple. A Monocryl 6-0 continuous running suture complements the closure in the periphery of the areola graft. The bolster dressing (petrolatum gauze and cotton balls) is tied over the skin grafts (Fig. 18-24). Figure 18-25 shows the final result.

Step 5. Pearls and Pitfalls

1. Pearls

◆ Use capsulotomies and capsuloplasties to correct irregularities not corrected by the tissue expander.
◆ Avoid overdissection of the lower breast capsule to prevent migration of the expander to the abdomen. This problem is quite difficult to correct.

2. Pitfalls

◆ Malpositioning and curling of the tissue expander may lead to inadvertent puncture of the expander and deflation, requiring replacement.
◆ Extrusion is more common when the expansion is performed in previously irradiated tissues. Therefore, expansion in this situation should be performed slowly.
◆ Tight-fitting bras worn postoperatively may cause skin ischemia.
◆ Necrosis of the native skin flaps of the mastectomy and infection are the most serious complications that may lead to the abortion of the reconstruction. Necrosis must be dealt with aggressively and urgently to avoid the possibility of infection.

Bibliography

Hochberg J, Beck BS, Yuen CJ, et al: Reconstruction of the nipple-sparing total mastectomy. Plast Reconstr Surg 2006;118:147-148.
Hochberg J, Layeeque R, Klimberg S, et al: Botulinum toxin (BT) infiltration for pain control after mastectomy and subpectoral tissue expansion. Plast Surg Forum 2004;27:190.
Hochberg J, Margulies A, Yuen CJ, et al: Alloderm (acellular human dermis) in breast reconstruction with tissue expander. Plast Reconstr Surg 2005;116:126-127.
Layeeque R, Hochberg J, Klimberg S, et al: Botulinum toxin infiltration for pain control after mastectomy and expander reconstruction. Ann Surg 2004;240:608-613.
Margulies AG, Hochberg J, Klimberg S, et al: Total skin sparing mastectomy without the preservation of the nipple/areola complex. Am J Surg 2005;190:907-912.
Povoski SP, Hochberg J, Ardenghy M, et al: Aggressive surgical resection and reconstruction for locally recurrent and focally advanced breast cancer. Plast Surg Forum 2002;269-271.

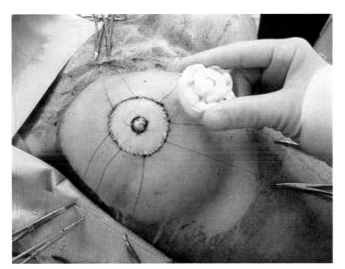

Figure 18-24

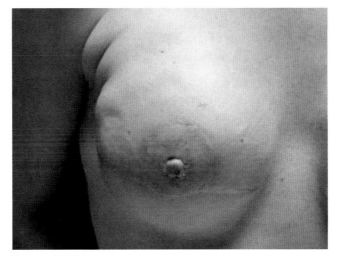

Figure 18-25

CHAPTER 19

TISSUE BREAST
RECONSTRUCTION

Donald P. Baumann and Steven J. Kronowitz

Common Goals of Breast Reconstruction

- Create breasts of equal volume and similar contour.
- Balance the inframammary folds.
- Conceal and maintain symmetry between scars on each breast.
- Provide medial fullness to the reconstructed breast to create cleavage.
- Design the autologous tissue flap to position the most vascularized region in the most critical aspect of the reconstructed breast (inferomedial aspect) and the least vascularized region laterally, adjacent to the axilla.
- Secure the reconstructed breast on the chest wall to avoid shifting into the axilla.
- Create a reconstructed breast with a soft, natural texture by optimizing the blood supply to the flap that will decrease the occurrence of fat necrosis and atrophy.
- Minimize donor site morbidity by limiting the harvest of muscle and fascia.

A. Latissimus Dorsi Myocutaneous Flap for Repair of a Partial Mastectomy Defect

Step 1. Surgical Anatomy

- The thoracodorsal vessels provide the main blood supply to the latissimus dorsi (LD) flap (Fig. 19-1).

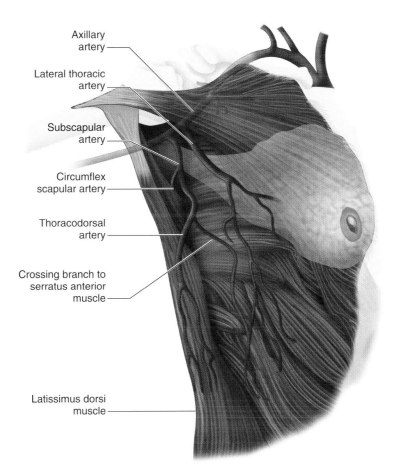

Axillary artery

Lateral thoracic artery

Subscapular artery

Circumflex scapular artery

Thoracodorsal artery

Crossing branch to serratus anterior muscle

Latissimus dorsi muscle

Figure 19-1

Step 2. Preoperative Considerations

♦ Depending on the location of the tumor, the relative defect size (defect volume/breast volume), and the need to resect breast skin, a breast deformity that results from segmental mastectomy can be repaired with either an LD myocutaneous flap or with oncoplastic techniques with rearrangement of the remaining breast tissue.

♦ LD flaps are well suited to reconstruct large lateral defects, especially in small-breasted patients (C-cup breast or smaller) because these patients often have insufficient remaining breast tissue to rearrange after the segmental mastectomy.

♦ An LD flap can also be used to reconstruct a postradiation deformity after breast-conserving therapy when autologous tissue is preferred. The use of a transverse rectus abdominis myocutaneous (TRAM) flap is not recommended so it can be preserved for future reconstruction needs in the event a total mastectomy should become necessary.

♦ An estimated 20% defect in the upper outer quadrant of the breast is shown in Figure 19-2.

♦ Given the small size of the breast, large defect size, and favorable location of the defect (adjacent to axilla and TD vessels), an immediate repair can be performed with a pedicled LD flap.

Step 3. Operative Steps

1. Preoperative Markings

♦ The patient is marked before surgery in the standing position. Breast markings include the sternal notch, midline, inframammary fold, and superior border of the breast. The anterolateral border of the LD is marked while the patient adducts her upper extremity (Fig. 19-3). The scapular tip, iliac crest, and posterior midline are then marked. The skin defect is estimated and transposed to the skin island of the flap. The location of the skin island of the flap is positioned overlying the LD to allow for an adequate arc of rotation into the breast defect. The skin paddle (outlined in red) is oriented within the patient's bra strap line so that the donor site can be concealed.

2. Intraoperative Patient Positioning

♦ The patient is positioned in the lateral decubitus position for flap harvest and donor site closure. Flap insetting is performed with the patient supine and then upright, with the upper extremities abducted 90 degrees and padded to avoid injury to the shoulder and brachial plexus.

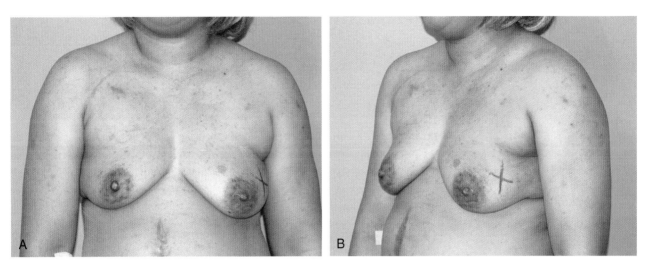

Figure 19-2

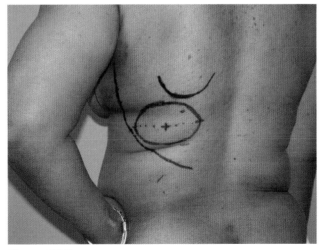

Figure 19-3

3. Flap Dissection

- The skin island is incised to the level of the LD fascia (Fig. 19-4, *A*).
- The anterior border of the LD muscle adjacent to the serratus anterior (SA) muscle, the posterior border adjacent to the trapezius muscle, along with the superior border adjacent to the teres muscles are identified to clarify the extent of the flap harvest.
- Dissection of the posterior surface of the LD is carried out by separating the muscle from the underlying SA (Fig. 19-4, *B*).
- Care must be taken to ligate the thoracolumbar perforators. Attention must be given to the location and course of the TD vascular pedicle, located on the undersurface of the muscle (superior anterior border), to avoid vascular compromise to the flap. When dissecting the flap toward the scapular tip, the plane of dissection must be just deep to the LD to avoid elevating the subscapular fat pad or serratus posterior muscle.
- Next, the LD is transected inferiorly, allowing the muscle to be elevated off the posterior chest wall and the dissection continued superiorly toward the TD pedicle.
- The other branches of the subscapular vessels to the SA, the circumflex scapular vessels, can be ligated to gain added vascular pedicle length for the flap's arc of rotation (Fig. 19-4, *C*).
- The TD nerve, situated medial to TD artery and vein, is transected to prevent postoperative muscle contraction that can detract from the aesthetic outcome of the repair.
- Similarly, the humeral origin of the LD can be divided to improve the arc of rotation and minimize muscle contracture. This region should be sutured to the lateral edge of the pectoralis major muscle to prevent undue tension or torsion on the TD vascular pedicle and recreate the anterior axillary fold, which leads to a more aesthetically pleasing result.
- A tunnel is created to transpose the flap into the segmental mastectomy defect (Fig. 19-5, *A*).

4. Donor Site Closure

- The donor site closure is performed after placement of closed-suction drains.
- The Scarpa fascial layer is closed with 2-0 absorbable sutures to decrease tension on skin closure.
- The subcutaneous layer is closed with 3-0 absorbable sutures and the dermal closure is performed with a running subcuticular 4-0 absorbable suture.
- The patient is then repositioned supine on the operating table for flap insetting.

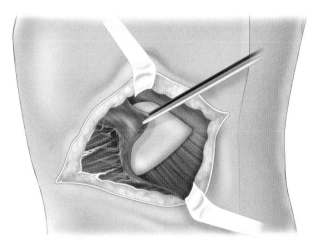

A. Dissection of latissimus muscle from underlying serratus anterior muscle and chest wall

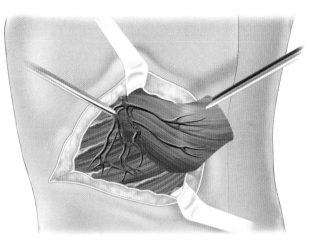

B. Exposure of thoracodorsal vessels and crossing branch to serratus anterior muscle

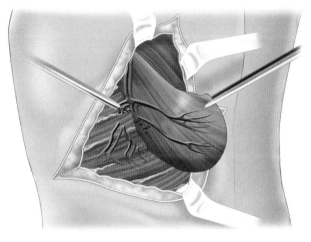

C. Ligation of crossing branch to serratus anterior muscle

Figure 19-4

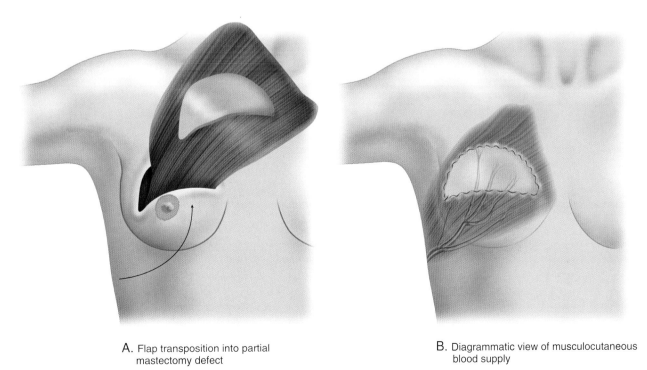

A. Flap transposition into partial mastectomy defect

B. Diagrammatic view of musculocutaneous blood supply

Figure 19-5

5. Flap Insetting

- The flap is delivered to the segmental mastectomy defect and its perfusion inspected. The patient is placed in the sitting position and the flap contoured to fill the volume of and plicated to the shape of the segmental mastectomy defect (Figs. 19-6, *A* and *B* and see Fig. 19-5, *B*)
- Alternatively, if there is no skin defect, the skin island of the flap can be de-epithelialized and placed underlying the native breast skin to provide additional soft tissue coverage (the de-epithelialized skin will not atrophy, like the LD muscle; Figs. 19-6, *C* and *D*)
- A tension-free inset of the skin island is then performed over closed-suction drains.

Step 4. Postoperative Care

- After surgery, the patient is maintained with the ipsilateral arm abducted 30 degrees on a pillow to avoid compression of the vascular pedicle along its transaxillary course. The flap is monitored during the hospitalization for color, temperature, and capillary refill.
- As the operative site heals, the flap tissue integrates into the breast parenchyma (Figs. 19-6, *E* and *F*). The LD muscle continues to atrophy over the next year or so.

Step 5. Pearls and Pitfalls

- The skin island should be kept small (minimizing the tension of closure results in a more cosmetically acceptable scar) and concealed (patients can wear more revealing apparel).
- Remember to transect the TD nerve to avoid LD muscle contraction during daily activities.
- Premature drain removal confers a significant risk for seroma formation at the donor site.
- Do not compress the vascular pedicle as it traverses through the tunnel to the defect in the breast.
- After insetting the flap, abduct the ipsilateral extremity to ensure this motion does not place undue tension on the vascular pedicle.
- When planning an LD flap after a previous axillary dissection, muscle function is tested (patient extends her shoulders while pushing into hips to contract the LD muscle) to confirm the vascular pedicle is intact (the TD nerve lies adjacent to the TD vessels; the assumption is that if nerve is intact, so are vessels). Previous TD vessel injury could preclude flap transfer.

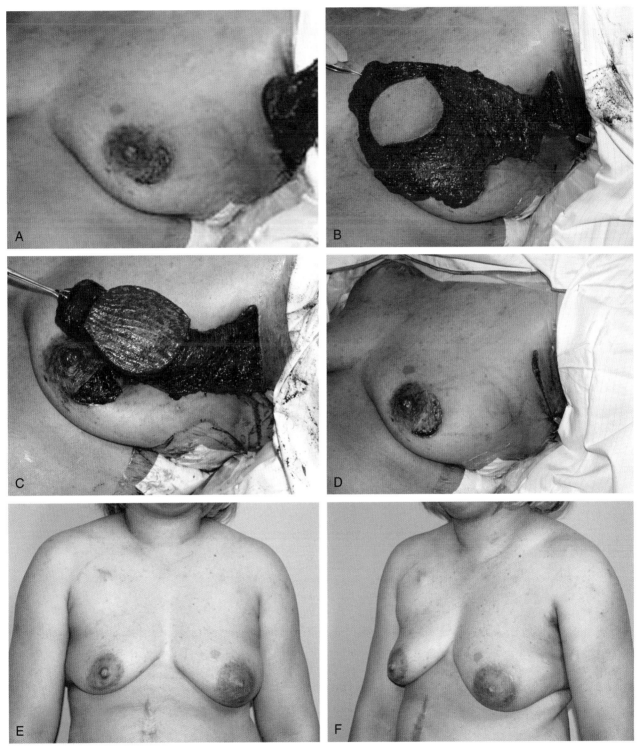

Figure 19-6

B. Latissimus Dorsi Flap with Breast Implant for Total Breast Reconstruction after Mastectomy

Step 1. Surgical Anatomy

- See Figure 19-1.

Step 2. Preoperative Considerations

- An LD flap with an implant is ideal to reconstruct a total breast defect in a thin patient who does not require radiation therapy.
- This method of reconstruction is favored in patients with low body mass indexes and insufficient abdominal tissue for a lower abdominal flap.
- An LD flap is also useful in patients who have undergone a previous abdominal surgery that precludes the use of a lower abdominal flap or in those who are obese.
- Compared with a lower abdominal flap, an LD flap has the advantages of shorter operative time, a quicker recovery, and no requirement for microsurgery.
- The use of an LD flap for bilateral reconstruction also has the advantage of not requiring that both breasts be reconstructed simultaneously, as in the case of lower abdominal flaps.
- The decision to proceed with a reconstruction using an LD flap plus a breast implant must be based on many factors, including the breast pathology, clinical stage, and the need for adjuvant radiation therapy; if the latter is required, a delayed approach to breast reconstruction is preferred to minimize complications and improve the overall cosmetic outcome.
- An LD flap reconstruction is limited by the amount of skin available to restore a large mastectomy skin defect. With delayed breast reconstruction, the skin requirement often exceeds that available from the LD flap because of the need to primarily close the donor site.
- The nipple-areolar defect that results from a skin-sparing mastectomy provides the ideal opportunity to minimize donor site morbidity with an LD flap.
- In patients who have had prior axillary surgery, it is critical to assess the motor function of the LD muscle as a potential indicator of an intact TD pedicle. Preoperative Doppler ultrasonography can be performed to evaluate blood flow in the TD pedicle.
- In unilateral LD reconstruction, the contralateral breast must be evaluated because it is ideal to have an implant in this breast as well to optimize symmetry. This usually is done as a contralateral mastopexy with breast implant augmentation.
- An advantage of the LD flap plus an implant is that it enables the reconstructive surgeon to match the breast tissue in the previously augmented contralateral breast. The LD serves as the breast tissue and the use of breast implants in both breasts tends to result in a symmetric appearance (Fig. 19-7).

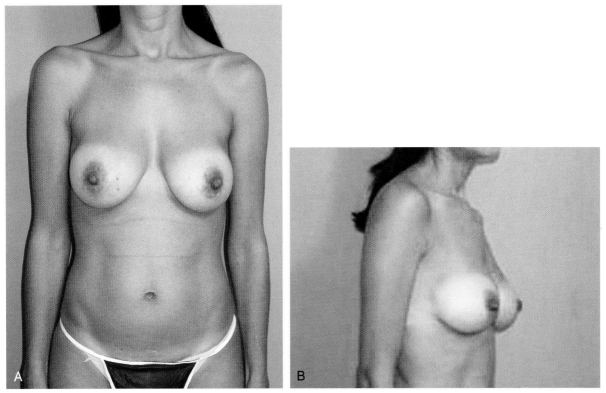

Figure 19-7

Step 3. Operative Steps

1. Preoperative Markings

- The patient is marked preoperatively as described earlier (see Fig. 19-3).
- If the breast is absent, such as in a delayed reconstruction, the inframammary fold and superior breast border are transposed from the contralateral normal breast.
- The skin island is usually positioned centrally in the breast in the vicinity of the nipple-areolar complex.
- The location of the flap skin island on the back overlying the LD is checked to ensure it will allow for an adequate arc of rotation to the breast defect. The skin island is oriented in line with the patient's bra strap so that donor scar closure can be concealed (Fig. 19-8).

2. Intraoperative Patient Positioning

- The patient is positioned in the lateral decubitus position for flap harvest and donor site closure. Flap insetting is performed with the patient supine and then upright, with the upper extremities abducted 90 degrees and padded to avoid injury to the shoulder and brachial plexus.
- When immediate reconstruction is performed at the time of mastectomy, the patient remains in the supine position to initiate the dissection of the TD vessels before being repositioned to the lateral decubitus position to perform the flap harvest.
- Before the patient is repositioned, the mastectomy defect is temporarily closed and covered with a plastic occlusive dressing.

3. Flap Harvest

- The mastectomy defect is assessed and a template of the skin defect is created to aid in designing the skin island of the flap (see Fig. 19-4).
- As discussed for the harvest of the LD flap for repair of a segmental mastectomy defect, the skin island is incised, the anterior aspect of the muscle is freed from the overlying skin and subcutaneous tissue, and the posterior muscle dissection is initiated anteriorly between the anterior border of the LD and the underlying SA. The dissection then proceeds from inferior to superior, with meticulous dissection of the vascular pedicle in the axilla. After completing the flap dissection, the flap is passed through the axilla into the mastectomy defect to allow for closure of the back wound (Figs. 19-9 and 19-10).

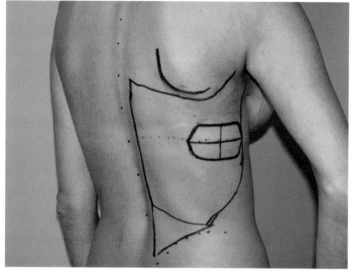

Figure 19-8

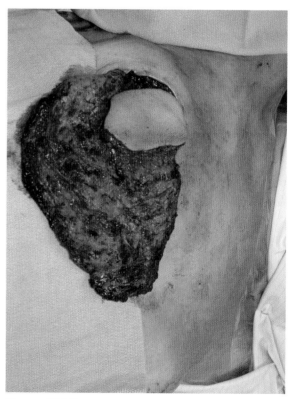

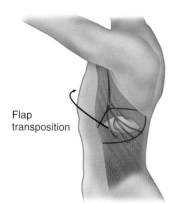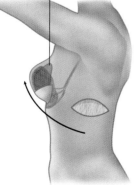

Location for implant

Flap
transposition

Figure 19-9

Figure 19-10

4. Flap Insetting

♦ A subpectoral pocket is developed to allow placement of the implant in the subpectoral plane. This creates a smooth contour in the upper pole and minimizes the prominence of the breast implant superiorly.

♦ The LD flap (inferior border of muscle) is then inset with a 3-0 absorbable suture along the superior and medial border of the breast.

♦ Next, a disposable breast implant sizer is placed behind the prepared submuscular (pectoralis major and LD muscles) pocket (Fig. 19-11).

♦ The LD muscle is then inset to the lateral chest wall, defining the lateral edge of the reconstructed breast.

♦ The implant sizer is injected with saline to the desired volume and the patient is placed in the sitting position. The shape, projection, contour, and location of the reconstructed breast are compared with the contralateral breast.

♦ Modifications to the flap inset are made as needed and the implant sizer is exchanged for a permanent breast implant. The remaining inferior muscle flap is allowed to drape over the lower pole and conform to the previously defined inframammary fold. The skin island is inset with a subcutaneous layer of 3-0 absorbable sutures and a running layer of 4-0 absorbable sutures for intradermal closure (Fig. 19-12).

Step 4. Postoperative Care

♦ After surgery, the patient is maintained with the ipsilateral arm abducted 30 degrees on a pillow to avoid compression of the pedicle along its transaxillary course.

♦ The patient wears a surgical bra and the visible portion of the flap is used to assess skin perfusion. The bra should be loose to avoid compression of the vascular pedicle and used mainly to secure fluffed gauze in the lateral aspect of the reconstructed breast to assist in maintaining the position of the implant and avoid axillary migration.

♦ After surgery, trained staff assess the flap's color, temperature, and capillary refill.

♦ As seen in this patient 18 months after reconstruction, the LD continues to atrophy over time and the underlying implant plays a more prominent role in the reconstruction (Fig. 19-13).

Step 5. Pearls and Pitfalls

♦ Confirm TD pedicle continuity before committing to flap harvest.

♦ Place the breast implant under both the pectoralis major and LD muscles to minimize implant rippling in the superior and medial aspects of the reconstructed breast.

♦ Avoid donor site seroma formation with prolonged use of closed-suction drains.

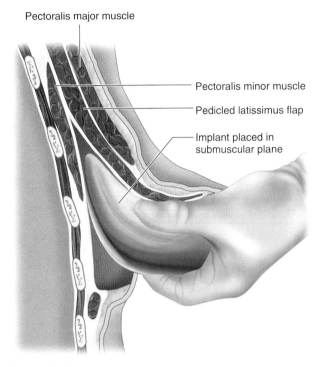

Pectoralis major muscle

Pectoralis minor muscle

Pedicled latissimus flap

Implant placed in
submuscular plane

Figure 19-11

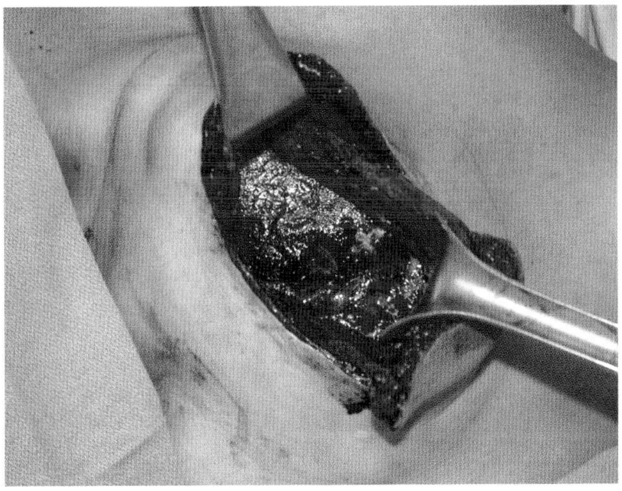

Figure 19-12

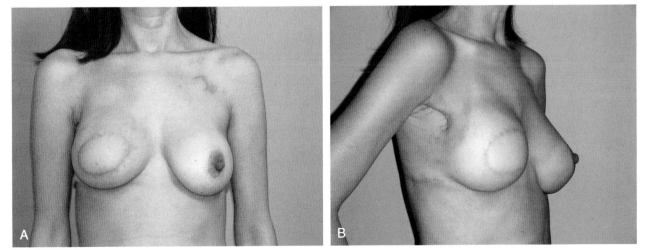

Figure 19-13

C. Lower Abdominal Flaps: Transverse Rectus Abdominis Myocutaneous (TRAM) Flap and Deep Inferior Epigastric Perforator Flap

Step 1. Surgical Anatomy

- The superior epigastric artery and vein are the terminal branches of the internal mammary system (Fig. 19-14).
- The deep inferior epigastric artery and vein that originate from the iliac vessels provide the dominant blood supply to the tissues of the lower abdominal wall. These vessels are connected through a variable number of intramuscular "choke anastomoses" (connecting branches) in the rectus abdominis muscle at the umbilical region that allow for perfusion of the lower abdominal tissue through the superior epigastric system. This provides the basis of perfusion of the pedicled TRAM flap.
- The deep inferior epigastric vessels originate from the iliac vessels (inguinal region) and enter the rectus muscle inferolaterally after giving off a medial branch to the rectus muscle (see Fig. 19-14).
- The vessels then travel along the undersurface of the muscle until they enter the substance of the muscle, giving off perforating branches that pierce the anterior rectus sheath to supply the overlying skin and subcutaneous tissue of the lower abdominal region (Fig. 19-15).
- Similarly, the medial branch to the rectus muscle that originated from the main trunk of the deep inferior epigastric vessels supplies the medial row of perforating blood vessels. These perforating vessels provide blood flow to the subcutaneous tissue and skin of the lower abdominal flap (see Fig. 19-15).

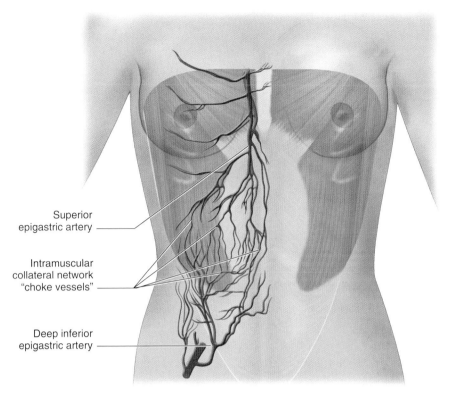

Superior
epigastric artery

Intramuscular
collateral network
"choke vessels"

Deep inferior
epigastric artery

Figure 19-14

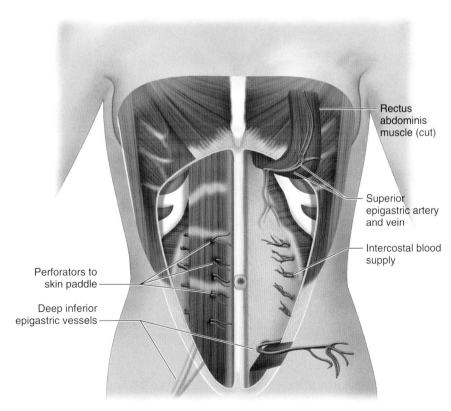

Rectus
abdominis
muscle (cut)

Superior
epigastric artery
and vein

Intercostal blood
supply

Perforators to
skin paddle

Deep inferior
epigastric vessels

Figure 19-15

- Vascular supply of a unilateral TRAM flap is classified into four zones on the basis of perfusion to the overlying skin and subcutaneous tissues: zone 1 overlies the ipsilateral rectus sheath; zone 2 is lateral to and on the same side of the abdominal wall as zone 1; zone 3 overlies the contralateral rectus sheath across the midline; and zone 4 is lateral to and on the same side as zone 3 (Fig. 19-16).
- When either pedicled or free TRAM flaps are transferred to the chest wall, zone 1 has the best perfusion and zone 4 the worst. However, because of variable watershed regions of blood supply to the lower abdomen, these zones of perfusion can differ from patient to patient.

1. Variations of Lower Abdominal Flaps

- The lower abdominal adipose tissue can be used to reconstruct a breast in several different ways. Tissue can be transferred as a pedicled flap (Fig. 19-17, *A*), in which the blood supply to the flap remains attached to the rectus abdominis muscle, or as a microvascular free flap, in which the flap is completely freed from the deep inferior epigastric vessels and then anastomosed to recipient vessels located on the chest wall (most commonly, internal mammary or TD artery and vein) using microsurgical techniques.
- A pedicled TRAM flap requires harvest of the entire rectus abdominis muscle to include blood supply from the superior epigastric artery and vein. The advantage of this flap design is that it does not require microsurgical skills; however, there can be significant donor site morbidity owing to the need to extensively repair the abdominal wall after harvest of the flap. The blood supply to the pedicle is not the dominant supply to the lower abdominal adipose tissue (deep inferior epigastric vessels) and depends on the number of choke anastomoses (connections) at the umbilical region, which can alter the perfusion to the flap and result in higher rates of fat necrosis than in microsurgical TRAM flaps (see Fig. 19-14).
- Although a microsurgical TRAM flap requires expertise in microsurgery, it requires less rectus abdominis muscle (only the lower one third) than a pedicled TRAM flap because it does not need to remain attached to the rectus muscle while being tunneled to the chest wall. A variant of the free TRAM flap that preserves a lateral or medial strip of rectus muscle, the so-called muscle-sparing microvascular TRAM flap, further reduces the amount of rectus muscle that needs to be harvested with the flap while providing a similar degree of perfusion to the flap (Fig. 19-17, *B*).
- A deep inferior epigastric perforator (DIEP) flap (Fig. 19-17, *C*), which comes from the same area as a TRAM flap, involves harvesting only the perforating blood vessels that branch off from the deep inferior epigastric vessels (located in the rectus abdominis muscle) and perforate the lower abdominal adipose tissue. The DIEP flap avoids having to harvest any rectus muscle or fascia with the lower abdominal tissue flap because the perforating blood vessels, as well as the deep inferior epigastric vessels, are dissected free from the rectus abdominis using a longitudinal muscle-splitting incision.

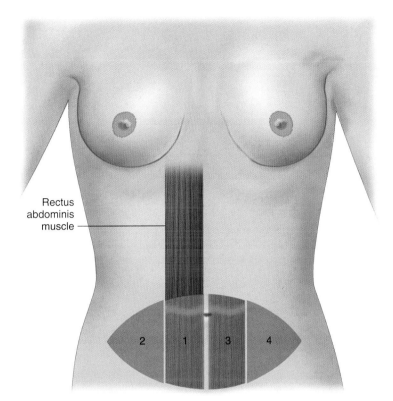

Rectus
abdominis
muscle

Figure 19-16

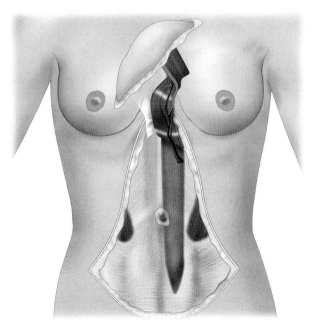

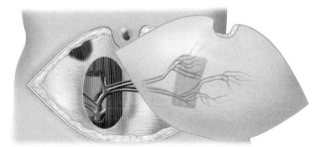

B. Muscle-sparing TRAM flap

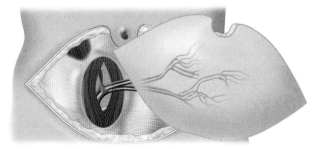

C. DIEP flap

A. Pedicled TRAM flap

Figure 19-17

Step 2. Preoperative Considerations

- Microsurgical free tissue transfer has enabled creation of reconstructed breasts with an optimal blood supply and resultant decrease in postoperative fat necrosis of the flap. The lower abdominal donor site offers abundant skin and subcutaneous tissue of a texture that replicates the tissue quality of the breast.
- The decision to proceed with autologous breast reconstruction must be based on many factors, including the patient's physiologic age, breast pathology, clinical stage, and the potential need for adjuvant radiation therapy. Although there are no clearly defined age criteria for free tissue transfer, patients with significant comorbidities may not be optimal candidates for this approach. If the need for adjuvant radiation therapy is anticipated, a delayed approach to breast reconstruction is preferred to minimize complications and improve the eventual cosmetic outcome of the breast reconstruction.
- In unilateral autologous tissue reconstruction, the contralateral breast should have adequate volume to match the free autologous tissue transfer because the use of a unilateral breast implant can lead to asymmetry between the breasts, with gravitational effects predominantly leading to ptosis of the autologous reconstructed breast. However, the need for a contralateral mastopexy or reduction mammoplasty is not uncommon in many patients undergoing unilateral autologous tissue reconstruction.
- There has been an increasing trend away from using the TD vessels and toward the internal mammary vessels as recipient vessels for an immediate microvascular tissue transfer, which allows for reoperative axillary surgery to be performed without concern for injury to the vascular pedicle. This would be important in the clinical scenario of an axillary sentinel lymph node that was negative intraoperatively but was subsequently found to be positive on permanent pathology.

Step 3. Operative Steps

1. Preoperative Markings

- The patient is marked preoperatively in the standing position (Fig. 19-18).
- The lower abdomen flap is outlined as an ellipse extending from the suprapubic area inferiorly, to the anterior superior iliac spine laterally, and to the supraumbilical area superiorly.
- The patient is positioned supine on the examination table with the knees flexed, and the borders of the lower abdominal flap are approximated to assess the resultant tension on the donor site closure.
- The markings are evaluated for symmetry at a distance and preoperative photographs are obtained to assist in finalizing the operative plan.

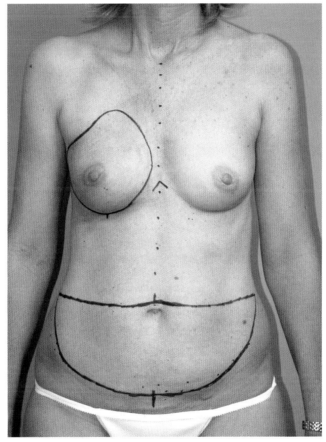

Figure 19-18

2. **Intraoperative Patient Positioning**

- The patient is positioned supine with the upper extremities abducted to 90 degrees and padded.
- Semi-Fowler positioning is used to decrease the tension of the abdominal donor site closure.
- Care is taken to secure the patient's head, endotracheal tube, and arms in anticipation of sitting the patient in the upright position during the insetting of the reconstructed breast.

3. **Harvest of the Lower Abdominal Flap**

- The inferior lower abdominal markings are incised initially and dissection is carried down to the anterior fascia of the abdominal wall (anterior fascial layer of rectus abdominis and external oblique muscles). The superficial inferior epigastric (SIE) veins are preserved along the lower border of the flap to serve as potential donor veins (microsurgical anastomoses) for the flap if it exhibits signs of venous congestion after transfer to the chest wall. If a large-caliber SIE artery is found along with an SIE vein, consideration can be given to perform an SIE artery flap. The superior lower incision is then taken down to the anterior rectus sheath and external oblique fascia. The umbilicus is then dissected away from the flap with a wide vascular cuff (Fig. 19-19).
- The dissection of the undersurface of the flap is then performed from lateral to medial toward the anterior rectus sheath until the lateral row of perforators from the underlying rectus abdominis muscle is identified bilaterally. If a hemi (one-half) lower abdominal flap is planned, the flap is incised in the midline and the medial row of perforators is identified. If the tissue across the midline is to be included with the flap (depends on volume needs of the reconstructed breast), the medial perforators are dissected by freeing the adipose tissue from the midline fascia without transection of the overlying skin and adipose tissue. All perforating blood vessels from both rectus muscles are subsequently evaluated using Doppler ultrasonography for their location, luminal diameter, and flow.
- The selected perforators are then assessed by placing Acland microsurgical occluding clamps on the perforators not selected for inclusion with the flap to be certain that the selected perforator(s) will provide adequate perfusion to the flap. Once the perforators have been appropriately selected, the flap harvest can proceed either as a fascia-sparing, pedicled TRAM flap, a fascia-sparing microvascular TRAM flap, a fascia-sparing, muscle-sparing microvascular TRAM flap, or a DIEP flap, depending on the volume of tissue required, perforator anatomy, and the surgeon's preference.

4. **Harvest of Pedicled TRAM Flap**

- The anterior rectus fascia is incised around the previously dissected perforators to spare as much fascia as possible. The rectus abdominis muscle is then freed from its encasement in the rectus sheath with careful dissection of the muscle from the tendinous inscriptions. The deep inferior epigastric pedicle is identified, dissected, and ligated at its origin from the iliac vessels (Fig. 19-20).

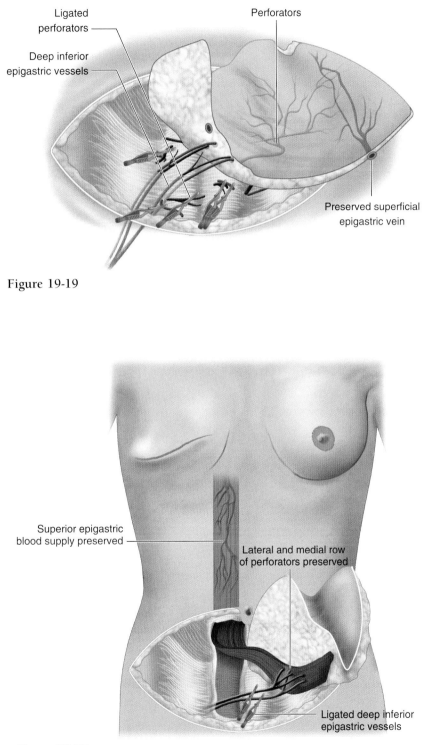

Ligated perforators

Deep inferior epigastric vessels

Perforators

Preserved superficial epigastric vein

Figure 19-19

Superior epigastric blood supply preserved

Lateral and medial row of perforators preserved

Ligated deep inferior epigastric vessels

Figure 19-20

◆ Preserving adequate length of these vessels is imperative should additional lateral supply or venous drainage from the flap be required after transfer to the chest wall.

◆ The anterior rectus sheath is then incised superiorly along the muscle length to the costal margin. Next, the rectus muscle is further freed from the rectus sheath and divided inferiorly below the entry point of the deep inferior epigastric vessels (Fig. 19-21, *A*).

◆ A subcutaneous tunnel is then created through the superomedial aspect of the abdominal donor site to allow transfer of the flap to the mastectomy defect without undue tension or constriction. The flap is then delivered to the mastectomy defect and shaped into the reconstructed breast (Fig. 19-21, *B*).

5. Harvest of Microvascular TRAM Flap

◆ Once the perforator anatomy has been delineated, the decision as to whether to perform a microvascular TRAM flap or a DIEP flap can be made.

◆ The decision to perform a microvascular TRAM flap as opposed to a DIEP flap is based on the finding of inadequate perforators (small size, few in number, or poor flow or perfusion to the flap). As with a pedicled TRAM flap, multiple perforators are harvested with a microvascular TRAM flap, including perforators from both the medial and lateral rows.

◆ In a manner similar to that described for a pedicled TRAM flap, the anterior rectus fascia is incised around the selected perforators in order to spare anterior rectus sheath fascia. At the inferolateral aspect of the rectus abdominis muscle, the deep inferior epigastric vascular pedicle is identified and dissected toward its origin from the iliac artery and vein (Fig.19-22, *A*). Next, the rectus muscle is divided at the superior and inferior margin. The deep inferior epigastric vascular pedicle is then divided at its origin from the external iliac vessels. The flap is then completely freed from the body and positioned on the chest wall for microsurgical anastomosis to the already prepared recipient vessels (Fig. 19-22, *B*).

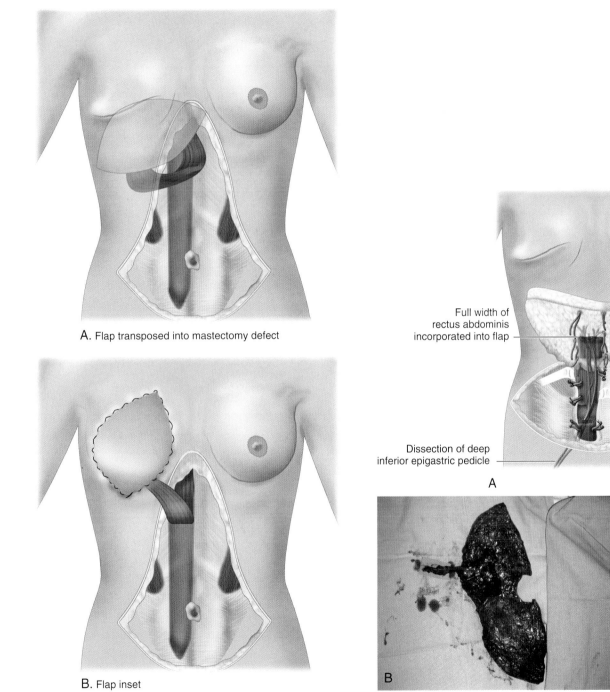

A. Flap transposed into mastectomy defect

B. Flap inset

Figure 19-21

Full width of
rectus abdominis
incorporated into flap

Dissection of deep
inferior epigastric pedicle

A

B

Figure 19-22

Case Example: Free TRAM Flap

◆ A 43-year-old woman presented with left-sided ductal carcinoma in situ (Figs. 19-23, *A*). Pre-operative markings were made for lower abdominal TRAM flap (Fig. 19-23, *B*). The left-sided internal mammary perforating artery and vein through the third intercostal space were used as recipient vessels, instead of the internal mammary vessels proper. Microsurgical anastomoses were done of the left internal mammary artery perforator to the right deep inferior epigastric artery and the left internal mammary perforating vein to the right deep inferior epigastric vein (Fig. 19-23, *C*). The anterior rectus sheath fascia, which was excised with the harvested TRAM flap, was replaced with an inlay allograft of human cadaver dermis. Figure 19-23, *D* shows the patient 2 years after reconstruction of the left breast with a microvascular TRAM flap.

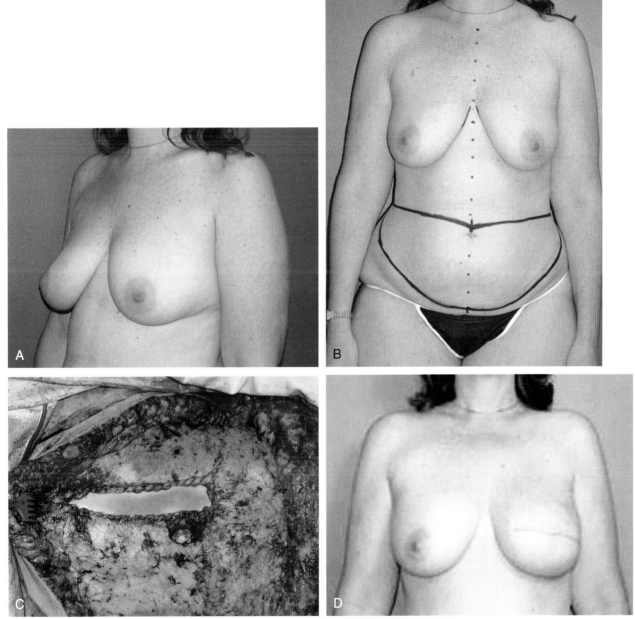

Figure 19-23

6. **Harvest of Muscle-Sparing TRAM Flap**

♦ Once the perforator anatomy has been established, a muscle-sparing TRAM flap can be designed. If medial-row perforators are selected, the lateral muscle can be spared with its intercostal neurovascular supply left intact. If the lateral row of perforators is selected, the medial muscle can be preserved. The intercostal branches enter the rectus muscle laterally, contributing sensory and motor innervation as well as vascular branches that anastomose with the deep inferior epigastric vessels. In muscle-sparing TRAM flaps, preservation of the intercostal nerves maintains the function of the rectus muscle that remains after harvest of the flap (Fig. 19-24). As with a non–muscle-sparing TRAM flap, the harvest of the anterior rectus fascia is minimized by incising medially and laterally to incorporate only the selected perforators, thus sparing as much fascia as possible for closure.

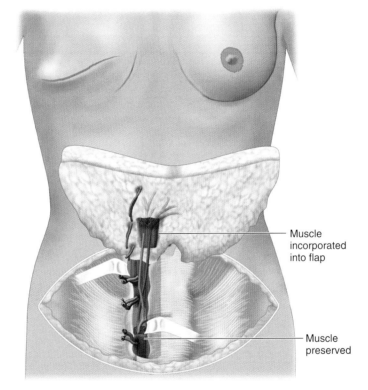

Muscle
incorporated
into flap

Muscle
preserved

Portion of muscle surrounding perforators is incorporated into flap design

Figure 19-24

7. Harvest of DIEP Flap

- Once the perforator anatomy has been established and adequate perforators (large size, good flow, and adequate perfusion to flap) identified, a DIEP flap can be designed.
- DIEP flaps can be designed with one or multiple perforators depending on intraoperative assessment of flap perfusion and clustering of perforator location. Each selected perforator is meticulously dissected, sparing the anterior rectus sheath with careful intramuscular dissection (Fig. 19-25, *A*).
- Care is taken not to denervate the rectus abdominis muscle. The intramuscular dissection is performed to trace the perforating artery and vein back to the deep inferior epigastric artery and vein. These vessels, which will serve as the vascular pedicle to the flap, are dissected to their origin from the external iliac vessels to obtain a pedicle of adequate length and caliber for the microvascular anastomosis (Fig. 19-25, *B*).

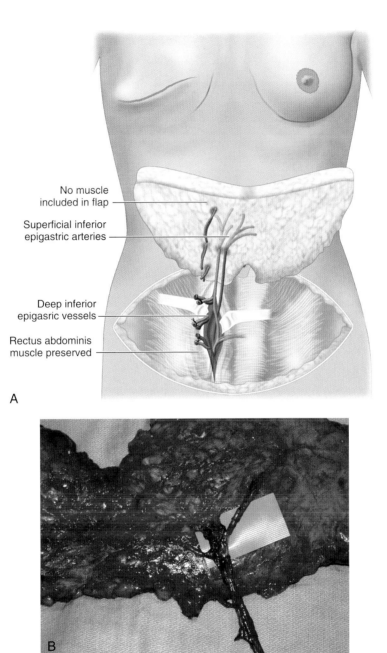

No muscle
included in flap

Superficial inferior
epigastric arteries

Deep inferior
epigasric vessels

Rectus abdominis
muscle preserved

A

B

Figure 19-25

Case Examples: DIEP Flaps

◆ A 41-year-old woman presented with left-sided breast cancer (Fig. 19-26, *A*). Preoperative markings were made for a lower abdominal DIEP flap, just as for a TRAM flap (Fig. 19-26, *B*). The DIEP flap after harvest is shown in Fig. 19-26, *C*. The result is a flap with no muscle or abdominal fascia, which allows for primary repair of the abdominal fascia without any significant disruption. Figure 19-26, *D* and *E* show the patient 3 months after reconstruction of the left breast with a right-sided DIEP flap.

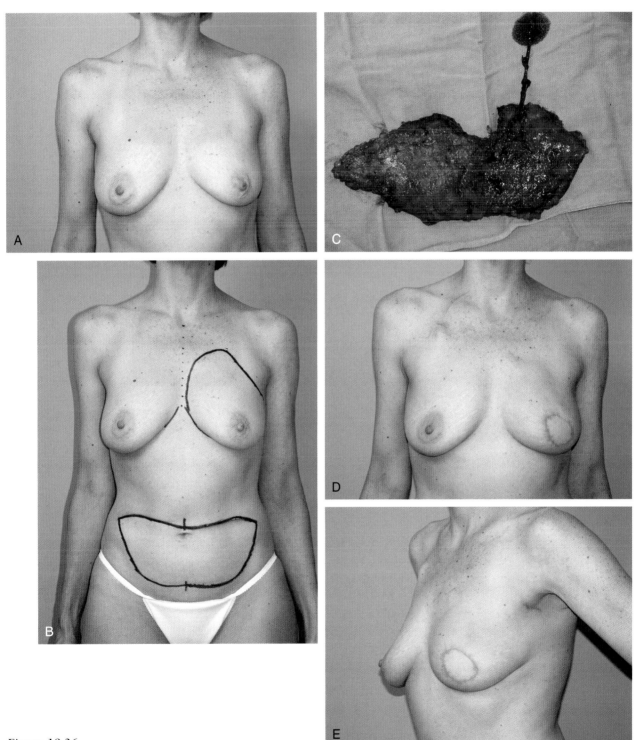

Figure 19-26

◆ A 31-year-old woman with angiosarcoma of the left breast underwent preoperative radiation therapy before mastectomy and immediate breast reconstruction (Figs. 19-27, A and B). Preoperative markings were made for a lower abdominal DIEP flap, just as for a TRAM flap (Fig. 19-27, C). Figure 19-27, D shows an in situ view of the multiple perforators supplying the flap from the deep inferior epigastric vessels. The flap after harvest (Fig. 19-27, E). Figures 19-27, F and G show the patient 1 year after reconstruction of the left breast with a right-sided DIEP flap.

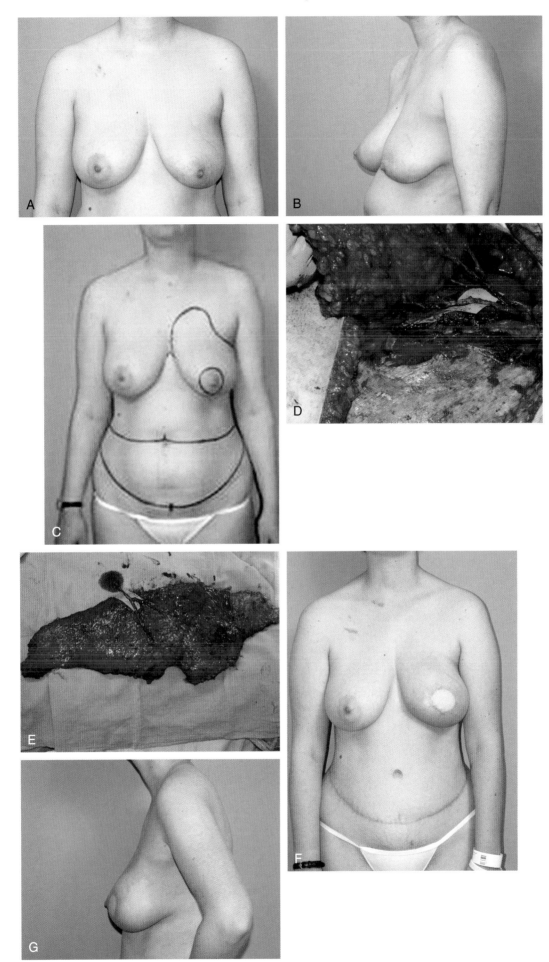

Figure 19-27

8. Preparation of Recipient Vessels for Microvascular Anastomosis

- The internal mammary vessels are preferred over the TD vessels as recipients for microvascular breast reconstruction. The internal mammary vessels have the advantage of allowing flap inset and positioning more medially on the chest wall, and are not involved in the operative field in the event the patient requires additional axillary nodal removal because of a positive sentinel lymph node on the permanent pathology.
- The internal mammary vessels are usually accessed through the third intercostal space.
- The overlying pectoralis major is divided along its fibers and the perichondrium overlying the costal cartilage is incised, enabling the costal cartilage to be separated from the posterior perichondrium.
- Next, a lateral incision is made through the cartilage and the medial sternocostal ligaments are disrupted, allowing for removal of the cartilage. Meticulous dissection is then performed to dissect the posterior perichondrium away from the internal mammary vessels, with special care taken to ligate the intercostal and cutaneous branches.
- When there is only a single internal mammary vein (IMV), it is usually located medial to the internal mammary artery (IMA). The left IMV is often smaller than the right IMV. When two IMVs are present, the second vein is usually positioned lateral to the IMA (Fig. 19-28).
- The internal mammary vessels are then dissected from each other and the surrounding adventitial tissue in preparation for microvascular anastomosis. Great care must be taken in the previously irradiated patient.

9. Flap Transfer and Revascularization

- Once the flap is evaluated for in situ perfusion, the pedicle is clamped with Acland clamps and ligated, and the deep inferior epigastric artery is irrigated with heparinized saline until clear effluent returns through the vein. The flap is then temporarily secured to the chest wall.
- With the aid of an operating microscope or surgical loupes, end-to-end microvascular anastomoses of the arteries (IMA to deep inferior epigastric artery) and veins (IMV to deep inferior epigastric vein) are then performed, using 9.0 nylon suture. The 11th intercostal nerve is also anastomosed to intercostal nerves on the chest wall with 10-0 nylon.
- Venous microvascular coupling devices or end-to-side microvascular anastomoses are sometimes used.
- On completion of the microsurgery, the Acland clamps are removed and perfusion to the flap is reestablished. Careful inspection for patency and blood flow is performed by gross examination and hand-held Doppler ultrasound probe, and confirmed by observing distal dermal bleeding (Fig. 19-29).

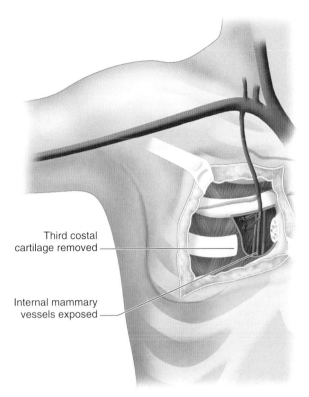

Third costal
cartilage removed

Internal mammary
vessels exposed

Figure 19-28

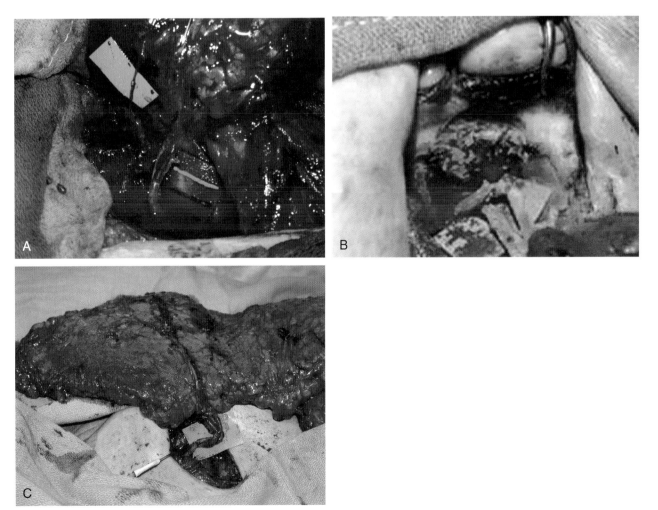

Figure 19-29

10. Flap Insetting

♦ The flap is then introduced into the mastectomy defect, with care taken to position the vascular pedicle without kinking or compression.

♦ For unilateral breast reconstruction, the flap can be based on either the ipsilateral or contralateral vascular pedicle. If the flap is based on the contralateral vascular pedicle, the flap is inset vertically to allow the areas of maximal blood supply (zones 1 and 2) to be positioned in the medial and inferior aspects of the reconstructed breast and the lesser-perfused region (zone 3) to be positioned either underneath zone 1 (increased lower pole projection) or in the lateral aspect (increased lateral breast and axillary volume, especially pertinent to patients who required a complete nodal dissection with axillary irradiation) of the reconstructed breast (Figs. 19-30 and 19-31).

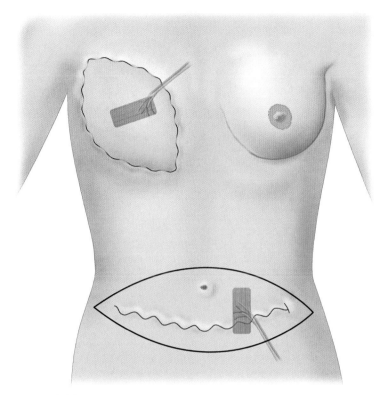

Figure 19-30

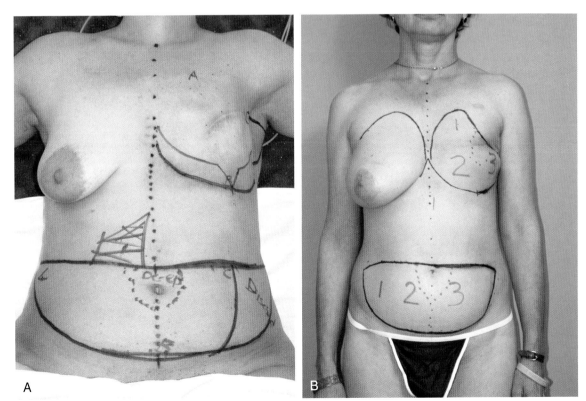

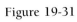
Figure 19-31

- Alternatively, if a horizontal inset is preferred to reconstruct a wider-shaped breast, the lower abdominal flap should be based on the ipsilateral vascular pedicle and rotated 180 degrees to inset (Figs. 19-32 and 19-33). With the horizontal orientation, there can be some soft tissue deficiency in the superior aspect of the reconstructed breast.
- With either orientation, the flap can be plicated to maximize projection in the lower pole of the reconstructed breast. The mastectomy flaps are then evaluated and trimmed as needed. The skin island of the flap is then marked to fit the mastectomy skin defect, and the remaining skin is de-epithelialized.
- Drains are placed superiorly and inferiorly in the mastectomy pocket, with care taken to avoid placing the drains adjacent to the vascular pedicle.
- The flap is then inset with 3-0 absorbable deep dermal inverted sutures; a running intradermal 4-0 absorbable suture completes the skin closure.
- A hand-held Doppler ultrasound probe is used to locate the transcutaneous arterial and venous signals for postoperative monitoring.

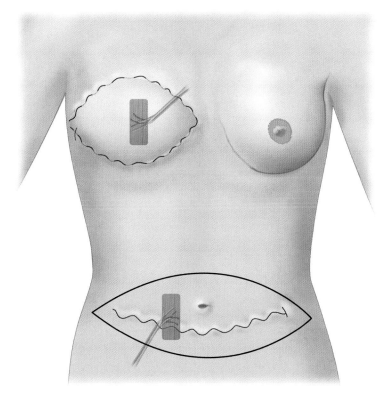

Figure 19-32

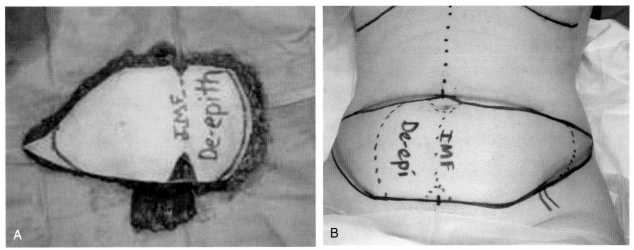

Figure 19-33

11. Closure of the Abdominal Donor Site

♦ Closure of the anterior rectus sheath fascial defect is accomplished with interrupted or running no. 1 nonabsorbable sutures.

♦ Care is taken to incorporate the cut edge of the aponeurosis of both the internal and external oblique muscles into the closure. This prevents musculofascial laxity that can later result in bulge formation.

♦ If the fascial defect can be closed primarily, the contralateral aspect of the lower abdominal wall usually will need to be plicated in order to centralize the umbilicus to the midline of the abdominal wall. The contralateral plication can be difficult in this situation because the fascia is already tight from closing the primary defect and can result in tearing of the fascia, which may weaken its integrity.

♦ If there is tension and primary fascial closure is not feasible, a synthetic mesh inlay or allograft can be used to replace the resected fascia of the anterior rectus sheath (Figs. 19-34 and 19-35).

♦ Patients who undergo breast reconstruction using a DIEP flap can usually have primary tension-free repair of the fascial incision without plication of the contralateral lower abdominal wall because the umbilical position is maintained in the midline (Figs. 19-36 and 19-37).

♦ The upper abdominal skin flap is then minimally undermined to the costal margin to allow for a tension-free skin closure. This also provides access to plicate the upper midline of the abdominal wall, which maintains a smooth contour to the abdominal wall.

♦ Skin closure along the lower abdominal crease is then performed after placement of drains.

♦ The Scarpa fascial layer is closed with 2-0 absorbable sutures to minimize tension on the skin closure.

♦ The skin layer is closed with 3-0 absorbable subcuticular inverted sutures; a running intradermal 4-0 absorbable suture is used for skin-edge approximation.

♦ The umbilical stalk, which remains attached to the abdominal wall throughout the flap harvest, is then delivered through the abdominal skin flap and inset into its anatomic position with absorbable sutures.

Step 4. Postoperative Care

♦ The patient is maintained in the semi-Fowler position to minimize tension on the abdominal skin closure. The patient wears a loose-fitting surgical bra.

♦ The visible portion of the flap is assessed for skin perfusion using a hand-held Doppler ultrasound probe.

♦ The flap is also monitored hourly for color, temperature, and capillary refill by trained staff.

♦ If at any time there is an interruption of vascular flow, either arterial or venous, the patient is returned to the operating room for emergent reexploration.

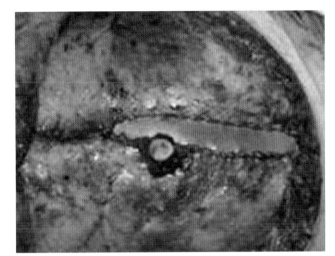

Figure 19-34

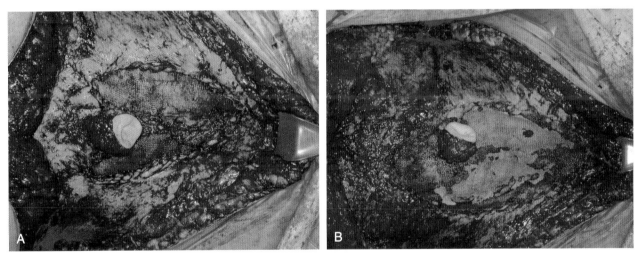

Figure 19-35

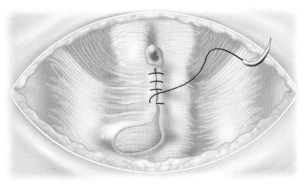

Primary fascial closure of abdominal donor site

Figure 19-36

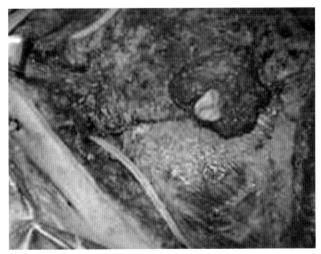

Figure 19-37

Step 5. Pearls and Pitfalls

- For a pedicled TRAM flap, be sure to create a tunnel of adequate width to avoid compression of pedicle. After flap transfer, decompress the deep inferior epigastric vein and anastomose for venous supercharging as needed.
- The left IMV is smaller than the right IMV.
- Be meticulous when dissecting irradiated vessels.
- With DIEP flaps, preserve the SIE vein in the event the flap becomes venous congested and requires supercharging to provide additional venous drainage.
- Incorporate both the internal and external oblique muscle aponeuroses during abdominal closure to avoid bulge formation.

D. Gluteal Artery Perforator (GAP) Flap

Step 1. Surgical Anatomy

- Figure 19-38 shows the anatomic considerations for a gluteal flap.

Step 2. Preoperative Considerations

- The ideal candidate for a gluteal flap is a patient who does not want to pursue implant reconstruction and does not have adequate abdominal tissue.
- Thin patients must have the appropriate body habitus to allow for sufficient tissue harvest from the gluteal region.
- Obese patients who usually are not considered candidates for an abdominal flap are also usually not eligible for a gluteal flap.
- The blood supply is a single perforator from the superior or inferior gluteal vessel, depending on where the selected perforator enters the flap.
- The redesigned gluteal flap shown in the case example allows for the reconstruction of a larger and better-contoured breast than with the standard elliptical flap.

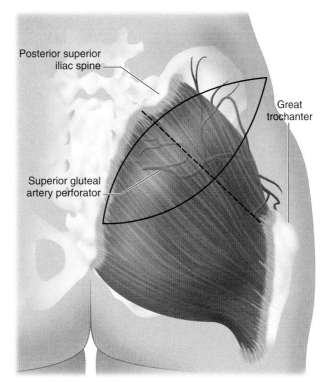

Figure 19-38

1. Preoperative Markings

- The patient is marked in the prone position. A line is drawn between the posterior superior iliac spine and the greater trochanter. The gluteal artery is found approximately one third of the distance from the posterior iliac spine along this line (Fig. 19-39). Cutaneous perforators can be identified with a hand-held Doppler ultrasound probe along this line. A curvilinear skin island is outlined within the vascular territory of the identified perforators. The flap is oriented so that the superior and medial aspects of the breast flap correspond to the medial and inferior aspects, respectively, of the gluteal donor site. This orientation allows the regions of maximal blood supply to correspond to the more visible aspects of the reconstructed breast (Fig. 19-40).

2. Intraoperative Patient Positioning

- There are two position changes required during the procedure. The patient is initially positioned supine for the dissection of the internal mammary recipient vessels and then again later after the flap harvest for the microsurgery and flap insetting.
- After preparation of the internal mammary vessels, which serve as the recipient vessels for gluteal flaps, the patient is repositioned to the prone position for flap harvest.

3. Flap Harvest

- The redesigned gluteal flap is harvested from the contralateral buttock. The patient is positioned in the prone position for harvest, not the corkscrew position, to avoid back-related injury. The skin island of the flap is incised down to the gluteal fascia; however, in the superolateral aspect of the flap on the buttock, only the adipose tissue located below the Scarpa fascial layer is harvested to create a circumferential flap with regard to blood supply. The circumferential blood supply allows for adequate perfusion of the curvilinear skin island.
- Next, the deep gluteal fascia is identified and incised. Subfascial dissection begins at the inferomedial aspect of the flap, which allows for easier identification of the perforators as they penetrate the gluteal muscles. Usually one to three perforators can be identified; the determination of which perforator to use is based on caliber and location relative to the skin island. The entire gluteal flap can be raised on a single perforator of adequate caliber. Perforators positioned laterally from the flap's long axis will produce a longer vascular pedicle.
- Once the perforator is selected, it is traced proximally. Meticulous intramuscular dissection is carried out, with care taken to ligate all intramuscular side branches. Extended proximal dissection on the pedicle is carried out to obtain an artery of appropriate caliber for anastomosis with the IMA. Subsequent dissection is complicated by a dense venous network that requires tedious vascular control. Once an adequate pedicle caliber is obtained, the flap is ready for transfer (Fig. 19-41). The flap is evaluated for in situ perfusion while it is still attached to its native vascular supply in the buttock.

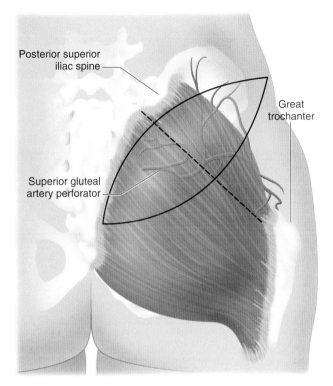

Figure 19-39

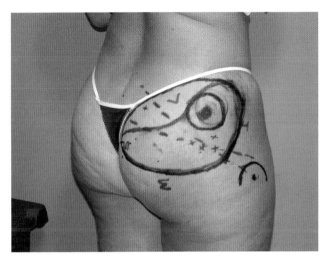

Figure 19-40

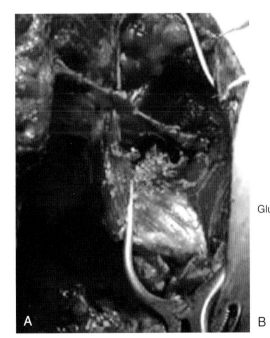

Figure 19-41

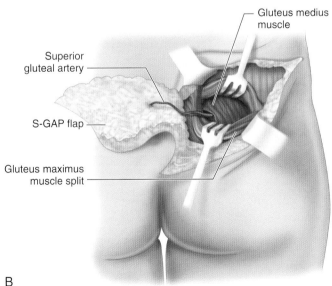

◆ Next, the pedicle is ligated and the deep gluteal artery is irrigated with heparinized saline until there is clear return through the vein. The flap is then placed on cold ischemia during donor site closure and repositioning of the patient (Fig. 19-42).

4. Closure of Donor Site

◆ The gluteal donor site is closed in layers over suction drains. The Scarpa fascial layer is closed with 2-0 absorbable sutures to alleviate any tension on the skin closure. The skin layer is closed with 3-0 absorbable subcuticular inverted sutures, and a running intradermal 4-0 suture is used for skin closure.

5. Flap Transfer and Revascularization

◆ Next, the patient is positioned supine on the operating table.
◆ The flap is then transferred and secured to the chest wall. Vascular control of the internal mammary vessels is obtained with Acland clamps. The donor and recipient vessels are prepared for microsurgery and sewn with the aid of the operating microscope or surgical loupes. The microvascular anastomoses between the gluteal artery and IMA and the gluteal vein and IMV are usually performed in an end-to-end fashion with 9-0 nylon (Fig. 19-43). On completion, the Acland clamps are removed and the anastomoses are inspected for patency and blood flow. Adequate flap reperfusion is confirmed by observing distal dermal bleeding.

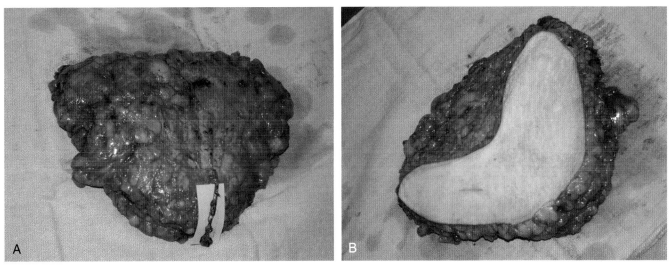

Figure 19-42

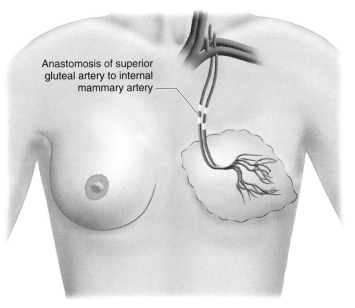

Figure 19-43

6. **Flap Insetting**

- The flap is then introduced into the mastectomy defect, orienting the pedicle without torsion.
- The gluteal subcutaneous fat is more fibrodense than that of the lower abdominal wall. With the standard elliptical flap, this can be problematic because of kinking of the perforator, but with the redesigned flap, the shape is built into the design. As a result, it is not necessary to shape the flap for inset. The flap requires only minimal plication to complete the shape of the reconstructed breast.
- The mastectomy flaps are then evaluated and trimmed as needed. The skin island of the flap is marked to the dimension of the mastectomy skin defect and the remaining flap skin is de-epithelialized. Drains are placed superiorly and inferiorly in the mastectomy pocket, away from the pedicle. The flap is then inset with 3-0 absorbable deep dermal inverted sutures; a running intradermal absorbable suture completes the epidermal closure. A hand-held Doppler ultrasound probe is used to locate transcutaneous arterial and venous signals, which are marked for postoperative monitoring.
- Figure 19-44 shows preoperative and postoperative views of the reconstructed breast and the donor site 3 months after revision.

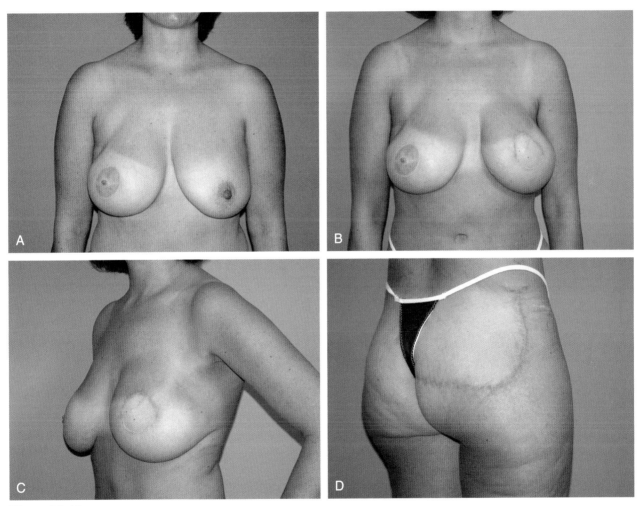

Figure 19-44

Case Example

- A 26-year-old woman (Fig. 19-45, *A*) with a 32C breast size and minimal abdominal adipose tissue and laxity (nulliparous) presented with right-sided breast cancer (stage IIA). A modified radical mastectomy and a delayed-immediate approach to breast reconstruction was planned because she was considered preoperatively to require postmastectomy radiation therapy (PMRT). After mastectomy a subpectoral, fully inflated tissue expander (400 mL) was placed to preserve the breast skin envelope. The tissue expander remained inflated during the 6-week interval between mastectomy and the start of PMRT.
- The expander was completely deflated during PMRT (6 weeks) and reinflated (Fig. 19-45, *B*) 2 weeks after the completion of PMRT to the predeflation volume (400 mL). The expander was removed at the time of the redesigned gluteal artery perforator flap reconstruction.
- Figure 19-45, *C* shows an intraoperative view of the patient in prone position with the redesigned gluteal artery perforator flap design marked on the left buttock. The black curvilinear line indicates the outline for the skin island. The red oval line indicates the sub-Scarpa fascial layer superomedial extension and subcutaneous inferolateral extension of the flap. The red "X" marks indicate audible Doppler signals at the preferred locations in the flap. The trochanter is marked in black on the lateral hip.
- Figures 19-45, *D* and *E* show the flap after harvest.
- Figure 19-45, *F* shows the patient after being repositioned supine with the flap temporarily in the axilla after completion of the microsurgery. The long pedicle length provided with the redesigned gluteal artery perforator flap allows for the flap to be positioned within the axilla during microsurgery. This makes the microsurgery easier because the thick gluteal flap does not interfere with the delicate hand movements required. The longer pedicle also makes it possible to use other recipient vessels (e.g., the TD vessels) while still positioning the flap medially on the chest wall.
- Positioning the perforator at the inferolateral aspect of the flap on the buttock (Fig. 19-45, *G*), placing the perforator near the internal mammary vessels on the chest wall, and the extended dissection of the gluteal vessels beyond the gluteal fascia all contribute to the long pedicle length. As shown, the perforator is located along the inferomedial aspect of the reconstructed breast, which avoids the full weight of the flap compressing the perforator against the underlying chest wall.
- Figure 19-45, *H* shows the redesigned gluteal artery perforator flap on the chest wall during insetting to create the breast form. The flap has been rotated 90 degrees counterclockwise from its orientation on the contralateral buttock, but has not yet been placed in the breast skin envelope. The superolateral border of the flap (buttock) has been rotated in a clockwise direction and plicated over the sub-Scarpa's fascial layer to enhance the vertical dimension and inferolateral aspect of the reconstructed breast. The superomedial aspect of the flap (buttock), the portion of the flap that includes only the tissue below the Scarpa fascial layer, will be positioned in the axillary region of the reconstructed breast, where it will supplant the axillary volume in this patient who underwent a level I and II axillary lymph node dissection as well as axillary radiation.
- Figures 19-45, *I* and *J* show the patient 2 weeks after a skin-preserving, delayed right breast reconstruction with a left-sided redesigned gluteal artery perforator flap.

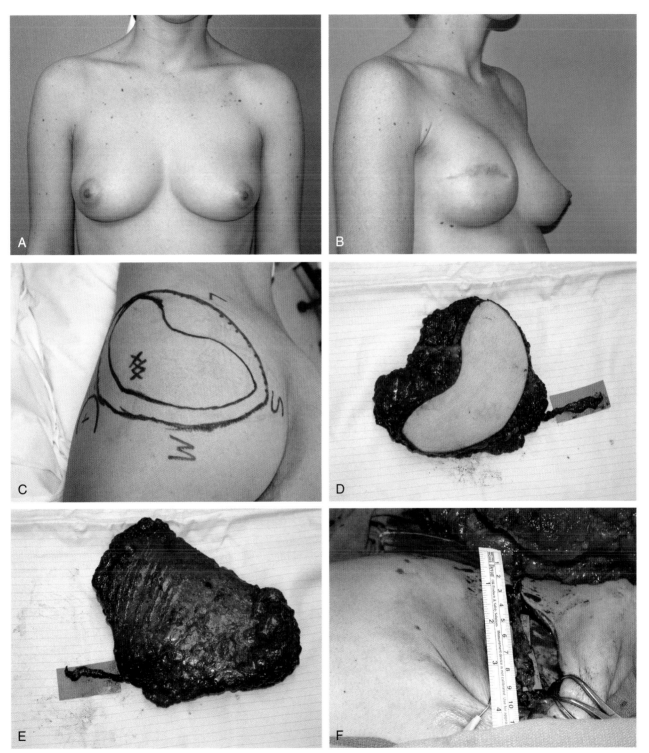

Figure 19-45

Step 4. Postoperative Care

- The patient uses several pillows for sitting to avoid undue pressure on the gluteal closure, but otherwise requires no specific bed positioning.
- The perfusion of the flap is assessed hourly, as previously indicated.
- The patient is maintained in a girdle to assist in recontouring the buttock region and to avoid seroma formation. Drains are maintained for 2 to 3 weeks to minimize the risk of seroma formation. Surgical revision of the donor site is deferred for 6 months to ensure sufficient tissue laxity to allow for advancement and de-epithelialization of the inferior skin flap underlying the superior skin flap.

Step 5. Pearls and Pitfalls

- Continue the proximal dissection of the inferior or superior gluteal artery until a large-caliber luminal diameter is available. A small arterial diameter significantly complicates the microsurgery and carries a higher rate of failure for these flaps.
- Avoid using a medially located perforator because this will limit the length of the donor vessels and lead to tension on the vascular pedicle when the patient is in an upright position, with a subsequently higher risk for flap failure.
- Avoid placing the patient in the corkscrew position to save time because this position for extended periods may be associated with subsequent back-related problems.

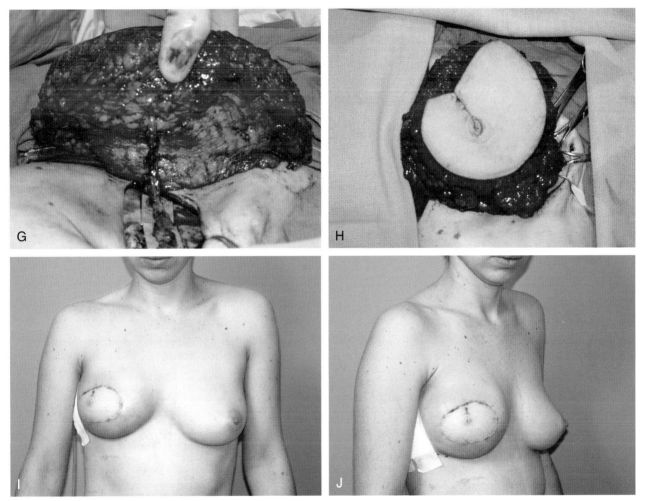

Figure 19-45, cont'd

Bibliography

A. Latissimus Dorsi Myocutaneous Flap for Repair of a Partial Mastectomy Defect

Clough KB, Kroll SS, Audretsch W: An approach to the repair of partial mastectomy defects. Plast Reconstr Surg 1999;104:409-420.
Hamdi M, Wolfli J, Van Landuyt K: Partial mastectomy reconstruction. Clin Plast Surg 2007;34:51-62.
Kronowitz SJ, Feledy JA, Hunt KK, et al: Determining the optimal approach to breast reconstruction after partial mastectomy. Plast Reconstr Surg 2006;117:1-14.
Levine JL, Soueid NE, Allen RJ: Algorithm for autologous breast reconstruction for partial mastectomy defects. Plast Reconstr Surg 2005;116:762-767.
Munhoz AM, Montag E, Fels KW, et al: Outcome analysis of breast-conservation surgery and immediate latissimus dorsi flap reconstruction in patients with T1 to T2 breast cancer. Plast Reconstr Surg 2005;116:741-752.

B. Latissimus Dorsi Flap with Breast Implant for Total Breast Reconstruction after Mastectomy

Munhoz AM, Aldrighi C, Montag E, et al: Periareolar skin-sparing mastectomy and latissimus dorsi flap with biodimensional expander implant reconstruction: Surgical planning, outcome, and complications. Plast Reconstr Surg 2007;119:1637-1649.
Munhoz AM, Montag E, Fels KW, et al: Outcome analysis of breast-conservation surgery and immediate latissimus dorsi flap reconstruction in patients with T1 to T2 breast cancer. Plast Reconstr Surg 2005;116:741-752.
Spear SL, Boehmler JH, Taylor NS, et al: The role of the latissimus dorsi flap in reconstruction of the irradiated breast. Plast Reconstr Surg 2007;119:1-9.
Tarantino I, Banic A, Fischer T: Evaluation of late results in breast reconstruction by latissimus dorsi flap and prosthesis implantation. Plast Reconstr Surg 2006;15;117:1387-1394.

C. Lower Abdominal Flaps: Transverse Rectus Abdominis Myocutaneous (TRAM) Flap and Deep Inferior Epigastric Perforator (DIEP) Flap

Bajaj AK, Chevray PM, Chang DW: Comparison of donor-site complications and functional outcomes in free muscle-sparing TRAM flap and free DIEP flap breast reconstruction. Plast Reconstr Surg 2006;117:737-746.

Kronowitz SJ, Hunt KK, Kuerer HM, et al: Delayed-immediate breast reconstruction. Plast Reconstr Surg 2004;113:1617-1628.

Kronowitz SJ, Kuerer HM: Advances and surgical decision-making for breast reconstruction. Cancer 2006;107:893-907.

Kronowitz SJ, Robb GL, Reece G, et al: Optimizing autologous breast reconstruction in thin patients. Plast Reconstr Surg 2003;112: 1768-1778.

Nahabedian MY, Momen B, Galdino G, et al: Breast reconstruction with the free TRAM or DIEP flap: Patient selection, choice of flap, and outcome. Plast Reconstr Surg 2002;110:466-477.

Saint-Cyr M, Robb GL, Chang DW, et al: Changing trends in recipient vessel selection for microvascular autologous breast reconstruction: An analysis of1483 consecutive cases. Plast Reconstr Surg 2007;119:1993-2000.

Serletti JM: Breast reconstruction with the TRAM flap: pedicled and free. J Surg Oncol 2006;94:532-537.

D. Gluteal Artery Perforator (GAP) Flap

DellaCroce FJ, Sullivan SK: Application and refinement of the superior gluteal artery perforator free flap for bilateral simultaneous breast reconstruction. Plast Reconstr Surg 2005;116:97-103.

Guerra AB, Metzinger SE, Bidros RS, et al: Breast reconstruction with gluteal artery perforator (GAP) flaps: A critical analysis of 142 cases. Ann Plast Surg 2004;52:118-125.

Hamdi M, Blondeel P, Van Landuyt K, et al: Bilateral autogenous breast reconstruction using perforator free flaps: A single center's experience. Plast Reconstr Surg 2004;114:83-90.

Heitmann C, Levine JL, Allen RJ: Gluteal artery perforator flaps. Clin Plast Surg 2007;34:123-130.

CHAPTER 20

UTILITY OF REDUCTION MAMMOPLASTY TECHNIQUES IN ONCOPLASTIC SURGERY

Gail S. Lebovic

Step 1. Surgical Anatomy

- ◆ Once the assessment has been completed regarding tumor size and location, attention is turned to the details of aesthetic qualities of the existing breasts, and the patient's desires. Symmetry, sensation, degree of ptosis, skin tone, stretch marks, and the like are all evaluated, noted, and discussed with the patient and documented with photography.
- ◆ Markings are placed on the patient before surgery with the patient in the upright position. Important anatomic landmarks include the following:
  - ▲ Suprasternal notch
  - ▲ Breast meridian
  - ▲ Inframammary fold
  - ▲ Superior areolar point (SAP)
  - ▲ New SAP
  - ▲ Distance to new SAP
- ◆ If the nipple–areolar complex (NAC) is to be preserved, it must be determined whether this can be accomplished on a tissue pedicle or if the NAC will need to be transferred as a free graft. If the new SAP is more than 10 to 11 cm from the existing SAP, the NAC will in many cases need to be removed and transplanted as a free nipple graft (particularly if the tissue is dense and firm). In the fatty, pendulous breast, the NAC tends to be more mobile, and often can be moved a greater distance while maintaining its attachment to the superior pedicle.
- ◆ The superior pedicle reduction mammoplasty relies on the following arterial blood supply (Fig. 20-1):
  - ▲ Lateral branches of the intercostal arteries
  - ▲ Lateral thoracic artery
  - ▲ Perforating branches off the internal mammary artery
  - ▲ Dermal plexuses of small arteries (mainly to the skin and NAC)
- ◆ In general, even a very large resection will not disrupt these arteries—hence the reliability of a good outcome in most cases when using this technique.

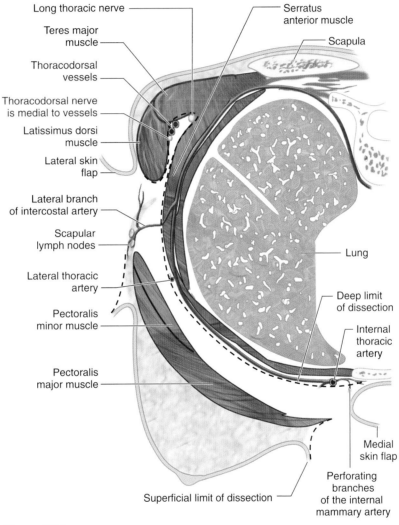

Figure 20-1

♦ Sensation to the breast is complex and consists of innervations of the skin and the NAC. The anterior cutaneous branches of the first through seventh intercostal nerves primarily innervate the skin overlying the medial aspect of the breast, whereas the lateral cutaneous branches of the second to the seventh intercostal nerves innervate the lateral aspect. The NAC derives its innervation from the anterior and lateral cutaneous branches of the fourth intercostal nerve, with contributions by the cutaneous branches of the third and fifth intercostal nerves.

♦ Before surgery it is of paramount importance to discuss potential changes in sensation to the skin overlying the breast and in particular the NAC with the patient. Although the surgical approach discussed here usually does not cause a loss of sensation to the nipple, changes may occur and patients should be prepared for and reconciled to this possibility.

Step 2. Preoperative Considerations

1. Patient Selection

♦ Reduction mammoplasty can be very useful in breast conservation surgery in appropriate patients. This technique is particularly helpful in patients with large or pendulous breasts, and with lesions located in the central and lower hemisphere of the breast (Figs. 20-2, *A* and *B*). Local tissue flaps are used to reconstruct the breast shape and the NAC is reconstructed with standard techniques. In selected cases the NAC can be preserved and relocated to its new position. The contralateral breast can be reduced or lifted at the same surgery and, if necessary, adjuvant therapy can be administered to the affected side after the healing period.

♦ Patient selection is critical, and a complete work-up including history and physical examination, detailed clinical breast examination, and thorough bilateral breast imaging (bilateral mammography, ultrasonography, and magnetic resonance imaging [MRI]) should be obtained before surgery. Preoperative *BRCA* testing should also be done in high-risk patients because if the result is positive, a different surgical approach may be considered.

♦ MRI is particularly useful in patients with newly diagnosed cancer to confirm the size and location of the tumor in the breast, and to determine any other evidence of disease (i.e., multifocal or contralateral lesions). Suspect lesions should be sampled for biopsy using minimally invasive techniques before definitive surgical resection.

♦ Three-dimensional MRI can be very helpful with preoperative planning.

♦ Marking the site of the tumor with the patient standing and lying down is important to determine whether the tumor bed will be excised with a generous margin within the boundaries of the reduction mammoplasty.

♦ Although there are numerous methods by which reduction mammoplasty can be performed, this chapter focuses on the superior pedicle or Wise pattern reduction mammoplasty. This procedure is the most straightforward for the surgeon in practice to learn and perform reliably.

♦ Additional medical problems and lifestyle issues such as smoking should be taken into account before surgery. These issues may increase the risk of complications such as delayed wound healing and infection.

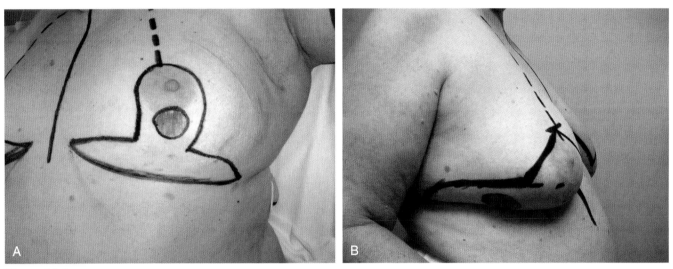

Figure 20-2

2. Preoperative Surgical Markings

- For preoperative marking, use a permanent marking pen (e.g., Sharpie) and an accurate measuring tape marked in centimeters.
- Begin with the patient facing you in the standing position. Sit in front of the patient.
- Mark the midline by drawing a vertical line from the suprasternal notch to the umbilicus (Fig. 20-3, A).
- Next, mark the breast meridian. This is done by measuring from the midline to the mid-clavicular point (usually 7 to 8 cm from the midline; Fig. 20-3, B).
- A vertical line is drawn from the mid-clavicular point down to the nipple (Fig. 20-4).
- Next, the new SAP is marked by placing a hand beneath the breast and resting the middle finger in the inframammary fold. A point is projected forward onto the breast and marked with the pen. This is the "new" SAP (Fig. 20-5).

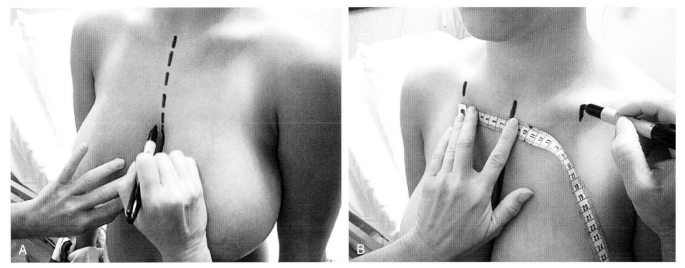

Figure 20-3

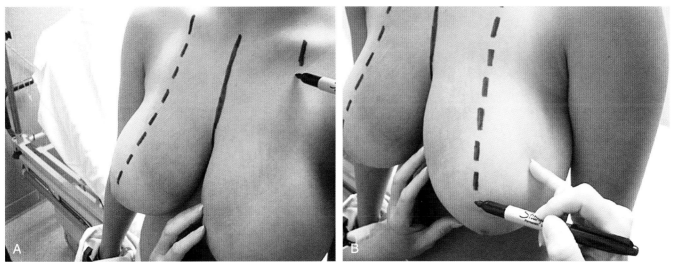

Figure 20-4

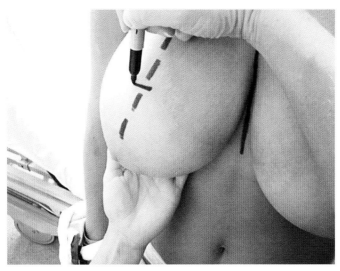

Figure 20-5

- From this point, measure and mark 10 cm medially (Fig. 20-6, *A*) and laterally (Fig. 20-6, *B*) from the new SAP.
- Mark the inframammary fold with the marking pen; this can be done at any point while marking the patient (Fig. 20-7, *A*).
- Mark a vertical reference line below the breast 8 to 9 cm from the midline. This will correspond to the breast meridian above and will be the point for approximating the breast once the resection is complete (Fig. 20-7, *B*).
- With the patient standing facing forward, grasp the breast firmly and pull the breast toward the midline. Draw a vertical line to connect the new SAP to the points previously marked at 10 cm, which are lined up with the reference point for the breast meridian beneath the breast (Fig. 20-8, *A*). Similarly, pull the breast laterally (Fig. 20-8, *B*) (*do not pull as firmly* when marking the medial aspect of the breast because this will result in a flattened shape of the breast).

Medial   Lateral

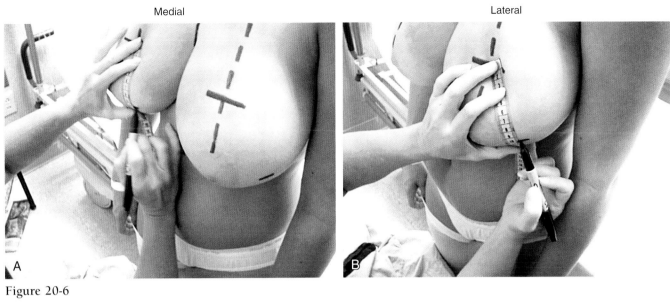

Figure 20-6

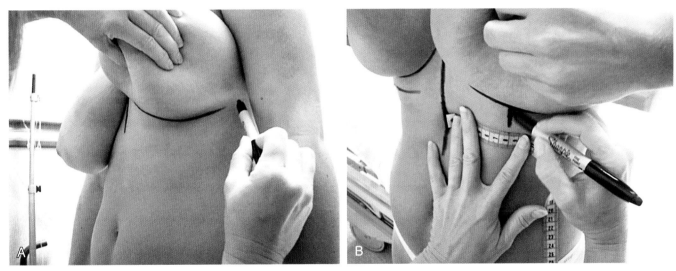

Figure 20-7

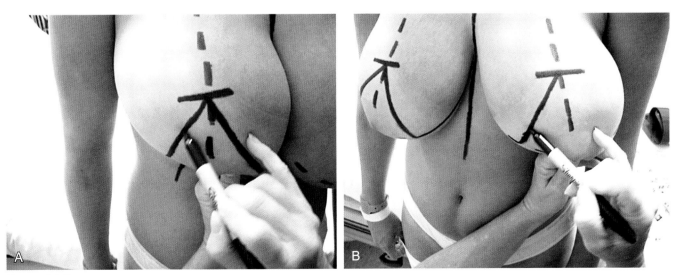

Figure 20-8

♦ Connect the vertical line to the inframammary fold medially (Fig. 20-9, *A*) and laterally (Fig. 20-9, *B*).
♦ Once the preoperative markings are complete, photographs are taken (Fig. 20-10) and the patient may proceed to the operating room.

3. Surgical Preparation

♦ We recommend wide skin preparation with povidone-iodine scrub and paint, followed by wide draping with sterile drapes. Caution the scrub nurse not to erase the skin markings.
♦ A Foley catheter is placed because most cases take 3 to 4 hours.
♦ We also use thigh-high TED antiembolism hose and compression devices during the case, and administer 1 g of cefazolin intravenously before surgery (in patients with penicillin allergy, we use ciprofloxacin 400 mg intravenously).
♦ The markings are then reinforced using methylene blue dye or a surgical marking pen.

Step 3. Operative Steps

♦ Dissection begins by scoring the outline of the areola using a "cookie cutter" nipple sizer (most common size is 4.2 cm). The NAC is placed on four-way stretch and the outline for the new areola is then made. The scalpel is used to score the area.
♦ A no. 22 scalpel blade (on a no. 4 handle) is used and dissection is carried down through the epidermis to the level of the deep dermis. Electrocautery is then used for the remainder of the dissection. This helps to significantly decrease the amount of blood loss during surgery.
♦ Next, the inframammary incision is made in the same fashion, and the dissection is carried down to the pectoralis major fascia using electrocautery (Fig. 20-11). The electrocautery typically is set to 40 to 45 (blend and spray). We use the coagulation mode for dissection rather than the cutting mode because this also helps decrease bleeding.
♦ The inferior segment of the breast is elevated off the pectoralis muscle fascia using electrocautery. Next, the medial and lateral incisions are made in the skin and the breast tissue is dissected free down to fascia. On completing this dissection, the inferior wedge of tissue will be free from the remaining superior pedicle with the NAC still attached (Figs. 20-12, *A* and *B*).
♦ Local anesthesia (1% lidocaine mixed with 0.25% bupivacaine, 1:1 dilution) is injected into the underlying muscle, and a 15-Fr round drain is placed through a stab wound incision at the lateral lower edge of the breast and secured to the skin with a single suture.

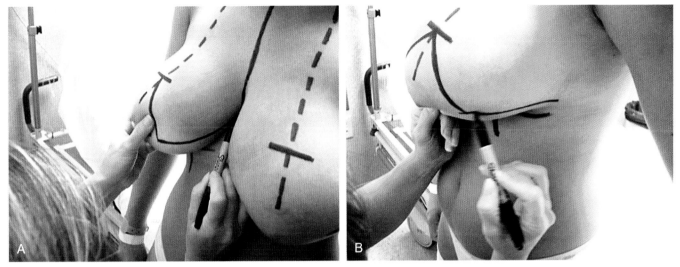

Figure 20-9

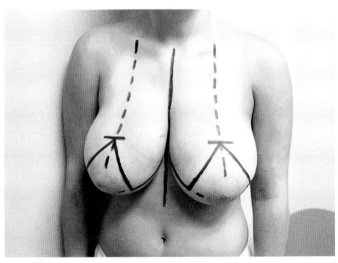

Figure 20-10

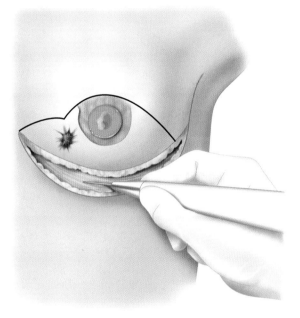

Figure 20-11

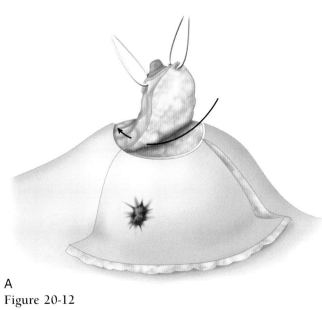

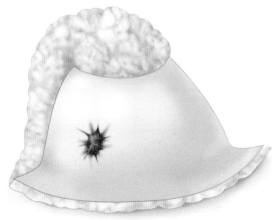

A

B

Figure 20-12

- Temporary closure is performed using skin staples. It is best to begin at the lateral edge, using firm medial pulling to approximate the skin edges. Skin staples are placed every 2 cm until the edge of the lateral flap is reached. Then the medial segment is secured, but when approximating the medial segment, the breast tissue is not pulled as firmly as the lateral aspect. This helps to preserve the conical shape of the breast, rather than giving it a flattened appearance (Fig. 20-13).

- If this technique is used for a **central** lumpectomy with a tumor adjacent to the NAC (partial mastectomy), the NAC and central pedicle of the breast is excised down to the pectoral muscle en bloc (Fig. 20-14). Next, the lateral and medial segments of the remaining breast tissue are brought together medially and laterally, and the deep tissues are approximated with a number of interrupted 3-0 Vicryl sutures.

- In either situation, the vertical incision is then closed temporarily with skin staples and the patient is placed in the sitting position to determine the position of the new SAP. In most patients, the NAC can be repositioned without difficulty. However, in some cases, the distance to the new SAP is greater than 10 cm, which usually is the limiting factor in raising the NAC on a pedicle. If this is the case, the NAC may need to be transposed as a free nipple graft, and it is secured in the same manner as a full-thickness skin graft.

- Once the new position for the SAP is determined, the segment of excess skin surrounding the NAC is de-epithelialized. The medial and lateral skin flaps adjacent to the vertical incision are undermined 4 to 5 mm to mobilize the NAC on the superior pedicle (Figs. 20-15 and 20-16). All bleeding is controlled and the wounds are irrigated and checked once again (see Fig. 20-12).

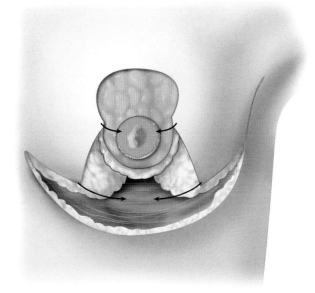

Figure 20-13

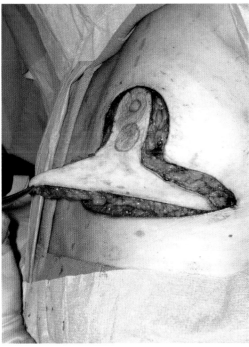

Figure 20-14

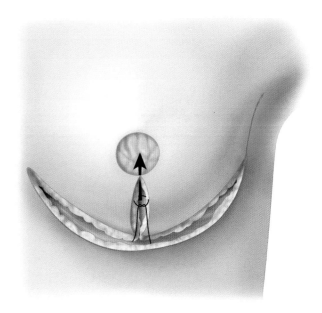

Figure 20-15

- The inframammary and vertical incisions are then sutured closed in a complex layered fashion beginning with 3-0 or 4-0 polydioxanone (PDS) or Vicryl. The first layer is placed in the deep dermis, and a buried knot is used. Next, a 3-0 Prolene is used to close the skin, and any fine details of skin approximation can be performed with 5-0 nylon suture. The Prolene stitch is left in place for 3 weeks during the healing process (Figs. 20-15 and 20-16).

1. Case Examples: Specific Application of Breast Reduction to Oncoplastic Surgery

Case 1

- In this patient (Fig. 20-17), an occult tumor located in the 6 o'clock position of the right breast was entirely removed within the inferior breast segment during the course of a routine reduction mammoplasty. The patient subsequently underwent radiation therapy, with some skin changes still evident.

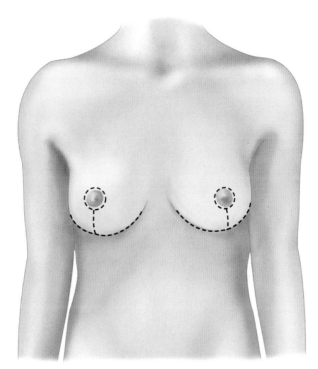

Figure 20-16

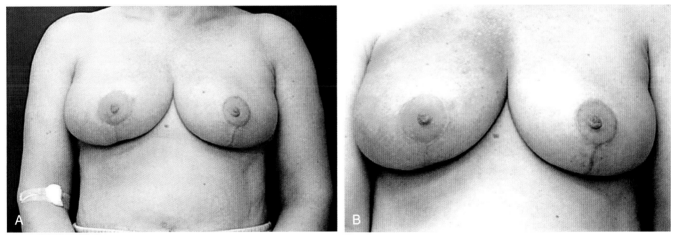

Figure 20-17

Case 2

◆ In this patient (Fig. 20-18), a central tumor of the left breast encroaching on the NAC was resected along with the NAC. The breast was then reconstructed using the local tissue flaps of the breast in the same manner as a breast reduction. She underwent postoperative radiation therapy and a subsequent nipple reconstruction. Note shrinkage of left breast following radiation.

Case 3

◆ This patient presented with ductal carcinoma in situ of the left breast and a family history of breast cancer (Fig. 20-19). Work-up revealed isolated disease in the left breast, and *BRCA* testing was negative. She had a skin-sparing mastectomy of the left breast with a two-stage breast reconstruction using a tissue expander, which was subsequently changed to a subpectoral saline-filled implant. She also had a right breast reduction and left NAC reconstruction.

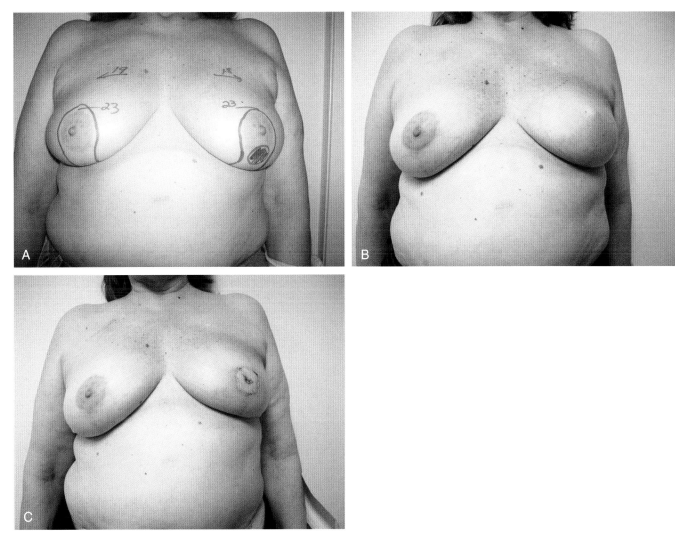

Figure 20-18

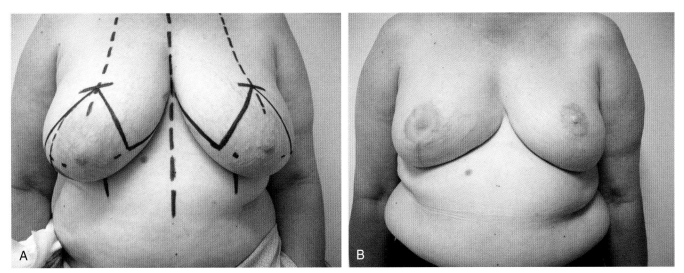

Figure 20-19

Case 4

◆ This patient had a long history of symptomatic macromastia and was found to have an invasive tumor in the inferior lateral aspect of the right breast (Fig. 20-20). She underwent right central partial mastectomy with reconstruction using the techniques described in this chapter, along with a left breast reduction. Ultrasound-guided wire localization and sentinel node biopsy were also performed at the time of surgery.

Step 4. Postoperative Care

◆ On completion, the chest is carefully cleaned and sterile dressings consisting of large petrolatum gauze (Xeroform; Covidien, North Haven, Conn) are placed directly over the incisions. Next, a sterile cotton roll is used for a soft layer of cushioning and then a breast binder or elastic bandage wrap is used for compression dressing. This should be firm but not tight. The skin under the drains is padded with cotton.

◆ Patients are placed on prophylactic antibiotics and remain on oral antibiotics for at least 2 weeks after surgery. The drains are removed when they are draining less than 20 mL over 24 hours. A supportive compression dressing (e.g., a sports bra) is worn 24 hours a day for the next 4 to 6 weeks.

◆ Exercise is limited to walking only during the first several weeks after surgery. These restrictions can be lifted as the patient progresses.

◆ The patient is not allowed to shower until the drains are removed.

◆ Regular activity is generally resumed 4 to 6 weeks after surgery.

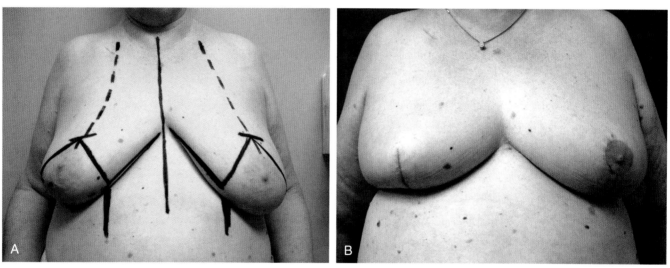

Figure 20-20

Step 5. Pearls and Pitfalls

- ◆ Thorough preoperative evaluation of each patient is critical, including MRI of both breasts.
- ◆ Before trying this procedure, it is recommended that surgeons learn the procedure by taking a course in oncoplastic surgery, practice the procedure in the cadaver laboratory, and scrub on a number of cases with an experienced surgeon in order to feel comfortable with the technique.
- ◆ This technique can be combined with other essential procedures such as preoperative wire localization, intraoperative ultrasonography, and sentinel lymph node biopsy.
- ◆ Sit the patient up several times during surgery to check symmetry (ensure the patient is secured to the table, and the table is working before induction of anesthesia).
- ◆ Prophylactic antibiotics can be discontinued after 7 to 14 days if there is no sign of infection.

Bibliography

Association of Breast Surgery at BASO, BAPRAS: Oncoplastic breast surgery: A guide to good practice. Eur J Surg Oncol 2007;33(Suppl): S1-S23.

Clough KB, Lewis JS, Couturaud B, et al: Oncoplastic techniques allow extensive resections for conserving therapy of breast carcinomas. Ann Surg 2003;237:26-34.

Clough KB, Nos C, Salmon RJ, et al: Conservative treatment of breast cancers by mammoplasty: A new approach to lower quadrant tumors. Plast Reconstr Surg 1995;96:363-370.

Lebovic GS, Laub DR, Berkowitz RL: Aesthetic approach to simple and modified radical mastectomy. Contemp Surg 1994;44:15-19.

Lebovic GS, Silverstein M, Laub DR: Oncoplastic surgery and breast health care. Semin Breast Dis 2004;7:140-147.

Petit JY, Rietjens M, Garusi C, Perry C: Integration of plastic surgery in the course of breast-conserving surgery for cancer to improve cosmetic results and radicality of tumour excision. Recent Results Cancer Res 1998;152:202-211.

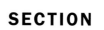

Extensive Resections

CHAPTER 21

CHEST WALL RESECTION

John Harrison Howard, Ching-Wei D. Tzeng,
R. Jobe Fix, and Kirby I. Bland

Step 1. Surgical Anatomy

- The chest wall, including skin, subcutaneous tissue, musculature, ribs, and parietal pleura, with potential extension into visceral pleura and lung parenchyma, can be removed for resection of locally recurrent breast cancer. Figure 21-1 labels major anatomic structures of the chest wall from an external view.
- Care should be taken to avoid injuring the intercostal neurovascular bundles at the superior and inferior edges of the resection by extending margins to the superior aspect of resected ribs.
- The internal mammary artery (IMA) should be preserved for reconstructive pedicle flaps or as inflow for free flaps if possible. The IMA is shown in Figure 21-2, along with major anatomic features from an internal view.

Step 2. Preoperative Considerations

- Indications for operation include isolated chest wall recurrence (Fig. 21-3), curative intent, or palliation for painful, nonhealing, ulcerated lesions.
- Absolute contraindications to resections with curative intent include systemic disease or multifocal recurrence.
- Relative contraindications include advanced age, short disease-free interval, poor pulmonary function, and high operative risk.
- Preoperative imaging and staging are essential for evaluation of chest wall anatomy, tumor invasion into the lung, metastatic disease, pleural effusion, and preoperative planning. Magnetic resonance imaging, positron emission tomography, and computed tomography are standard imaging modalities. Bronchial washings may be appropriate to rule out direct lung invasion if the imaging results cause suspicion.
- Resection extending beyond four ribs will usually require rigid chest wall reconstruction with a mesh and methyl methacrylate sandwich. Mesh alone may be sufficient for smaller defects with less risk of flail chest.

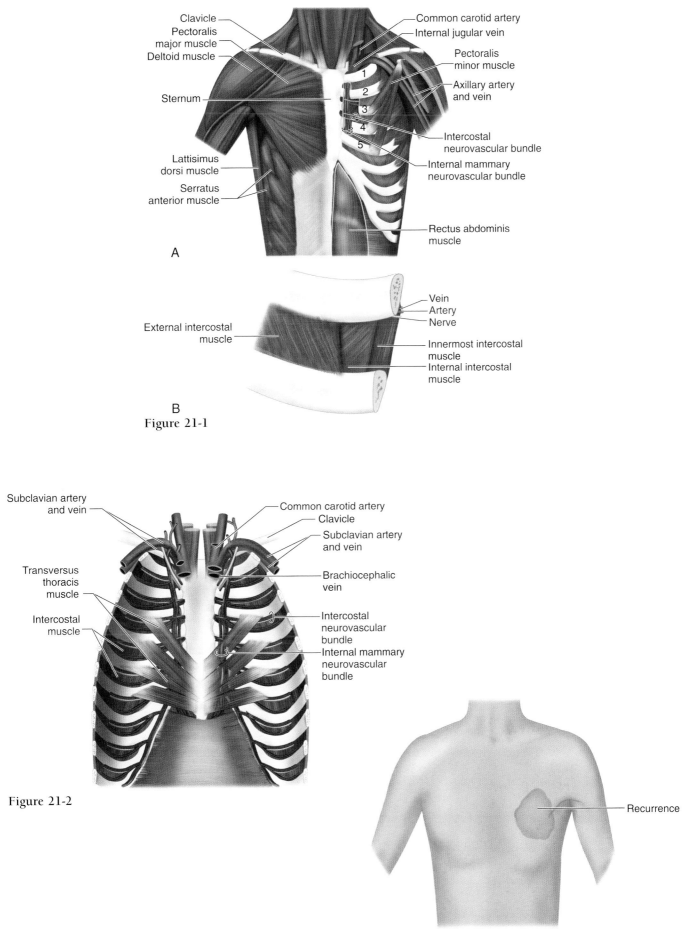

Clavicle
Pectoralis
major muscle
Deltoid muscle
Sternum
Lattisimus
dorsi muscle
Serratus
anterior muscle
Common carotid artery
Internal jugular vein
Pectoralis
minor muscle
Axillary artery
and vein
Intercostal
neurovascular bundle
Internal mammary
neurovascular bundle
Rectus abdominis
muscle

A

External intercostal
muscle
Vein
Artery
Nerve
Innermost intercostal
muscle
Internal intercostal
muscle

B

Figure 21-1

Subclavian artery
and vein
Transversus
thoracis
muscle
Intercostal
muscle
Common carotid artery
Clavicle
Subclavian artery
and vein
Brachiocephalic
vein
Intercostal
neurovascular
bundle
Internal mammary
neurovascular
bundle

Figure 21-2

Recurrence

Figure 21-3

- ◆ Recurrence location as well as the patient's operative history will affect flap choice for defect coverage. A latissimus pedicle flap is the most versatile and is usually the most readily available. Flaps from previously radiated fields should be avoided if possible.
- ◆ Preoperative planning between oncologic and reconstructive surgeons should help elucidate flaps that will be available after oncologic resection.

Step 3. Operative Steps

1. Incision

- ◆ The patient should be intubated with a double-lumen endotracheal tube. Positioning may be either supine or lateral decubitus, depending on location of recurrence and flap choice. Areas of potential flaps and skin graft donor sites should also be prepared and draped.
- ◆ Margins of 2 cm should be drawn around the planned area of resection. Margins should extend one intercostal space above and below the mass to the superior aspects of ribs. Circumferential full-thickness skin punch biopsies should be sent for frozen-section analysis to verify negative margins before incision (Fig. 21-4).
- ◆ Once preoperative negative margins are verified, extend the incision through the skin and the pectoralis muscles to the chest wall using electrocautery (Fig. 21-5).

2. Dissection

- ◆ Before entering the pleural space, the ipsilateral lung should be deflated. The thoracotomy should be initiated through the superior margin of the planned resection (Fig. 21-6).

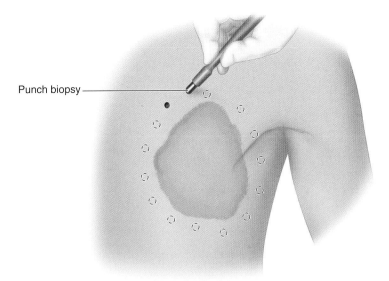

Punch biopsy

Figure 21-4

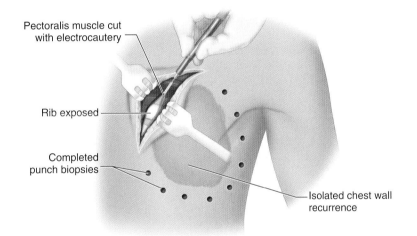

Pectoralis muscle cut
with electrocautery

Rib exposed

Completed
punch biopsies

Isolated chest wall
recurrence

Figure 21-5

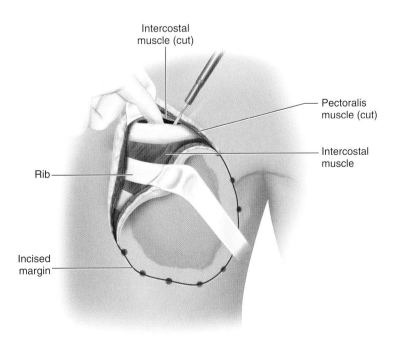

Intercostal
muscle (cut)

Pectoralis
muscle (cut)

Intercostal
muscle

Rib

Incised
margin

Figure 21-6

- On entering the thorax, pleural adhesions caused by previous radiation therapy or surgery should be bluntly dissected. If blunt dissection is inadequate, adhesiolysis should be performed with sharp dissection to avoid the formation of a bronchopulmonary fistula (Fig. 21-7). If the parietal pleura is grossly adherent to the interior surface of the chest, a complete pleurectomy may be necessary. Repair any pneumonotomies by oversewing with 3-0 nonabsorbable polypropylene sutures.
- After lysis of adhesions, the incision should be extended around the margin edges through the intercostal muscles. Double-ligate intercostal neurovascular bundles with 2-0 silk stick ligatures (Fig. 21-8).

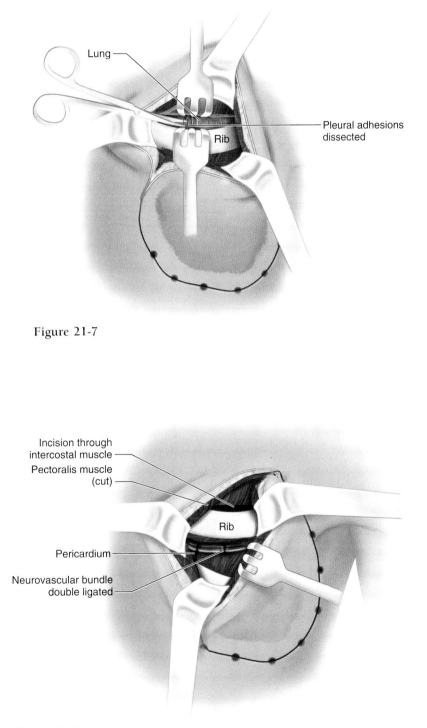

Figure 21-7

Figure 21-8

- As the incision is extended around the margins of the resection, the periosteum of the ribs should be elevated with a Doyen rib raspatory before using a rib cutter (Fig. 21-9).
- If the margin extends medially to the sternum, a sternal saw may be used for partial or total sternotomy. The incision should be extended to the sternocostal margin where the IMA may be palpated, ligated, and divided. The sternum may then be divided while protecting the pericardium.

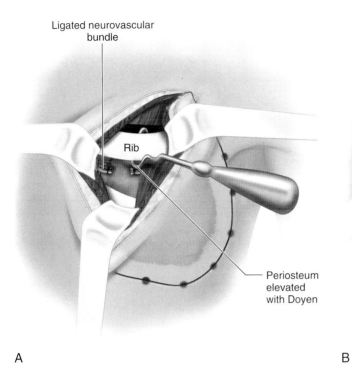

Ligated neurovascular
bundle

Rib

Periosteum
elevated
with Doyen

A

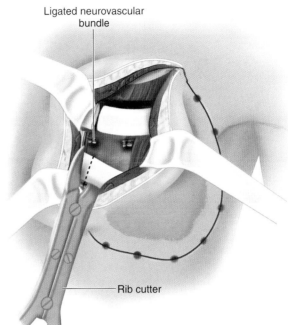

Ligated neurovascular
bundle

Rib cutter

B

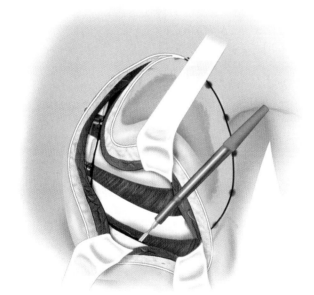

C

Figure 21-9

- ◆ The specimen should be removed en bloc, leaving the chest defect and exposed lung (Fig. 21-10, *A*). It is important to inspect the underlying lung for evidence of invasion. If invasive disease is detected grossly or by biopsy, a wedge resection of the involved lung should be performed (Fig. 21-10, *B*). The defect should be oversewn and tested for air leaks before closing the chest.
- ◆ Before closing the chest wall defect, two chest tubes should be placed. An angled chest tube is inserted inferior to the defect along the anterior axillary line and positioned anteromedially over the diaphragm. The second chest tube is inserted more posteriorly along the mid-axillary line and positioned toward the lung apex. Small-caliber tubes are usually sufficient to clear the resulting pneumothorax.

3. Reconstruction

- ◆ After measuring the defect, a methyl methacrylate and mesh sandwich should be shaped to fit the chest wall defect. The sandwich is layered as methyl methacrylate between two layers of mesh (or one large piece folded in half).
- ◆ The methyl methacrylate should be prepared and mixed on a back table. The methyl methacrylate should be shaped to be 1 cm thick and that circumferentially leaves a 1-cm margin short of the edges of the defect. This will avoid the potential for uncomfortable rubbing and clicking of the hardened methyl methacrylate against the ribs. As the methyl methacrylate is hardening, the mesh should be applied to both sides to form the sandwich. The hardening process is an exothermic reaction that has the potential to cause thermal injury to the lung. The sandwich should be allowed to harden and cool before being sewn into the chest wall defect.
- ◆ The methyl methacrylate and mesh sandwich is secured to the edges of the wound using either bone anchors or nonabsorbable 0 or no. 1 polypropylene sutures.

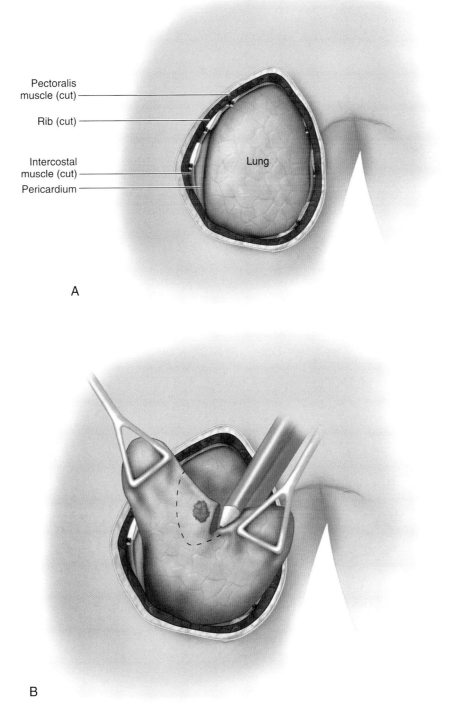

Pectoralis
muscle (cut)

Rib (cut)

Intercostal
muscle (cut)

Pericardium

Lung

A

B

Figure 21-10

◆ If sutures are used, the sandwich should be secured with horizontal mattress stitches placed in the intercostal spaces to avoid injury to the intercostal neurovascular bundles (Fig. 21-11). Sutures can alternatively encircle the ribs along the edges of resection. This method has a higher incidence of entrapping or injuring the intercostal neurovascular bundles while securing the mesh. Surgeon's knots should be tied on the anterior side of the mesh for either closure.

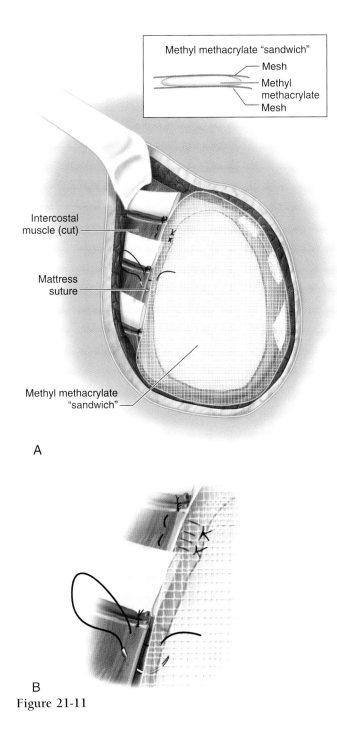

Methyl methacrylate "sandwich"
Mesh
Methyl methacrylate
Mesh

Intercostal muscle (cut)

Mattress suture

Methyl methacrylate "sandwich"

A

B

Figure 21-11

♦ After the methyl methacrylate and mesh sandwich is secured, reconstruction of the soft tissue defect can begin. A pedicled latissimus flap with a skin paddle is the most versatile flap for this area. Figure 21-12, *A* highlights the planned latissimus flap. Figure 21-12, *B* illustrates exposure of the latissimus muscle with the skin paddle. Figure 21-12, *C* shows the rotated flap covering the defect and sewn in place.

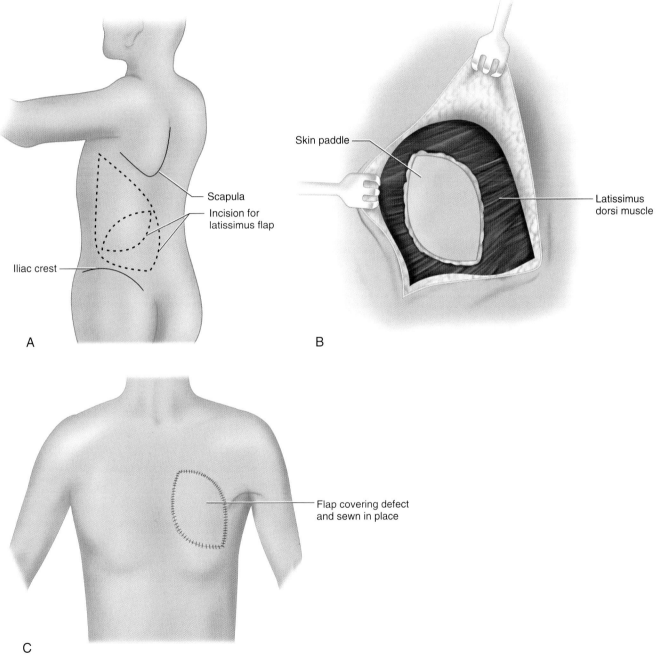

Scapula

Incision for
latissimus flap

Iliac crest

A

Skin paddle

Latissimus
dorsi muscle

B

Flap covering defect
and sewn in place

C

Figure 21-12

- An omental flap based on the right gastroepiploic artery may also be used to cover the defect. An upper midline laparotomy incision is used to approach the omentum. The omentum is transected from the splenocolic ligament to the base of the right gastroepiploic artery. Division and ligation of the vasa recta of the anterior and posterior leaves of the omentum are performed using 3-0 absorbable ties (Fig. 21-13).
- After exiting the midline incision, the omentum may be delivered to the chest by a retrosternal, transdiaphragmatic, or subcutaneous tunnel to the defect (Fig. 21-14). Care should be taken not to strangulate or twist the omental pedicle. Figure 21-15, A shows the omentum exposed. Figure 21-15, B shows the tunneled omentum in place. Planning of the defect coverage before the omentum is tunneled is optimal. Figure 21-15, C shows the flap covered with a split-thickness skin graft 3 weeks later.

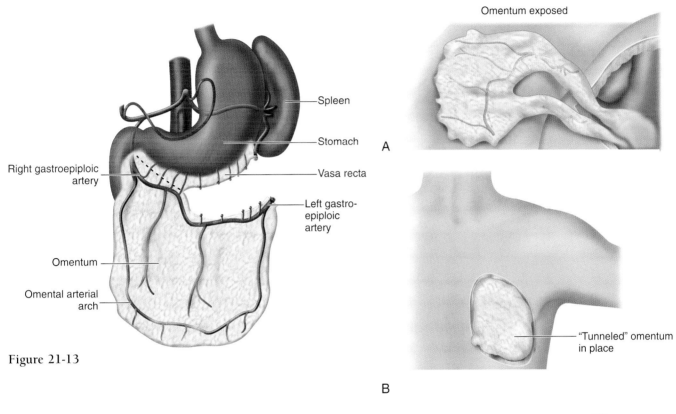

Figure 21-13

Right gastroepiploic artery

Omentum

Omental arterial arch

Spleen

Stomach

Vasa recta

Left gastro-epiploic artery

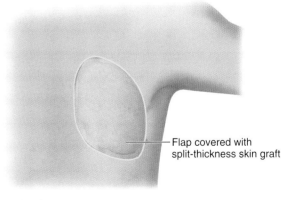

Omentum exposed

A

"Tunneled" omentum in place

B

Flap covered with split-thickness skin graft

C

Figure 21-15

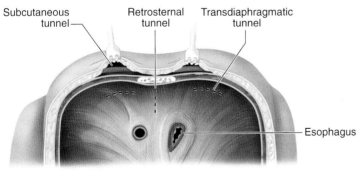

Subcutaneous tunnel

Retrosternal tunnel

Transdiaphragmatic tunnel

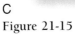

Esophagus

Figure 21-14

- Pedicled or free flaps using transverse or vertical rectus abdominis muscle flaps with skin paddles are possible alternatives for covering the defect. Free flaps may be anastomosed to the ipsilateral IMA as inflow (Fig. 21-16).
- Flaps should be closed in two layers. The deep dermal layer is closed with 3-0 absorbable sutures. A running subcuticular closure using absorbable 4-0 sutures is used for skin.
- Subcutaneous drains are also needed in the soft tissue reconstruction to prevent hematoma (Fig. 21-17). Internal Doppler probes may be placed for monitoring flap arterial supply.

Step 4. Postoperative Care

- Immediate postoperative extubation should be attempted in the operating room if possible. Minimized exposure to positive-pressure ventilation, especially in the setting of a lung resection, is optimal.
- Patients will require intensive care unit admission and may need ventilator management after surgery. Ventilator management should include preventive care for ventilator-associated pneumonia. Aggressive pulmonary toilet after extubation should be encouraged to prevent atelectasis and nosocomial pneumonia.
- Because of the extreme pain usually experienced with this procedure, postoperative epidural pain control should be considered.
- Wound care and flap management are necessary to monitor for flap ischemia or necrosis. Arterial supply can be evaluated by an internal Doppler ultrasound probe placed during surgery, a hand-held external Doppler probe, and capillary refill. Standard criteria can be used for removing chest tubes and subcutaneous drains.
- Complication rates for this procedure have been reported as high as 27% to 41%. Wound and pulmonary complications are the most common. Wound complications include infection, delayed healing, partial flap or skin graft necrosis, or complete flap loss. Pulmonary complications include reintubation, flail chest, or pleural infection. Despite the morbidity risk, the mortality rate for this procedure is low (<5%).
- A low threshold should be used for treating suspected wound or pulmonary infections.

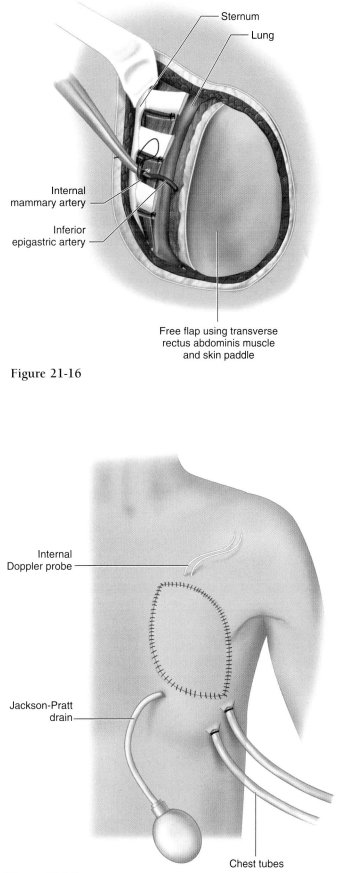

Sternum

Lung

Internal
mammary artery

Inferior
epigastric artery

Free flap using transverse
rectus abdominis muscle
and skin paddle

Figure 21-16

Internal
Doppler probe

Jackson-Pratt
drain

Chest tubes

Figure 21-17

Step 5. Pearls and Pitfalls

- ◆ Appropriate patient selection for chest wall resection is crucial. Curative intent requires ruling out systemic and multifocal disease.
- ◆ Preoperative evaluation of the patient's pulmonary function and reserve is important to minimize operative morbidity, especially if lung resection is anticipated.
- ◆ The complexity of these resections is often high because of previous operations (including past reconstructions), radiation, and patient comorbidities. Orchestrating preoperative collaboration between oncologic and reconstructive surgeons is critical for designing the best procedure for the patient.
- ◆ Preoperative skin biopsies around the planned margins of resection should be sent for frozen-section analysis before the initial incision because failure of the resection is usually from lymphovascular invasion of the skin. Frozen sections should also be sent from the deep resection margins before reconstruction begins.
- ◆ Ideally, margins should be at least 2 cm and should extend one intercostal space above and below the defect. Anatomic location may sometimes limit margins.
- ◆ Change the chest tube from suction to water seal as soon as possible to avoid venous congestion in chest wall flaps.

Bibliography

Beahm E, Hunt K, Pollock R: Surgical procedures for advanced local and regional malignancies of the breast. In Bland K, Copeland E (eds): The Breast, vol 2, 3rd ed. St. Louis, Saunders, 2004, pp 1235-1254.

Chang RR, Mehrara BJ, Hu QY, et al: Reconstruction of complex oncologic chest wall defects: A 10-year experience. Ann Plast Surg 2004;52:471-479; discussion 479.

Faneyte IF, Rutgers EJ, Zoetmulder FA: Chest wall resection in the treatment of locally recurrent breast carcinoma: Indications and outcome for 44 patients. Cancer 1997;80:886-891.

Fix R, Vasconez L: Use of omentum in chest-wall reconstruction. Surg Clin North Am 1989;69:1029-1046.

McCraw J, Arnold P: Latissimus dorsi. In McCraw and Arnold's Atlas of muscle and musculocutaneous flaps. Norfolk, Va, Hampton Press, 1986, pp 157-226.

Pameijer CR, Smith D, McCahill LE, et al: Full-thickness chest wall resection for recurrent breast carcinoma: An institutional review and meta-analysis. Am Surg 2005;71:711-715.

CHAPTER 22

FOREQUARTER AMPUTATION

Jennifer B. Manders, Jaime D. Lewis,
and Elizabeth A. Shaughnessy

Step 1. Surgical Anatomy

- Table 22-1 and Figure 22-1 detail the anatomic structures that must be identified to perform a forequarter amputation.

TABLE 22-1	**Important Anatomic Structures in Forequarter Amputation**
ANTERIOR CHEST (SEE FIG. 22-1, A)	**POSTERIOR CHEST**
Pectoralis major and minor muscles	Superficial (see Fig. 22-1, B)
Deltoid muscle	Serratus anterior muscle
Brachial plexus with axillary vein and artery	Deltoid muscle
Biceps brachii muscle	Trapezius muscle
Coracobrachialis muscle	Scapula
Coracoid process of the scapula	Infraspinatus muscle
Clavicle	Supraspinatus muscle
	Mid-depth (see Fig. 22-1, C)
	Levator scapulae muscle
	Rhomboid major muscle
	Rhomboid minor muscle
	Deep (see Fig. 22-1, C)
	Teres major muscle*
	Teres minor muscle*
	Deep and arm (see Fig. 22-1, C)
	Triceps muscle*

*Muscles constituting the rotator cuff.

Step 2. Preoperative Considerations

- Review of the anatomy of the shoulder girdle, including musculature, ligament and tendon insertions, and neurovascular structures, is essential.
- Because the normal anatomy may be obscured by or involved with a tumor, preoperative imaging with computed tomography (CT) or magnetic resonance imaging (MRI) may help with the identification of anatomic structures of interest. MRI of the brachial plexus is extremely useful to identify the proximal extent of tumor involvement. These imaging studies may then be used to develop an operative plan.

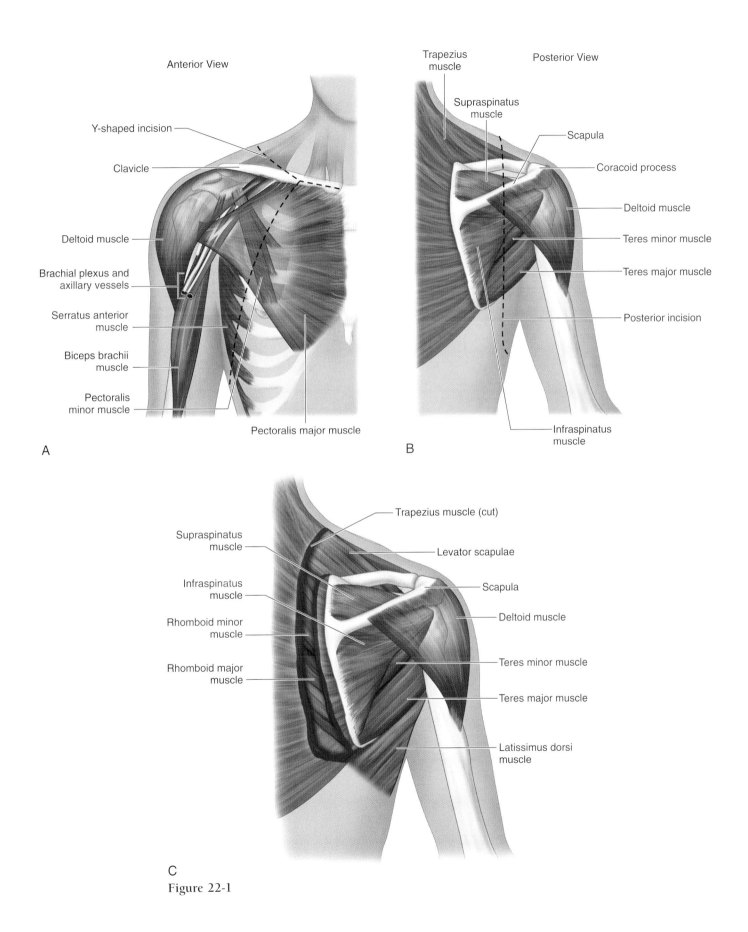

Anterior View

Y-shaped incision

Clavicle

Deltoid muscle

Brachial plexus and
axillary vessels

Serratus anterior
muscle

Biceps brachii
muscle

Pectoralis
minor muscle

Pectoralis major muscle

A

Posterior View

Trapezius
muscle

Supraspinatus
muscle

Scapula

Coracoid process

Deltoid muscle

Teres minor muscle

Teres major muscle

Posterior incision

Infraspinatus
muscle

B

Supraspinatus
muscle

Infraspinatus
muscle

Rhomboid minor
muscle

Rhomboid major
muscle

Trapezius muscle (cut)

Levator scapulae

Scapula

Deltoid muscle

Teres minor muscle

Teres major muscle

Latissimus dorsi
muscle

C

Figure 22-1

- On physical examination and imaging, attention should be paid to the surgical margins of resection. If the tumor extends beyond the clavicle, into the posterior triangle of the neck, or invades the chest wall, then residual disease after resection is likely.
- Patients should be counseled extensively about the risks and benefits associated with this procedure, and that anticipated survival and long-term prognosis are likely unaffected by forequarter amputation as a palliative or curative procedure.
- Phantom limb pain is often mild to moderate and usually controlled well with low-dose narcotics. Up to 60% to 90% of patients experience phantom limb pain, which may be exacerbated with previous exposure to chemotherapy or prolonged, uncontrollable preoperative pain.
- Metastatic work-up should include a bone scan and CT scans of the chest, abdomen, and pelvis. Thoracoscopy may be used to evaluate for the presence of pleural or parenchymal involvement.

Step 3. Operative Steps

1. Indications

- Forequarter amputation has been described historically as a useful procedure for locally advanced, high-grade bone and soft tissue sarcomas involving the shoulder girdle. More recently, its utility has been limited because of the increased use of neoadjuvant chemotherapy and radiation.
- Forequarter amputation may be of benefit in the case of locally advanced or recurrent metastatic carcinomas that affect the shoulder and are otherwise nonresectable by more common operations.
- Indications for the procedure may include the following:
  ▲ Local invasion along the rotator cuff and the scapula, including invasion into or ulceration of the axillary neurovascular bundle (brachial plexus or axillary vessels)
  ▲ Lymphangiosarcoma of the upper extremity (to include Stewart-Treves syndrome—resulting from long-term lymphedema after modified radical mastectomy with radiation)
  ▲ Salvage after failure of conservative management
  ▲ Severe, intractable pain with loss of limb function
  ▲ Local tumor-related complications: paralysis, tumor fungation, hemorrhage, sepsis, severe lymphedema, venous stasis with resultant limb necrosis, radiation-induced complications (severe brachial plexopathy)

2. Setup and Positioning

- The patient should be intubated with a double-lumen endotracheal tube.
- The patient should be placed in the lateral decubitus position, on a beanbag, with the affected side up. A pillow should be placed between the knees and, potentially, a roll placed under the dependent axilla (Fig. 22-2, A). Alternatively, if the hip is flexed, a bean bag can be skipped and the hip secured with tape to the table (Fig. 22-2, B). The affected extremity should be prepared in the field and covered with a stockinette per the surgeon's preference. The upper extremity is held by an assistant during the resection because dissection is both anterior and posterior. The extremity can then be maneuvered as necessary by resting the patient's bent elbow over the assistant's arm.

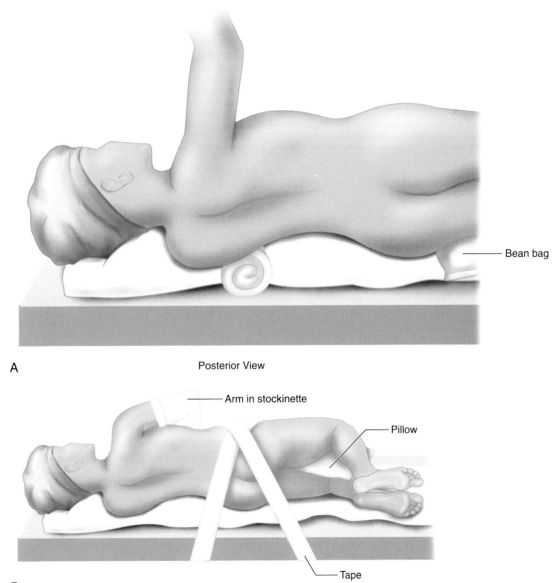

A   Posterior View

B
Figure 22-2

◆ Skin preparation of the upper extremity is performed circumferentially for its entire length, extending to the midline of the chest and back, and including the lateral thorax.

3. Operative Procedure

◆ Anterior exposure is performed to facilitate exploration of the infraclavicular portion of the brachial plexus and axillary vessels. This is begun with a **Y**-shaped incision below the clavicle, with one limb placed posteriorly across the clavicle onto the back (see Fig. 22-1, *A*) and one limb carried inferiorly along the deltopectoral groove, onto the chest wall, meeting in a loop under the arm (Fig. 22-3; see Figs. 22-1, *A* and *B*).

◆ The pectoralis major muscle is released from the humeral insertion, exposing the neurovascular bundle. The conjoined tendon (short head of biceps and the coracobrachialis), the coracobrachialis muscle, short head of the biceps brachii muscle, and pectoralis minor muscle are all subsequently released from the coracoid process, completing exposure of the neurovascular bundle (Fig. 22-4).

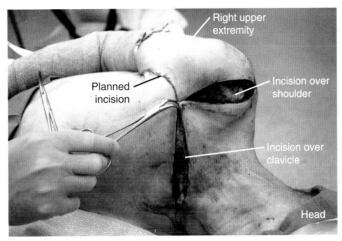

Figure 22-3

Anterior view

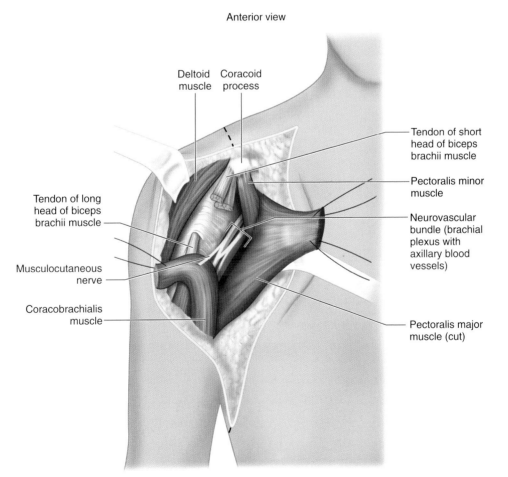

Figure 22-4

- ◆ Neurovascular encasement by tumor is then assessed. The subclavian artery and vein and the brachial plexus are individually doubly ligated and transected proximal to tumor and proximal to the planned clavicle resection (Fig. 22-5).
- ◆ The incision is extended posterolaterally over the shoulder, curving medially at the scapular tip, resulting in the construction of a medially based posterior fasciocutaneous flap. All muscles anchoring the scapula to the chest wall medial to the scapula (trapezius, and the deeper rhomboid major and minor muscles as well as the levator scapulae muscle) are released, after the arm is rotated anteriorly to place these muscles on tension. The serratus anterior muscle now anchors the upper extremity (Fig. 22-6).

Anterior view

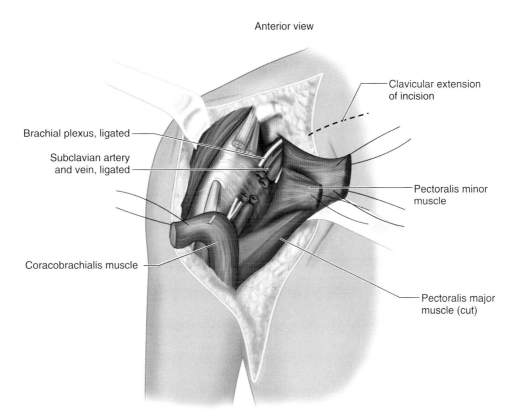

Clavicular extension
of incision

Brachial plexus, ligated

Subclavian artery
and vein, ligated

Pectoralis minor
muscle

Coracobrachialis muscle

Pectoralis major
muscle (cut)

Figure 22-5

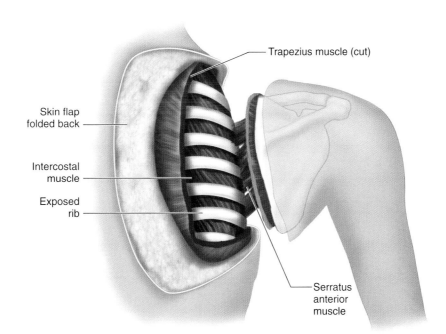

Trapezius muscle (cut)

Skin flap
folded back

Intercostal
muscle

Exposed
rib

Serratus
anterior
muscle

Figure 22-6

- The two skin incisions are connected under the axilla. The clavicle is osteotomized back one-third the distance from the acromion to the sternum (Fig. 22-7). The serratus anterior muscle is released from the scapula, usually along the rib insertion, and all remaining attachments to the humerus are divided. The arm is removed.
- The pectoralis major muscle is transected close to its origin or sutured to the chest wall (Fig. 22-8). Closed-suction drains are placed, and an epineural catheter can be inserted into the brachial plexus sheath, with delivery of a 0.25% bupivacaine bolus. A catheter delivering continuous bupivacaine can also be placed in the subcutaneous space. The flap is closed over the defect (Fig. 22-9).

Step 4. Postoperative Care

- The epineural catheter is kept in place until the patient is converted to oral pain medications. Neuropathic pain related to a brachial plexopathy or phantom limb pain not responsive to narcotics can be treated with γ-aminobutyric acid (GABA) receptor antagonists.
- Once incisions are healed, the patient can be fitted for a shoulder or arm prosthesis, or both. Physical and occupational therapy may be of great benefit for the patient, enabling her to resume activities of daily living.

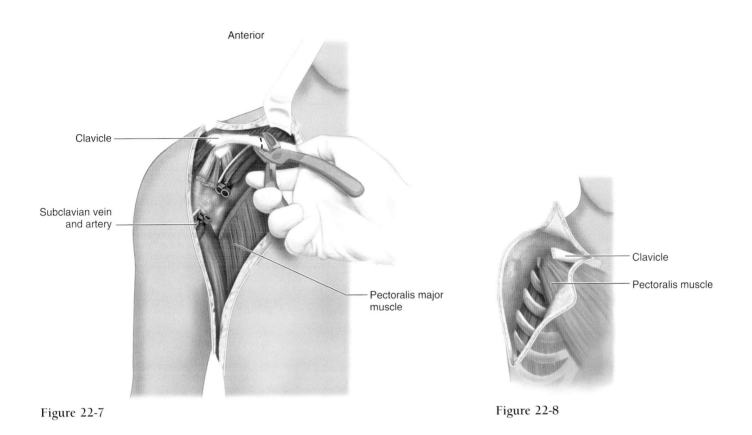

Anterior

Clavicle

Subclavian vein
and artery

Pectoralis major
muscle

Figure 22-7

Clavicle

Pectoralis muscle

Figure 22-8

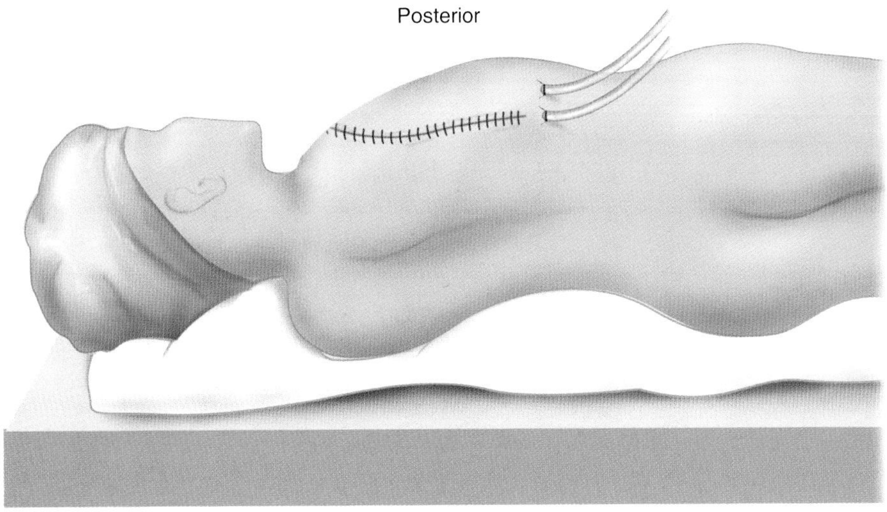

Posterior

Figure 22-9

Step 5. Pearls and Pitfalls

- Large defects caused by surgical resection can make the final wound edges difficult to reapproximate and may require the use of a split-thickness skin graft. If a posterior myocutaneous flap can be maintained without sacrificing surgical margins, this can aid in primary closure. Preoperative counseling and preparation of a potential harvest site should be included in surgical planning.
- Prostheses offered after forequarter amputation lack proprioception and precise movement. Shoulder pads help maintain normal contour, which is significantly affected by this radical procedure.
- Intervention with psychological counseling is extremely beneficial, especially in the preoperative setting, to help the patient prepare herself for the significant life change she will experience. Physical and occupational therapy should be instituted early in the patient's postoperative course. If available, contact with support groups or with other patients who have undergone forequarter amputation should be sought.

Bibliography

Bhagia SM, Elek EM, Grimer RJ, et al: Forequarter amputation for high-grade malignant tumours of the shoulder girdle. J Bone Joint Surg Br 1997;79:924-926.

Goodman MD, McIntyre B, Shaughnessy EA, et al: Forequarter amputation for recurrent breast cancer: A case report and review of the literature. J Surg Oncol 2005;92:134-141.

Moore KL: Clinically Oriented Anatomy, 3rd ed. Baltimore, Williams & Wilkins, 1992.

Sugarbaker PH: Forequarter amputation. In Sugarbaker PH, & Malawer MM (eds.), *Musculoskeletal surgery for cancer: principles and techniques*, pp. 306-316. New York, Thieme Medical Publishers, Inc., 1992.

Volpe CM, Peterson S, Doerr RJ, et al: Forequarter amputation with fasciocutaneous deltoid flap reconstruction for malignant tumors of the upper extremity. Ann Surg Oncol 2007;4:298-302.

Wittig JC, Bickels J, Kollender Y, et al: Palliative forequarter amputation for metastatic carcinoma to the shoulder girdle region: Indications, preoperative evaluation, surgical technique, and results. J Surg Oncol 2001;77:105-113.

SECTION 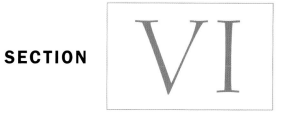 VI

Surgical
Techniques
to Assist
Irradiation

CHAPTER 23

MammoSite Balloon Catheter Placement and Other Brachytherapy Delivery Devices

Peter D. Beitsch

Step 1. Surgical Anatomy

- The placement of a MammoSite (Cytyc Surgical Products, Marlborough, MA) balloon requires a basic understanding of breast anatomy as well as a minimum level of ultrasonographic knowledge of the breast (Fig. 23-1).
- Cavity evaluation with ultrasonography is required to be able to measure skin-to-cavity distance (see Fig. 23-1) and to assess the entire lumpectomy cavity (Fig. 23-2) so the proper device and size can be selected. Skin-to-cavity distance is excellent at 18 mm with a fairly regular cavity of 36 mm × 25 mm (the cavity will conform to the expanded balloon).

Step 2. Preoperative Considerations

- The decision to place a MammoSite balloon or other brachytherapy device begins at the time of the initial evaluation of the patient with breast cancer.
- The size of the cancer itself as well as the tumor-to-breast size ratio is evaluated (a small breast may not be able to accommodate a MammoSite balloon, although the newer devices allow more flexibility). For MammoSite placement, a minimum distance of 5 mm from skin to lumpectomy cavity will be necessary after the lumpectomy. Other devices require less distance (potentially down to a 2-mm skin-to-cavity distance).
- The following are the generally accepted patient criteria for accelerated partial breast irradiation:
  - ▲ Age 50 years or older
  - ▲ Tumor size less than 3 cm
  - ▲ Negative margins

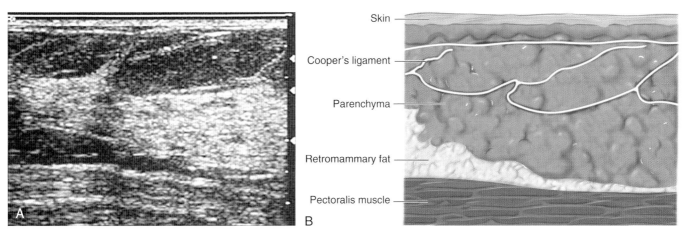

Figure 23-1

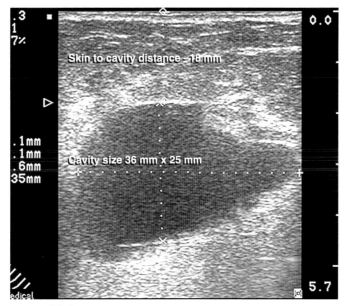

Figure 23-2

▲ Negative sentinel lymph node

▲ Ductal histology: infiltrating or ductal carcinoma in situ

◆ Discussing the possibility of accelerated partial breast irradiation before surgery, including a radiation oncology consult, will allow the patient to make a proper informed decision.

Step 3. Operative Steps

1. Intraoperative Placement

◆ Although most MammoSite balloons (and other brachytherapy devices) are placed postoperatively in the office, selected patients will have a balloon placed in the operating room. Reasons for intraoperative placement could include the following:

▲ Patient unable to tolerate minor procedures in the office because of fears or the need for very close monitoring

▲ Patient convenience during a re-lumpectomy for a close or positive margin

◆ The MammoSite placement begins after the lumpectomy and sentinel node biopsy (with intraoperative margin and sentinel node evaluation).

◆ A new lateral incision (or potentially medial or other incision) is made remote from the lumpectomy incision (Fig. 23-3).

◆ The trocar provided in the MammoSite kit (or a Kelly clamp or hemostat) is used to create a track into the lumpectomy cavity (Fig. 23-4).

◆ The deflated MammoSite balloon is placed through the incision into the track and advanced into the lumpectomy cavity. After the balloon is in the cavity, it is inflated to assess its position in the cavity (Fig. 23-5).

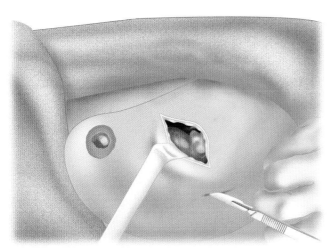

Figure 23-3

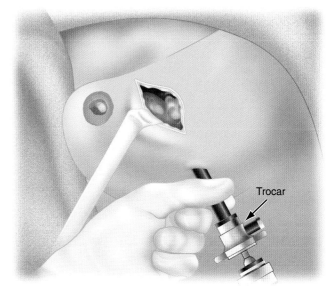

Figure 23-4

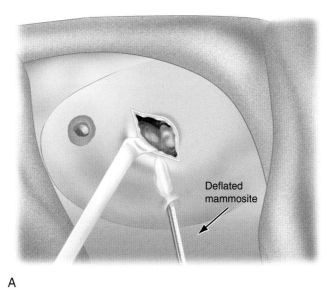

A

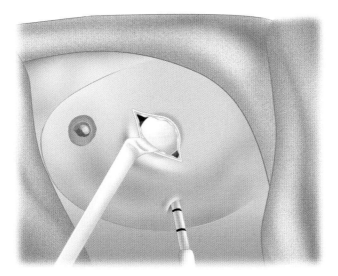

B

Figure 23-5

◆ The MammoSite balloon is deflated and the lumpectomy cavity is closed in layers to ensure a minimum of 5 mm and, ideally, greater than a full centimeter of tissue between the cavity and the skin (Fig. 23-6).

◆ Once the skin is closed, the balloon is reinflated (Fig. 23-7) and the skin-to-balloon distance is evaluated by ultrasonography (Fig. 23-8). The skin-to-balloon distance in Figure 23-8 is 16 mm, and the balloon diameter is 37 mm.

◆ The skin is closed and the usual sterile dressings are applied (Fig. 23-9).

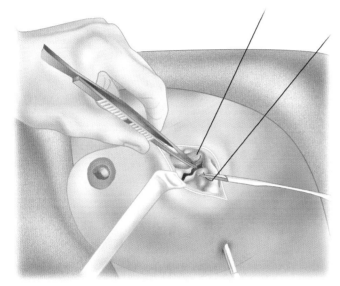

Figure 23-6

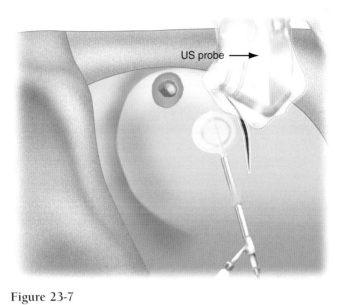

Figure 23-7

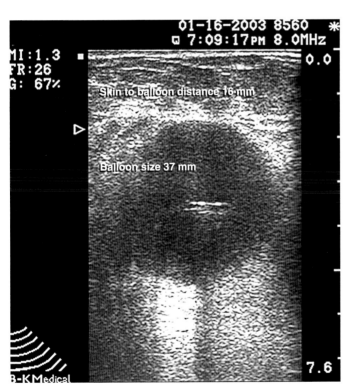

Figure 23-8

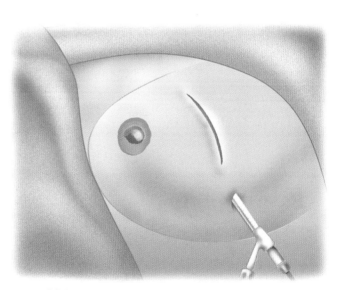

Figure 23-9

2. Postoperative Placement

Lateral Placement

- Most MammoSite balloons (and other brachytherapy devices) are placed in the office once the pathologic examination is complete. This ensures that the margins are negative and the sentinel lymph nodes are without metastases.
- Once the pathology requirements have been met, the first step is to evaluate the cavity and the skin-to-cavity distance (minimum 5 mm, and preferably >7 mm) to ensure the patient is still a candidate for MammoSite balloon placement. However, other devices require less skin-to-cavity distance and could be considered if spacing appears to be an issue (Fig. 23-10, *A*).
- The patient is then sterilely prepared and draped. A lateral stab incision (or occasionally medial or other locations) is made with a no. 11 blade (Fig. 23-10, *B*).
- The trocar provided in the MammoSite kit (or a Kelly clamp or hemostat) is used to create a track into the lumpectomy cavity. This is done under ultrasonographic guidance (Fig. 23-10, *C*).
- The uninflated balloon is placed through the skin nick, down the track, and into the cavity under ultrasonographic guidance (Figs. 23-10, *D* and *E*).
- The MammoSite balloon is inflated and a sterilely draped ultrasound probe is used to evaluate the skin-to-cavity distance and the balloon-to-cavity conformance (Fig. 23-10, *F*).
- A sterile dressing is then applied.

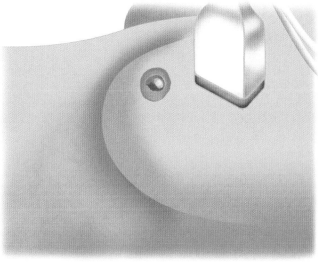

A

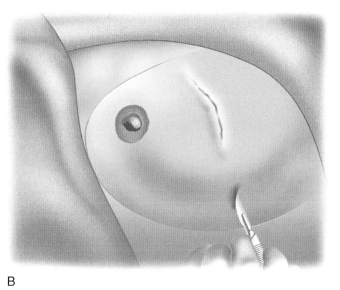

B

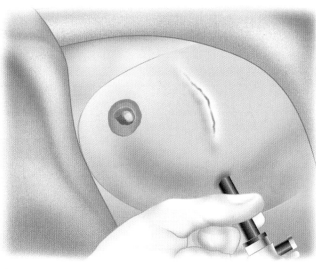

C

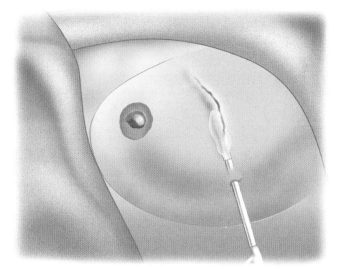

D

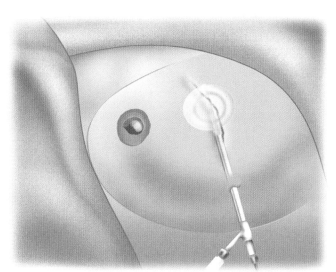

E

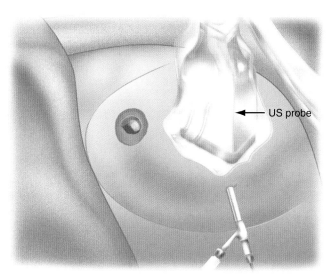

F

Figure 23-10

Scar Entry Technique

- To ensure adequate skin spacing, the cavity is evaluated by ultrasonography before deciding the patient is a MammoSite candidate (Fig. 23-11, *A*).
- The patient is then sterilely prepared and draped. A hemostat or Kelly clamp is used to slightly open the incision and then plunged into the cavity under direct ultrasonographic guidance (Fig. 23-11, *B*).
- The uninflated MammoSite balloon is placed through the incision into the cavity (Fig. 23-11, *C*).
- The balloon is inflated and the incision is sutured on either side to ensure the wound stays closed (Fig. 23-11, *D*).
- The balloon is evaluated by ultrasonography to ensure adequate skin spacing and good balloon-to-cavity conformance (Fig. 23-11, *E*).

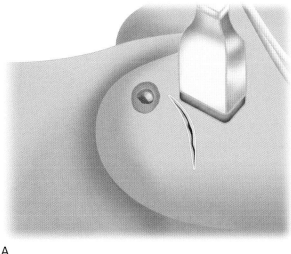

A

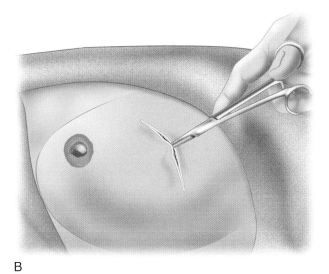

B

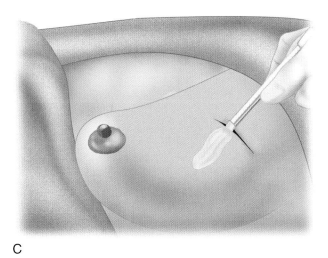

C

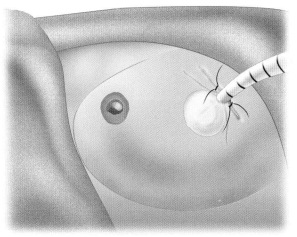

D

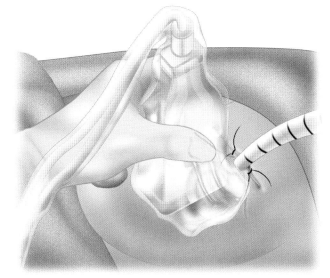

E

Figure 23-11

3. New Multicatheter Brachytherapy Delivery Devices

◆ All these devices allow treatment plans that reduce radiation dose to the skin and therefore allow a narrower skin-to-cavity distance.
  ▲ ClearPath (Renata Medical, Irvine, CA) is a single-entry, multicatheter device with a set of outer, nonfunctional struts to displace the breast tissue (similar to the balloon) and inner treatment struts (Fig. 23-12).
  ▲ Contura (SenoRx, Inc., Aliso Viejo, CA) is a single-insertion, multicatheter balloon device that has a stiff polyurethane balloon (which helps with cavity conformance) and five catheters contained within the balloon. There are also suction ports at the distal and proximal ends of the balloon to allow for aspiration of fluid around the balloon (Fig. 23-13).
  ▲ SAVI (Cianna Medical, Inc., Aliso Viejo, CA) is a single-entry, multicatheter device with 6, 8, or 10 struts that are in contact with the breast tissue (Fig. 23-14).

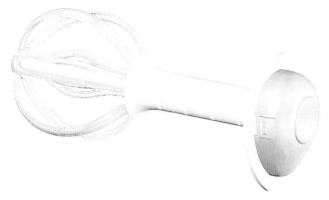

Figure 23-12
©Renata Medical, Irvine, CA.

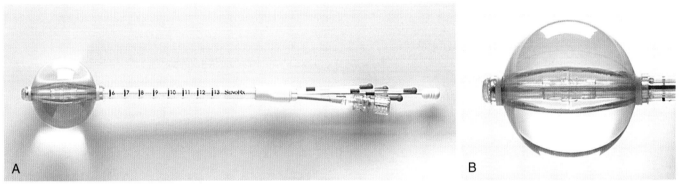

Figure 23-13
©SenoRx, Inc., Aliso Viejo, CA.

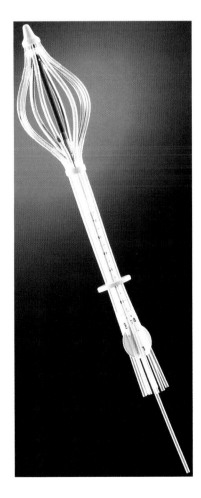

Figure 23-14
©Cianna Medical, Inc., Aliso Viejo, CA.

4. **Electronic Brachytherapy System**

 ◆ Current brachytherapy techniques all involve a radioactive source. Xoft (Sunnyvale, CA) has developed the Axxent, a miniaturized x-ray source that delivers a dose of radiation to the lumpectomy cavity similar to an iridium source (Fig. 23-15). The miniaturized x-ray source is delivered through a balloon device similar to a MammoSite balloon. The Xoft balloon has suction ports at the proximal and distal ends to allow for aspiration of fluid from around the balloon (Fig. 23-16).

Step 4. Postoperative Care

 ◆ After the last treatment (typically on Friday after the afternoon fraction), the balloon and multicatheter devices are removed by deflating the balloon or collapsing the multicatheters and pulling them out through the entry track. Steri-Strips are used to close the entry stab incision.
 ◆ Patients are usually seen in 1 to 2 weeks to evaluate the small incision and to assess the radiation effects.

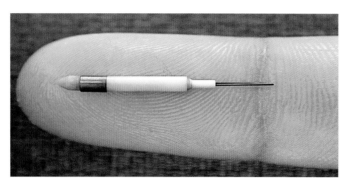

Figure 23-15
©Xoft, Inc., Sunnyvale, CA.

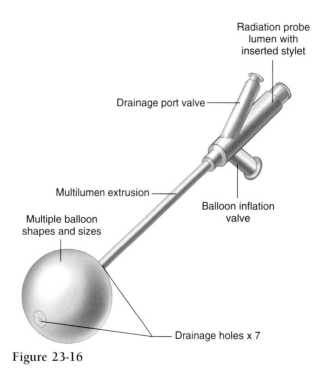

Figure 23-16

Step 5. Pearls and Pitfalls

◆ When placing a MammoSite (or any other device), there may be a significant amount of drainage from the small lateral incision. Discussing this with the patient will often save a midnight phone call.
◆ After placing a MammoSite balloon, fluid may be trapped between the balloon and the lumpectomy cavity wall. Gentle breast massage can be used to evacuate this fluid through the track and out the lateral stab incision.
◆ If the MammoSite is being placed in the operating room, sometimes the skin-to-balloon distance is inadequate. This can be solved by opening the wound, removing the thin skin flaps, and reapproximating more subcutaneous tissue before closing the skin.
◆ There is a finite amount of time between the lumpectomy surgery and the placement of the MammoSite or other brachytherapy device (usually less than 4 weeks). As the lumpectomy cavity heals, it will become progressively more fibrotic and less distensible, eventually disappearing entirely. This healing fibrosis may make symmetric deployment of the MammoSite balloon difficult (this may be less of an issue with the stiffer Contura polyurethane balloon or the multicatheter devices). Therefore, earlier placement of the MammoSite or other device is advisable.
◆ One of the advantages of brachytherapy is that all the radiation therapy is completed before the initiation of systemic therapy. However, to avoid radiation recall, chemotherapy should be delayed at least 3 weeks after completion of the brachytherapy.

Bibliography

Arthur DW, Vicini FA: Accelerated partial breast irradiation as a part of breast conservation therapy. J Clin Oncol 2005;23:1726-1735.

Chen PY, Vicini FA, Benitez P, et al: Long-term cosmetic results and toxicity after accelerated partial-breast irradiation. Cancer 2006;106:991-999.

Keisch M, Vicini F, Kuske RR, et al: Initial clinical experience with the MammoSite breast brachytherapy applicator in women with early-stage breast cancer treated with breast-conserving therapy. Int J Radiat Oncol Biol Phys 2003;55:289-293.

Kuske RR, Winter K, Arthur DW, et al: Phase II trial of brachytherapy alone after lumpectomy for select breast cancer: Toxicity analysis of RTOG 95-17. Int J Radiat Oncol Biol Phys 2006;65:45-51.

NSABP B-39, RTOG 0413: A randomized phase III study of conventional whole breast irradiation versus partial breast irradiation for women with stage 0, I, or II breast cancer. Clin Adv Hematol Oncol 2006;4:719-721.

Vicini FA, Antonucci JV, Wallace M, et al: Long-term efficacy and patterns of failure after accelerated partial breast irradiation: A molecular assay-based clonality evaluation. Int J Radiat Oncol Biol Phys 2007;68:341-346.

Vicini FA, Beitsch PD, Quiet CA, et al: First analysis of patient demographics, technical reproducibility, cosmesis, and early toxicity: Results of the American Society of Breast Surgeons MammoSite breast brachytherapy trial. Cancer 2005;104:1138-1148.

Zannis V, Beitsch P, Vicini F, et al: Descriptions and outcomes of insertion techniques of a breast brachytherapy balloon catheter in 1403 patients enrolled in the American Society of Breast Surgeons MammoSite breast brachytherapy registry trial. Am J Surg 2005;190:530-538.

In Vivo Intraoperative Radiation Therapy for Breast Cancer

Nancy Klauber-DeMore, Carolyn I. Sartor, and David W. Ollila

Step 1. Surgical Anatomy

- The adult breast lies between the second and sixth ribs and between the sternal edge and the mid-axillary line.
- Figure 24-1 demonstrates the major anatomic structures of the chest wall from an external view.

Step 2. Preoperative Considerations

- An increasing number of studies are attempting to decrease the overall treatment time for radiation after lumpectomy. To be considered for intraoperative radiation therapy (IORT) of the breast, the patient should be a breast-conservation candidate with an invasive ductal carcinoma with no extensive intraductal component. The tumor size should be 3 cm or less based on physical examination, mammography, and ultrasonography. The patient must be at least 48 years of age, and the tumor must be able to be visualized on ultrasonography.
- Exclusion criteria for breast IORT are invasive lobular carcinoma, ductal carcinoma in situ, extensive intraductal component, and pregnancy.
- The tumor is localized with a wire, and technetium sulfur colloid is injected for the sentinel lymph node biopsy.
- Breast ultrasonography is performed to define the target volume. Three distances are measured along the axis of the planned IORT delivery, usually the shortest distance from skin to tumor: (1) from the skin to the middle of the breast cancer, (2) from the skin to the posterior edge of the tumor, and (3) from the skin to the anterior surface of the pleural surface. These measurements will then be used by the treating radiation oncologist to determine dosimetry curves and the electron energy and applicator size required to deliver 15 Gy to the 90% isodose line covering the tumor with a 1-cm anteroposterior margin and a 2-cm lateral margin.

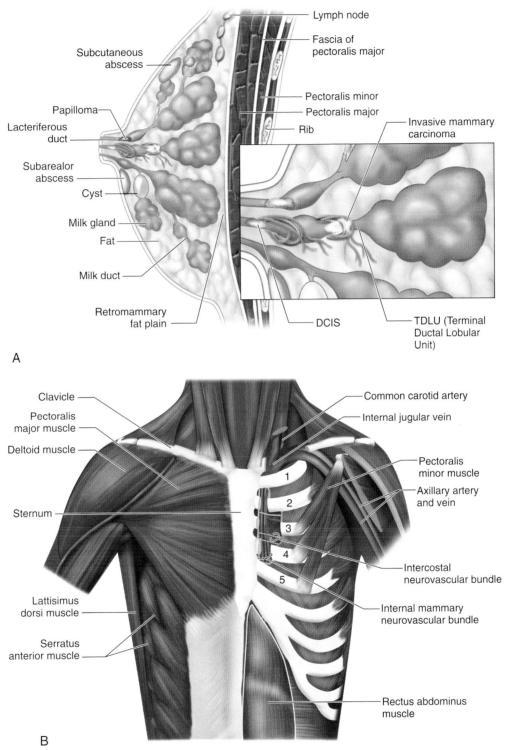

Lymph node

Fascia of
pectoralis major

Pectoralis minor

Pectoralis major

Rib

Invasive mammary
carcinoma

Subcutaneous
abscess

Papilloma

Lacteriferous
duct

Subarealor
abscess

Cyst

Milk gland

Fat

Milk duct

Retromammary
fat plain

DCIS

TDLU (Terminal
Ductal Lobular
Unit)

A

Clavicle

Pectoralis
major muscle

Deltoid muscle

Sternum

Lattisimus
dorsi muscle

Serratus
anterior muscle

Common carotid artery

Internal jugular vein

Pectoralis
minor muscle

Axillary artery
and vein

Intercostal
neurovascular bundle

Internal mammary
neurovascular bundle

Rectus abdominus
muscle

1
2
3
4
5

B

Figure 24-1

- The operating room table is turned 180 degrees so it can be moved under the Mobetron (IntraOp Medical Corporation, Sunnyvale, CA) machine. The patient is placed on the operating table in the supine position and general anesthesia is administered. A secure seatbelt is tightly fastened. Isosulfan blue (Lymphazurin) or methylene blue dye is injected peritumorally. The patient is prepared and draped in standard fashion.

Step 3. Operative Steps

1. Incision

- The incision needs to be large enough to encompass the diameter of the applicator used for the IORT. For example, if a 6-cm-diameter applicator is used, the incision must be at least 6 cm (Fig. 24-2).

2. Tumor Exposure

- The sentinel node biopsy is performed before IORT in standard fashion (see Chapter 10).
- An incision is made in the breast and very wide, thin skin flaps are raised (Fig. 24-3).

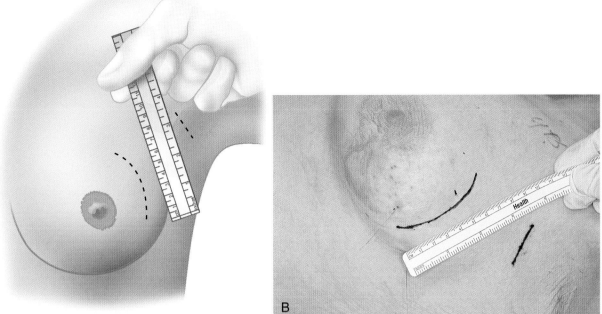

A

B

Figure 24-2

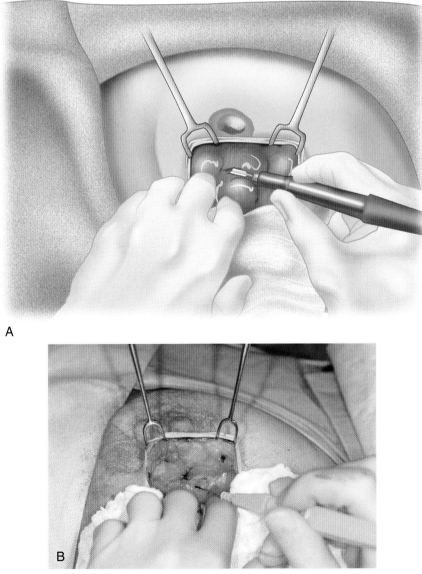

A

B

Figure 24-3

◆ A silk stitch is placed in the tumor and the stitch is kept long (Fig. 24-4). The stitch will be used later to position the tumor in the center of the applicator.

3. Delivery of Intraoperative Radiation Therapy

◆ IORT is delivered using a Mobetron device, which is a self-shielded, magnetron-driven, X-band linear accelerator specifically developed for IORT. This machine produces a megavoltage electron beam of energies ranging from 4 to 12 MeV. The radiation is delivered from the Mobetron to the tumor bed through an attached applicator.
◆ The sizes of applicators available for the Mobetron range from 3 to 10 cm in diameter. An applicator is selected that encompasses the tumor along with a 2-cm radial margin. The applicator is placed into the incision (Fig. 24-5).

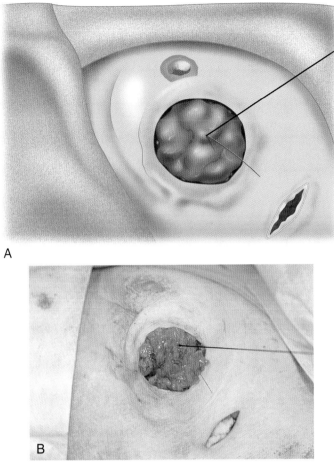

A

B

Figure 24-4

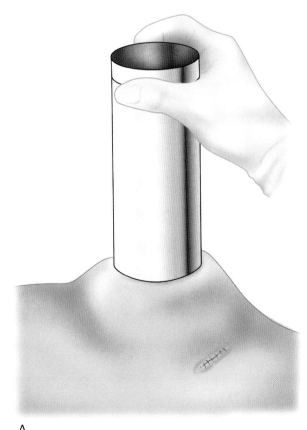

A

Figure 24-5

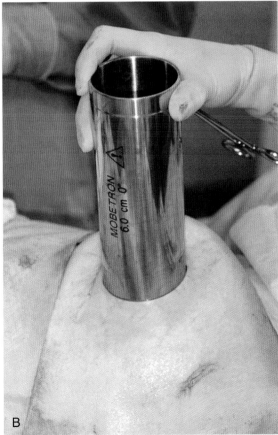

B

◆ The stitch is manipulated to place the tumor in the center of the applicator (Fig. 24-6).
◆ A moist, sterile gauze is placed between the skin and the radiation applicator to introduce a further tissue-equivalent barrier to absorb the low-energy electrons scattered by the applicator itself.
◆ The applicator is positioned such that there is a minimal air gap between the end of the applicator and the tumor. At the discretion of the radiation oncologist, a surface bolus (5 or 10 mm) may be attached to the end of the applicator before stabilization to improve surface dose.
◆ The applicator is then secured by a modified Bookwalter retraction system (Fig. 24-7). Visual inspection with the aid of a Surch-Lite lighted stylet (Aaron Medical, St. Petersburg, FL) is used

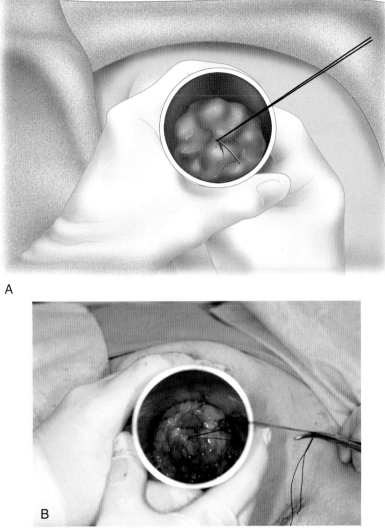

A

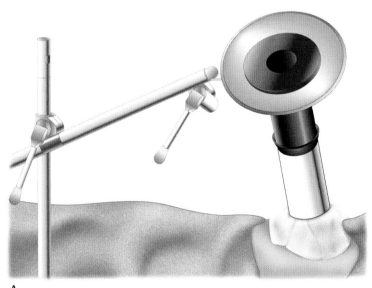

B

Figure 24-6

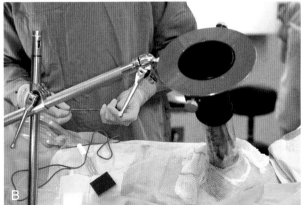

A

Figure 24-7

to confirm that the tumor remains in the center of the applicator (Fig. 24-8). Once immobilized by the Bookwalter retractor, there is no further movement of the applicator.

◆ A sterile shield is placed on the Mobetron (Fig. 24-9). Once the applicator has been positioned and stabilized appropriately, the operating room table is moved under the Mobetron such that the applicator is directly beneath the head of the machine (docking; Fig. 24-10).

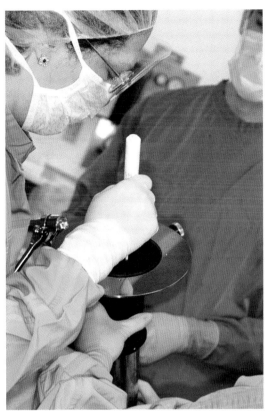

Figure 24-8

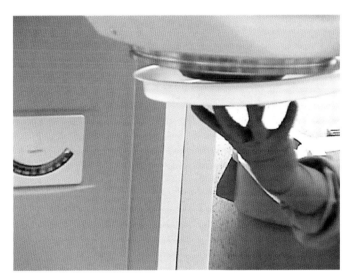

Figure 24-9

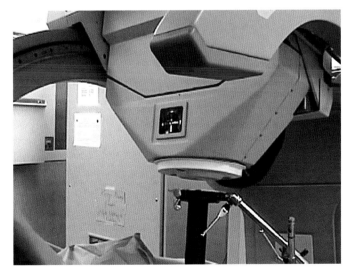

Figure 24-10

- ◆ Once the patient and the applicator have been placed under the Mobetron (Fig. 24-11), a geometric alignment of the treatment applicator with the gantry head of the Mobetron is achieved using a laser alignment system (Fig. 24-12).
- ◆ The operating room team moves to a substerile location outside of the operating room, and the anesthesiologist monitors the patient through a window in the substerile location while the radiation is delivered (Fig. 24-13).
- ◆ The patient is returned to her previous position and the Bookwalter retraction system is removed.

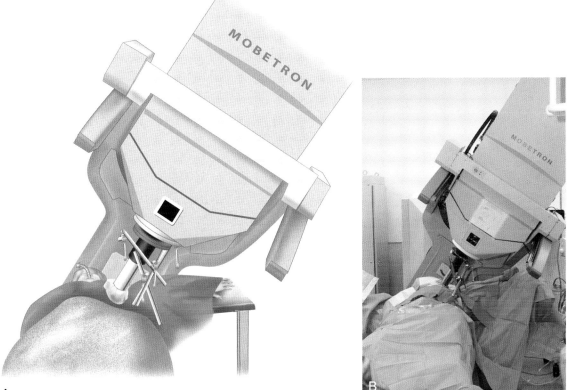

A

Figure 24-11

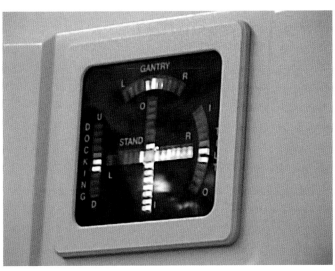

Figure 24-12

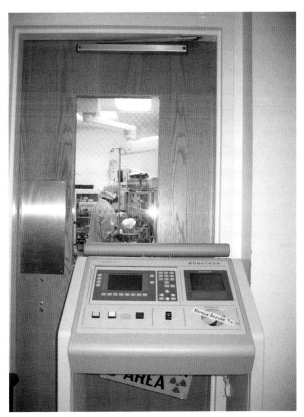

Figure 24-13

4. Segmental Mastectomy and Wound Closure

- The tumor is excised (see Chapter 15), appropriately marked for pathology (Fig. 24-14), and sent for specimen mammography.
- The incision is closed in standard fashion, such as with a simple interrupted 3-0 Vicryl suture and a running 4-0 Monocryl suture (Fig. 24-15).
- Sterile dressings and a surgical bra are applied.

Step 4. Postoperative Care

- Routine postoperative care is similar to care for a segmental mastectomy and a sentinel lymph node biopsy (see Chapters 11 and 15).

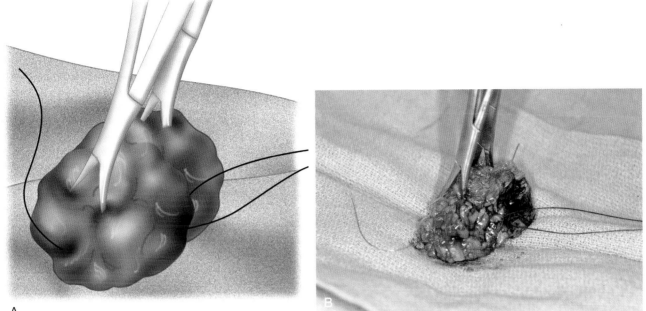

A

Figure 24-14

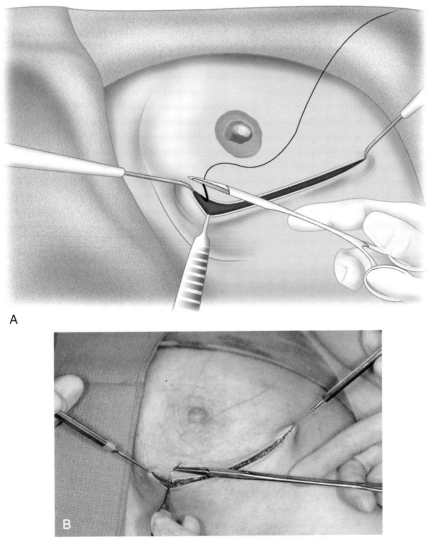

A

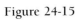

B

Figure 24-15

1. **Treatment of Patients Who Are Ineligible Based on Final Pathologic Evaluation**

◆ Because the resection is performed after irradiation, final pathologic characteristics will not be available at the time of treatment. If tumors are ultimately found to be larger than 3 cm, to have an extensive intraductal component, or to be node positive, then external-beam radiation therapy will follow, which is standard therapy. The IORT treatment serves as the boost.

◆ Patients who do not have tumor-free surgical margins (>1 mm) require a reoperative segmental mastectomy. If the patient has one or two tumor-involved surgical margins, she will be considered a candidate for a reoperative segmental mastectomy. The reoperative segmental mastectomy is performed in a standard fashion. If there is residual tumor with negative margins on reexcision, then whole-breast external-beam radiation is given for 5 weeks (the IORT that was previously given essentially serves as the radiation boost). If the reoperative segmental mastectomy fails to achieve complete tumor-free surgical margins, the patient is deemed a failure at breast preservation and proceeds to mastectomy.

Step 5. Pearls and Pitfalls

- General anesthesia must be administered for this procedure.
- Even if the tumor is palpable it should be wire localized, because this helps to ensure that the IORT is delivered directly over the tumor.
- Ensure that the operating table is rotated 180 degrees before administering general anesthesia. The table cannot fit under the Mobetron machine if it is not rotated.
- Ensure that the patient is securely fastened to the operating table with a seatbelt because the whole table may need to be tilted to achieve the correct positioning for delivery of the radiation.

Bibliography

Ollila DW, Klauber-DeMore N, Tesche LJ, et al: Feasibility of breast preserving therapy with single fraction in situ radiotherapy delivered intraoperatively. Ann Surg Oncol 2007;14:660-669.

Stitzenberg KB, Klauber-DeMore N, Chang XS, et al: In vivo intraoperative radiotherapy: A novel approach to radiotherapy for early stage breast cancer. Ann Surg Oncol 2007;14:1515-1516.

TARGETED INTRAOPERATIVE RADIATION THERAPY (TARGIT)

David R. McCready and Michael Andrew Henderson

Step 1. Surgical Anatomy

- Figure 25-1 demonstrates the relevant anatomy for intraoperative radiation therapy (IORT) treatment.

Step 2. Preoperative Considerations

- Small, screen-detected breast cancers in older women are ideal for IORT treatment.
- Mammography (Fig. 25-2, *A*) and ultrasonography (Fig. 25-2, *B*) show a lesion that is isolated and without extensive calcifications.
- Currently, patients are treated with orthovoltage (50-KeV) IORT only in the context of the TARGIT (targeted intraoperative radiation therapy) trial.
- Eligible patients who have a relatively low risk of local and distant relapse are selected for this randomized, controlled trial (Fig. 25-3). It is also important to obtain negative pathologic margins at the time of initial lumpectomy/partial mastectomy.
- Patients with the following characteristics appear to be ideal for IORT:
  - ▲ Biopsy-proven invasive ductal carcinoma
  - ▲ Age greater than 50 years
  - ▲ Tumor size less than 2 cm
  - ▲ Clinically negative nodes
  - ▲ Screen-detected disease
  - ▲ No malignant calcifications beyond tumor mass
- Patients with invasive lobular cancers are excluded from the study, as are those with an extensive intraductal component.
- Breast-specific preoperative work-up generally consists of the following:
  - ▲ History (usually asymptomatic; exclude those with concerning nipple discharge)
  - ▲ Physical examination (no signs of nodal disease, locally advanced cancer, or fixation to pectoralis major)
  - ▲ Mammography
  - ▲ Ultrasonography
  - ▲ Core biopsy
  - ▲ Axillary ultrasonography
  - ▲ Magnetic resonance imaging (selected patients)

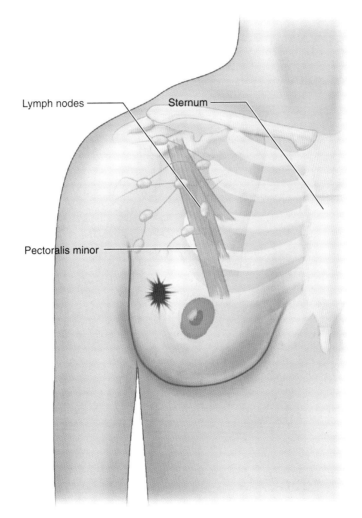

Figure 25-1

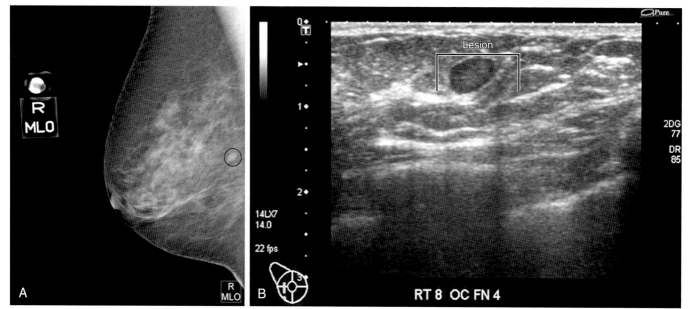

Figure 25-2

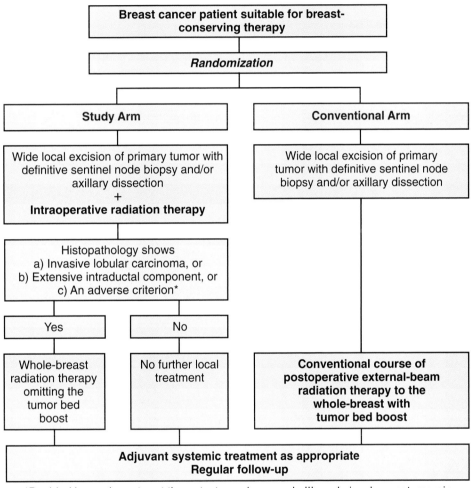

*Decided by each center at the outset - such as grade III, node involvement, margin
involvement, etc.

Figure 25-3

Step 3. Operative Steps

- ◆ IORT is ideally given at time of definitive breast surgery, but some centers deliver IORT to the lumpectomy cavity 1 to 3 days postsurgery when final pathology confirms negative margins and nonlobular histology.
- ◆ Before surgery, the breast has been injected with technetium-sulfur colloid for sentinel node mapping and a wire localization procedure has been performed to guide excision of nonpalpable tumors (Fig. 25-4).
- ◆ Preoperative antibiotics are given before incision.
- ◆ The procedure is performed under general anesthesia. Blue dye is injected around the tumor site. The sentinel node biopsy is performed first.
- ◆ Incisions are kept relatively small and placed directly over the tumor (Fig. 25-5). Drawing the incision before surgery with the patient upright can aid in cosmesis because different areas of the breast pull downward in different amounts depending on skin laxity and breast ptosis.
- ◆ Intraoperative ultrasonography can aid in locating small tumors. Skin is usually not excised unless the tumor is very superficial. The surgeon should attempt to leave 1 cm of subcutaneous tissue on the undersurface of the skin; thin flaps are discouraged (Fig. 25-6).

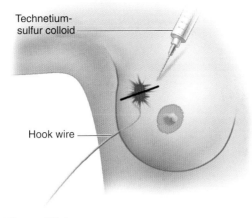

Figure 25-4

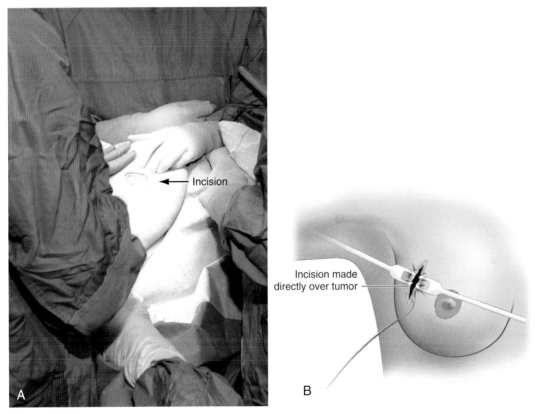

Figure 25-5

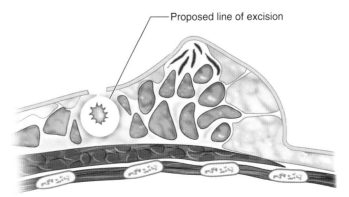

Figure 25-6

◆ Lumpectomies are best performed in a systematic fashion, starting with the superior portion followed by both medial and lateral sides, then the posterior margin down to pectoralis fascia, and finally the inferior margin. Meticulous hemostasis is important.

◆ Specimen radiography with mammography (or ultrasonography) is performed and close margins can be reexcised (Fig. 25-7). Margin assessment can be performed as needed by frozen-section analysis or touch imprint cytology as clinically or radiologically directed.

◆ The size of the cavity is estimated and the Intrabeam applicator (Carl Zeiss Meditec, Jena, Germany) is placed into the cavity. An appropriate size is selected to achieve a snug fit with a pursestring suture (Fig. 25-8). The purse string is best placed in breast tissue so it can ensure there are no gaps between applicator and tissue. Intraoperative ultrasonography can be used to ensure there are no gaps between applicator surface and cavity margin.

◆ Dosimetry is calculated so that 20 Gy is delivered at the surface of the applicator. The dose to breast tissue at a 1-cm depth from the cavity is about 5 Gy. Skin edges are everted if subcutaneous tissue is less than 1 cm thick.

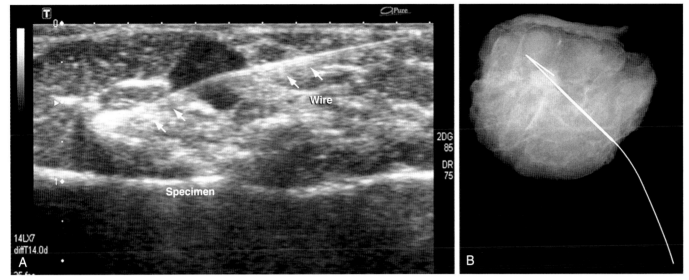

Figure 25-7

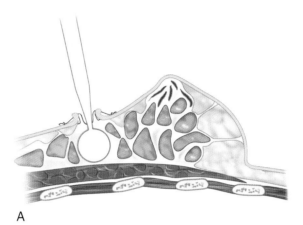

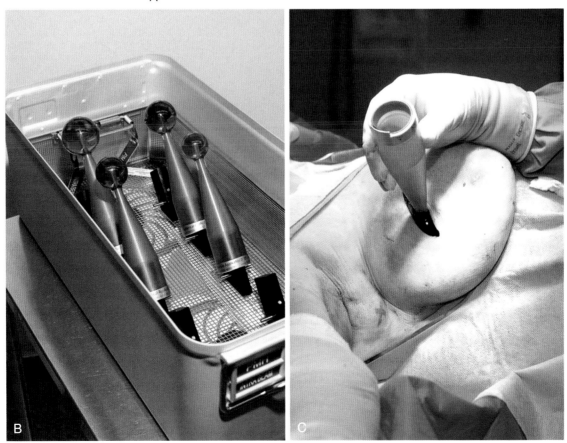

Figure 25-8

◆ The radiation delivery device is attached to the movable boom (Fig. 25-9), and the apparatus is sterilely draped with the applicator (Fig. 25-10).

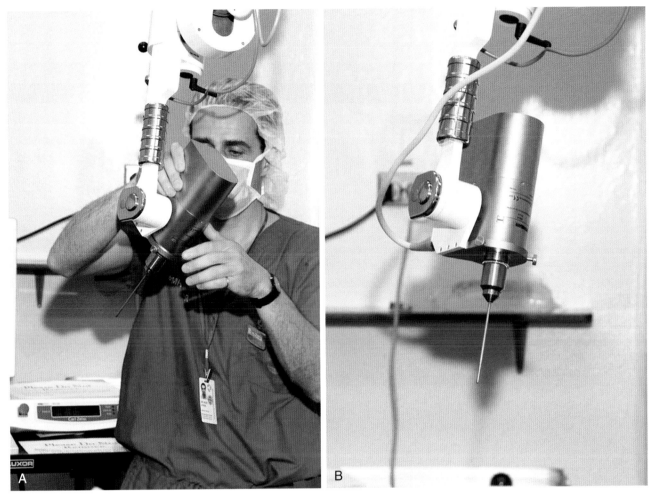

Figure 25-9

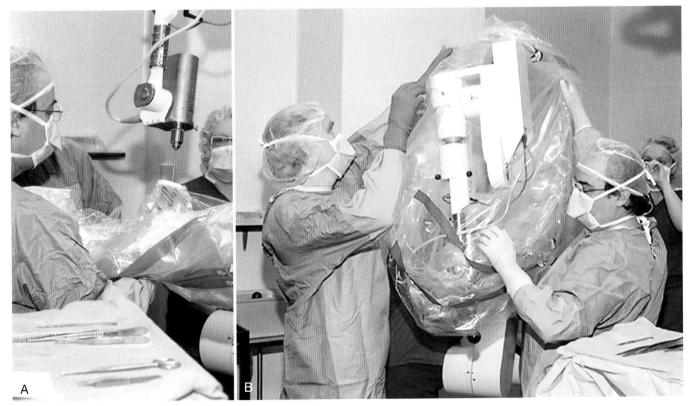

Figure 25-10

♦ The applicator is inserted into the cavity and the pursestring suture tied (Figs. 25-11 and 25-12). A posterior blocking shield can be used on the pectoralis fascia if the beam is directly aimed at the heart (Fig. 25-13).
♦ Duration of IORT is calculated based on applicator diameter (Table 25-1). Shielding is placed over the skin surface to reduce radiation scatter (Fig. 25-14), and the IORT is delivered (Fig. 25-15).

TABLE 25-1	Treatment Time for 20 Gy at the Applicator Surface	
APPLICATOR (MM)	TREATMENT TIME (MIN)
15	7.07
20	11.53
25	17.43
30	24.98
35	18.57
40	26.8
45	36.58
50	48.82

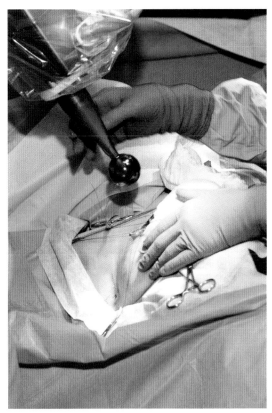

Figure 25-11

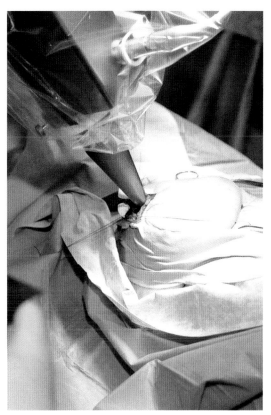

Figure 25-12

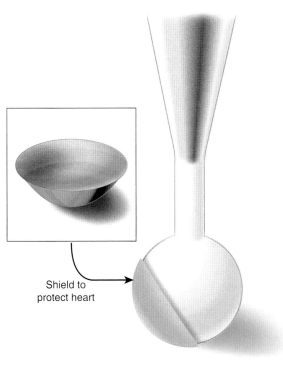

Shield to
protect heart

Figure 25-13

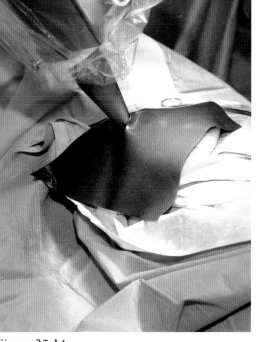

Figure 25-14

- During IORT, everyone leaves the room except the radiation therapist and anesthesiologist, who are behind a transparent lead glass shield and wearing appropriate shielding. The patient is ventilated and kept paralyzed during the IORT to minimize movement.
- On completion, the pursestring suture is cut, the applicator removed, and a visual inspection for bleeding performed. Subcuticular sutures are used to close the wound and Steri-Strips are applied (Fig. 25-16).

Step 4. Postoperative Care

- Postoperative care is the same as that given for lumpectomy (see Chapter 6).
- No special precautions are necessary.

Step 5. Pearls and Pitfalls

- Careful patient selection is crucial.
- The tumor should be centered within the specimen and a 1-cm margin of normal tissue obtained around the tumor. Larger excision cavities require larger applicators and correspondingly longer treatment times.
- The anterior margin is often the most difficult to control because a 1-cm buffer between the tumor and the specimen edge is the goal, but 1 cm of subcutaneous fat also should be left with the skin. The tumor margin is the first priority, and remaining skin can be managed by pursestring suture and skin eversion, or skin excision if necessary.
- The cavity must be in contact with applicator. Drape tape or OpSite (Smith & Nephew, London) can be used to hold the breast in an appropriate position (see Fig. 25-12).

Bibliography

Holmes DR, Baum M, Joseph D: The TARGIT trial: Targeted intraoperative radiation therapy versus conventional postoperative whole-breast radiotherapy after breast-conserving surgery for the management of early-stage invasive breast cancer (a trial update). Am J Surg 2007;194:207-210.

Schiller DE, Le LW, Cho, BCK, et al: Factors associated with negative margins of lumpectomy specimen: Potential use in selecting patients for intraoperative radiotherapy. Ann Surg Oncol 2007;15:833-842.

Vaidya JS, Baum M, Tobias JS, et al: Targeted intra-operative radiotherapy (TARGIT): An innovative method of treatment for early breast cancer. Ann Oncol 2001;12:1075-1180.

Vaidya JS, Baum M, Tobias JS, et al: Targeted intraoperative radiotherapy (TARGIT) yields very low recurrence rates when given as a boost. Int J Radiat Oncol Biol Phys 2006;66:1335-1338.

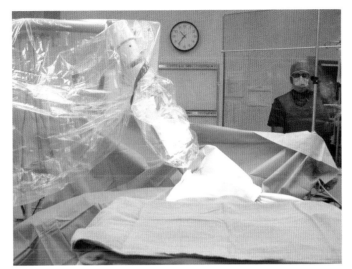

Figure 25-15

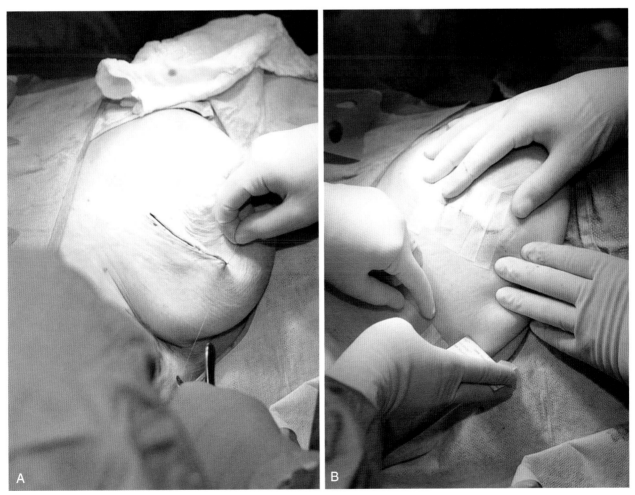

Figure 25-16

INDEX

Page numbers followed by *f* indicate figures; and those followed by *t* indicate tables.